A Simplified Approach To Electrocardiography

RICHARD JOHNSON, M.D.
Department of Medicine, University Hospital
State University of New York, Health Science Center
Stony Brook, New York

MARK H. SWARTZ, M.D., F.A.C.P.
Associate Professor of Clinical Medicine
Associate Director, Department of Electrocardiography
Director, Undergraduate Cardiovascular Education
The Mount Sinai Medical Center
New York, New York

W.B. SAUNDERS COMPANY
Philadelphia London Toronto Mexico City
Rio de Janeiro Sydney Tokyo Hong Kong

W. B. SAUNDERS COMPANY
Harcourt Brace Jovanovich, Inc.

The Curtis Center
Independence Square West
Philadelphia, PA 19106

Library of Congress Cataloging-in-Publication Data

Johnson, Richard, 1958–

A simplified approach to electrocardiography.

Includes index.

1. Electrocardiography. 2. Heart—Diseases—Diagnosis. I. Swartz, Mark H. II. Title. [DNLM: 1. Electrocardiography. 2. Heart Disease—diagnosis. WG 140 J68s]

RC683.5.E5J57 1986 616.1′207543 86–3963

ISBN 0–7216–1738–7

Editor: Dana Dreibelbis
Designer: Bill Donnelly
Production Manager: Bill Preston
Manuscript Editor: Roger Wall
Illustrator: Sharon Iwanczuk
Illustration Coordinator: Walt Verbitski

A Simplified Approach to Electrocardiography ISBN 0–7216–1738–7

Last digit is the print number: 9 8 7 6 5 4 3

To The Reader

This text is an introduction to learning electrocardiography. It is expected that some basic knowledge of electrocardiography exists; however, in-depth knowledge is not necessary.

The objective of this text-workbook is to help you gain some measure of confidence in interpreting electrocardiograms. This is accomplished by providing a review of the fundamentals of electrocardiography and by acquainting you with common electrocardiographic findings. Each electrocardiogram is presented in its entirety and is accompanied by a detailed objective analysis.

Part I of the text is a review of the essentials necessary for recognizing the basic complexes and patterns found in the electrocardiogram. The first four chapters of the text provide an introduction to the functional anatomy and basic electrophysiology of the heart. The remaining chapters in Part I review the principles necessary for using the electrocardiogram as a diagnostic tool. Because cardiac rhythm is of paramount importance, we have placed special emphasis on these sections.

The information in Part I is presented in a short, yet comprehensive format. You should not expect to gain a full understanding or be able to commit to memory all of this material upon the initial reading. Rather, the information should be used to review each of the tracings in part II. In this way, you will continually build a working knowledge of electrocardiography.

Pathophysiology has been included in appropriate sections in order to lay the groundwork for a better understanding of an electrocardiographic abnormality. Since electrocardiography is a graphic technique, a large number of tracings are shown. The text is also extensively illustrated with original diagrams that serve to summarize the important concepts. In addition, we have included sections on the clinical significance of electrocardiographic abnormalities as a means of stimulating thought, holding your attention and reinforcing the basic concepts.

Part II is a collection of electrocardiograms that you should attempt to analyze using the format outlined in the text. After completing a diagnosis, review the analysis given and the corresponding section of Part I.

In an attempt to provide the basics of electrocardiography in a more readable format, we have not used abbreviations in this book. Abbreviations tend to make a book more difficult to comprehend. However, since there are many common ones used in clinical practice, we have provided a list of acceptable abbreviations and their meanings in Appendix A.

This text is designed to teach the essentials of electrocardiographic interpretation. It is of special value to medical students who have for years struggled with the complexities of this subject. The book will also be of value to nursing students, nurses, physician assistants, electrocardiograph technicians and paramedical personnel, especially those who work in cardiac resuscitation units, emergency wards and intensive care units.

This book has been written with the student of electrocardiography in mind. The planning of this comprehensive text demanded a sense of selectivity and balance. One of us (R.J.) was a medical student when this text was developed and could appreciate the concerns and anxieties associated with learning this complex field. We have endeavored to make each concept understandable to both of us, so that anyone who reads the text will comprehend it. The collaboration of both student and physician has introduced an unusual blend, which we feel will make the subject of electrocardiography easier to understand.

R. J.

M. H. S.

Acknowledgements

We are indebted to Michael Lozano, Jr., a medical student at The Mount Sinai School of Medicine, who executed all of the illustrations. His careful and artistic approach to the anatomy of the heart has served to enhance the basic concepts discussed in the text. His illustrations speak eloquently for themselves, but we wish to pay tribute to his insight and imaginative collaboration.

We would also like to thank Kyung Suh, R. N., for having supplied some of the Holter monitor rhythm strips, which have enhanced our rhythm section.

Our warmest appreciation to Alma Lucas for her expert secretarial assistance, without whose help this book could not have been completed. She spent many painstaking hours in the typing of the numerous revisions necessary in the preparation of this manuscript.

We owe a special thanks to Dana Dreibelbis and the entire staff of W. B. Saunders Company for their invaluable assistance.

Preparation of this book consumed much of our time including evenings, weekends and holidays over the past 3 years. To Mark's wife, Vivian, and daughter, Talia, from whom this time was taken, his gratitude and love. To Richard's wife, Nora, his grateful appreciation and love for her indefatigable support and encouragement in bringing this book to fruition.

R. J.
M. H. S.

Contents

II Practice Tracings 117

I

Fundamentals

1

Functional Anatomy

The heart consists of two principal cell types. The first are *muscle cells,* also called *muscle fibers,* which have primarily contractile function and actually perform the mechanical work of contraction. The second are the *specialized cells* of the conducting system, which initiate the heart's rhythm and propagate the electrical impulse that stimulates the muscle cells to contract.

MUSCLE CELLS

Muscle fibers provide the bulk of the heart's four chambers. These chambers collect blood during their rest period, called *diastole,* then propel the blood into the cardiovascular system when the muscle fibers are stimulated to shorten during *systole.* Usually, diastole is long enough to allow the heart to fill adequately; however, at very rapid heart rates, this filling time may be severely shortened, resulting in less blood to pump during systole.

The structure of the chambers is shown in Figure 1–1. The atria are smaller than the ventricles and are located superiorly. Their function is to collect blood and to empty their contents into the ventricles just before ventricular systole. This provides the *"atrial kick"* to ventricular filling. The right atrium receives blood from the great veins during diastole. It is separated from the right ventricle by the *tricuspid valve.* This valve is a three-leafed structure that remains closed during most of diastole. However, when the blood in the right atrium reaches a certain filling pressure, the tricuspid valve is pushed open, and the blood from the right atrium empties into the right ventricle. Shortly thereafter, the atrium contracts, forcing all the remaining blood into the ventricle (i.e., the "atrial kick"). This occurs just prior to the onset of ventricular contraction.

The *left atrium* receives blood from the lungs and empties it into the left ventricle through the two-leafed mitral valve. The process of left atrial emptying is similar to that described for the right atrium.

The ventricles are located inferior to the atria, with the right ventricle anterior to the left ventricle. They are separated by the *interventricular septum.* The right ventricle's function is to receive venous blood from the right atrium and pump this deoxygenated blood to the lungs for oxygenation.

The lungs and the arteries in the lungs usually do not produce much vascular resistance, so the right side of the heart is considered a *low pressure system.* This means the right ventricle does not have to work against high pressures in order to pump blood to the lungs.

The left ventricle is normally the largest and most muscular chamber in the heart. It receives oxygenated blood from the left atrium that has returned from the lungs. It propels this blood into the aorta and the high pressure *systemic circulation.*

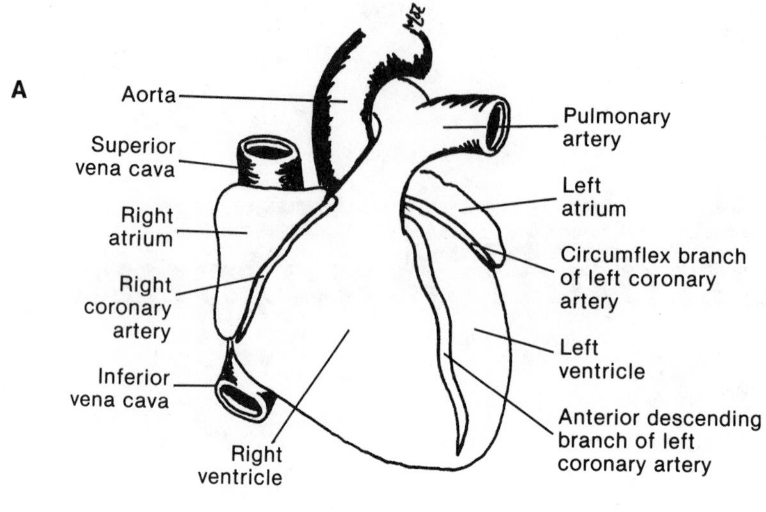

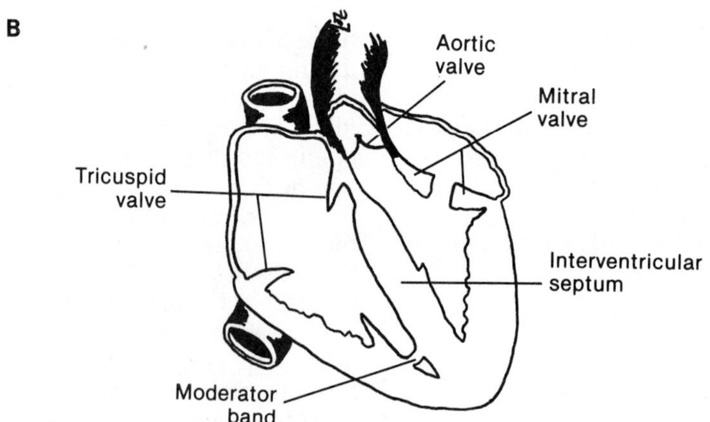

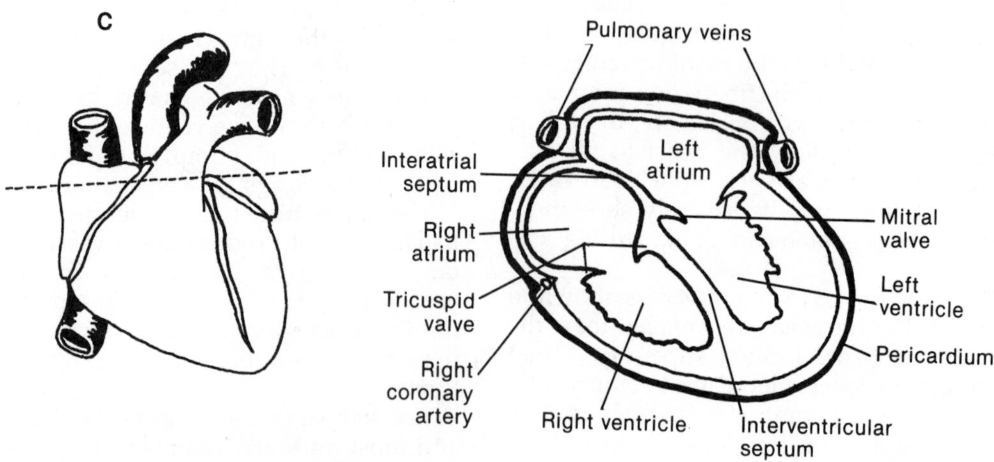

Figure 1–1. **Anatomical structures of the heart.** *A,* A normal heart without sectioning. *B,* A coronal section. *C,* Illustration of a cross section at the level of the atria, with the dotted line indicating the plane of section.

Each chamber of the heart is composed of three layers (Fig. 1–2). The *endocardium* is the layer closest to the inside of the chamber. The *myocardium* is the middle, main muscular layer (*myo* = muscle). This layer is thicker in the ventricles than in the atria and is thickest in the left ventricle. The *epicardium* is the outer layer. Coronary blood vessels course through it before diving deeper to supply the myocardium and endocardium.

One should be aware that each of these layers contains muscle cells, and the divisions are merely to help identify the inner, middle or outer layers of the heart. Also, the term myocardium is often used generically to indicate all of the muscle fibers within the heart.

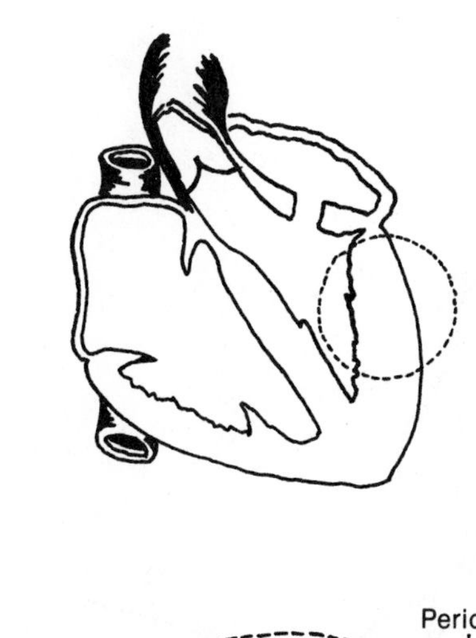

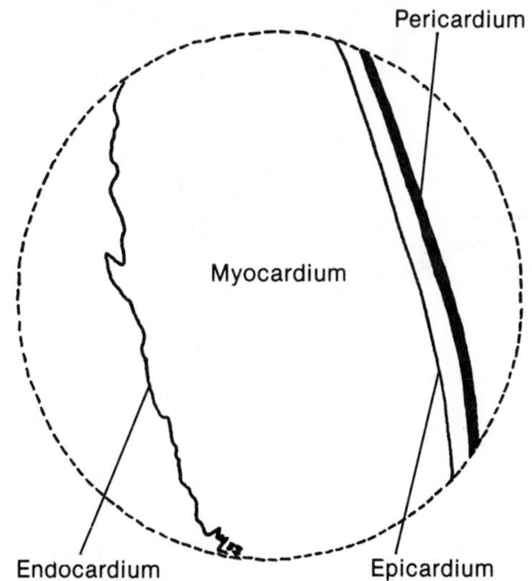

Figure 1–2. **Cross section through the myocardial wall.** The endocardium, myocardium, epicardium and pericardium are illustrated.

Surrounding the surface of the heart is a serous membrane called the *pericardium* (Fig. 1–2). The pericardium is composed of two layers of connective tissue, between which there is a small amount of fluid. This fluid is normally straw colored and sterile. The pericardium forms a protective sac around the heart, while the fluid reduces friction during the cardiac cycle.

Figure 1–3 illustrates the distinct microscopic features of cardiac muscle cells. Each cell has many striations and a single nucleus. *Intercalated discs* separate the muscle cells and provide a low resistance passageway for electrical impulses. The system of intercalated discs allows for an impulse in any part of the myocardium to spread throughout the heart. Thus, the heart is considered a *syncytium*.

SPECIALIZED CELLS

Cells of the conducting system are specialized cells that initiate and propagate electrical impulses. They do not perform the mechanical work of contraction, but they do coordinate the activity.

The electrical impulse for cardiac contraction is spontaneously generated in cells of the *sinoatrial node*, also called the sinus node (Fig. 1–4). The *sinus node* is an anatomical structure located near the junction of the superior vena cava and the right atrium. It is horseshoe shaped and lies just under the epicardium. Because of its subepicardial location, the sinus node is often affected by processes involving the pericardium.

Blood supply to the sinus node is provided by the *right coronary artery* in 60 per cent of patients. In most other cases it is supplied by the *left circumflex artery*. Innervation of the sinus node is provided both by the sympathetic autonomic nervous system, which speeds up the rate at which the sinus node will fire, and by the parasympathetic nervous system, which slows its rate of firing.

Once generated, the electrical impulse is conducted out of the sinus node to the atria, where it stimulates atrial muscle cells to contract. The impulse is also conducted to the atrioventricular node by three distinct *internodal pathways*. The largest of these tracts is called *Bachmann's bundle*. The impulse enters the atrioventricular node at its subendocardial location. The atrioventricular node lies on the right side of the *interatrial septum*, anterior to the coronary sinus.

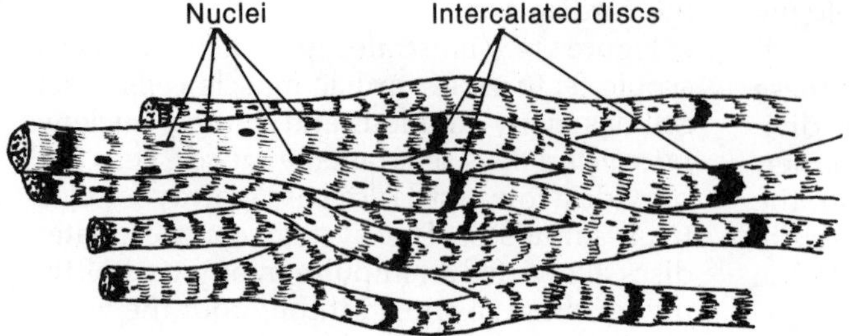

Figure 1–3. **Microscopic features of cardiac muscle cells.** Note the Y-shaped branchings as well as the overall parallel arrangement.

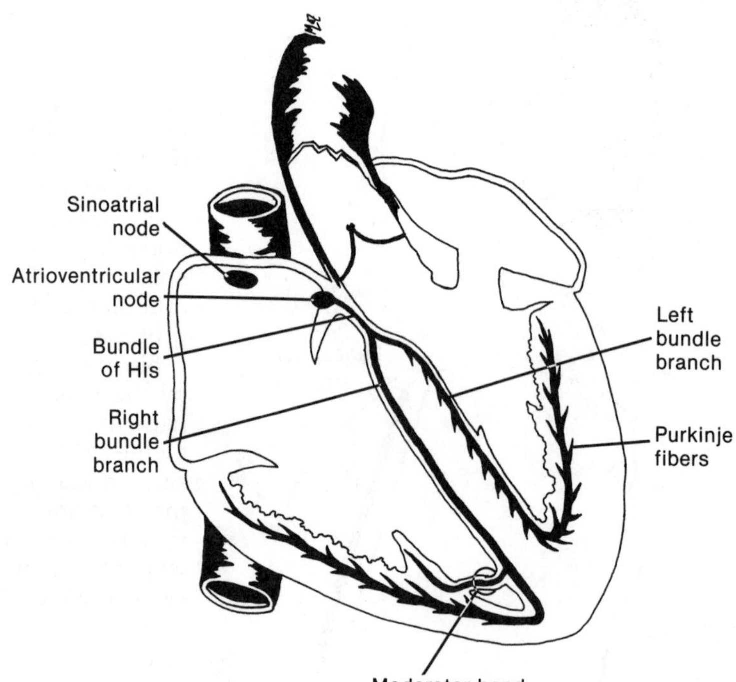

Figure 1–4. The conducting system of the heart.

The blood supply to the *atrioventricular node* is provided by the right coronary artery in 90 per cent of patients. In the remaining 10 per cent, the left circumflex artery provides the blood supply. The atrioventricular node normally functions to delay the transmission of the electrical impulse. This delay is enhanced by activation of the parasympathetic nervous system, which normally innervates the atrioventricular node.

Upon leaving the atrioventricular node, the electrical impulse continues to propagate down the conducting system to the *bundle of His*. The bundle of His proceeds down the interventricular septum, and at the inferior border of the membranous septum it bifurcates into the right and left bundle branches.

The *right bundle branch* is responsible for spreading the electrical impulse to the right ventricle. It propagates the impulse subendocardially along the right side of the septum, through the *moderator band* and finally to the right ventricular free wall.

The *left bundle branch* spreads the electrical impulse to the interventricular septum and the left ventricle. It travels in the subendocardium and divides into two branches: The *anterior superior fascicle* spreads the electrical impulse to the anterior superior segments of the left ventricle, while the *posterior inferior fascicle* propagates the impulse to the posterior-inferior segments of the left ventricle.

Once the electrical impulse has been propagated through the bundle branches, it reaches the *Purkinje fibers*. These fibers form a rapid conduction network within the myocardium and actually spread the impulse to all the muscle cells. Because the Purkinje fibers are located in the subendocardium, the electrical impulse first spreads from the endocardium to the myocardium and finally reaches the epicardial surface.

A summary of the normal route for propagating the electrical impulse is shown in Figure 1–4. Electrical activity originates in the sinus node, traverses the atria to the atrioventricular node, where the impulse is delayed, and then down the bundle of His through the bundle branches to the Purkinje network, which rapidly spreads the impulse throughout the ventricular myocardium (Fig. 1–5).

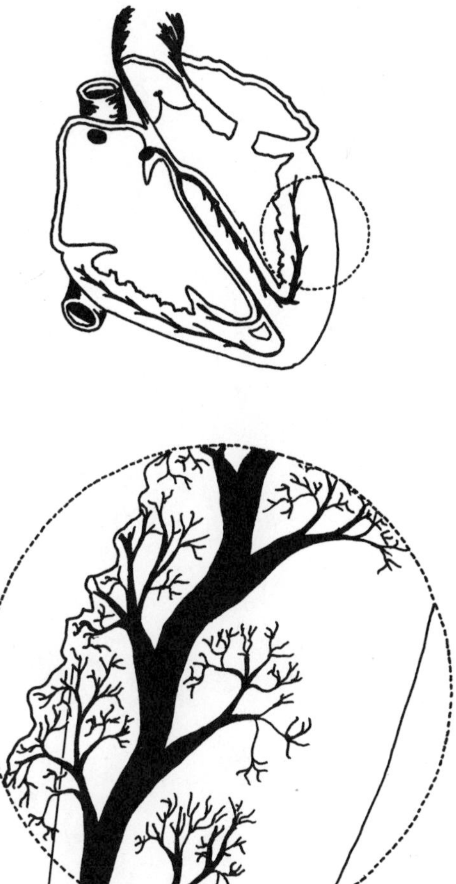

Figure 1–5. **Purkinje network.** The circled area is magnified to demonstrate the ramifications of the Purkinje network.

As the electrical impulse propagates down the specialized fibers of the conduction system, the myocardium around a given segment will be stimulated to contract. Essentially, the specialized cells of the conducting system provide the spark for the activation of the more massive myocardium. It is the electrical activity produced by myocardial activation that is recorded in the electrocardiogram. Activation of the atrial myocardium produces *P waves*, while the *QRS complex* is generated by the electrical activity of the ventricular myocardium.

2

The Action Potential

The electrocardiogram is a record of the electrical activity of the heart. This electrical action is caused by the movement of ions across the cell membranes of the heart. To better understand this electrical activity, a brief review of the basic electrophysiology of the myocardial cell is in order. The resting myocardial cell has an electrical charge of −90 millivolts. This charge is referred to as the *resting membrane potential*. This potential is generated by the Na^+-K^+ pump, which exchanges intracellular Na^+ for extracellular K^+, and creates a gradient of these ions across the cell membrane (Fig. 2–1). If the surface of a myocardial cell is stimulated, the permeability of the cell membrane to sodium suddenly increases. Sodium rushes into the cell and produces a large increase in its electrical activity. This process of activating the cell is referred to as *depolarization*. The process of returning the cell to its resting charge of −90 millivolts is called *repolarization*. The

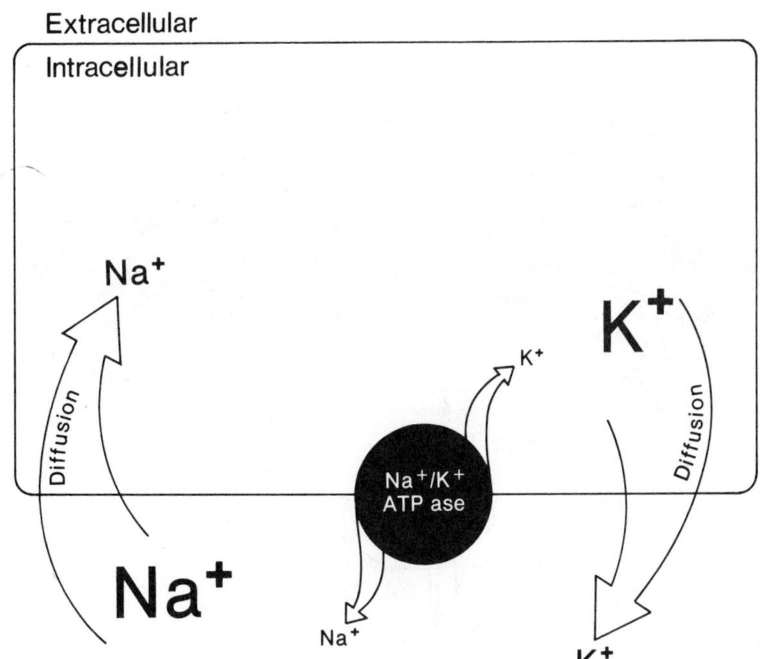

Figure 2–1. A diagram of the Na^+-K^+ pump, which exchanges intracellular Na^+ for extracellular K^+ and serves to establish a potential difference between the inside and the outside of the cell.

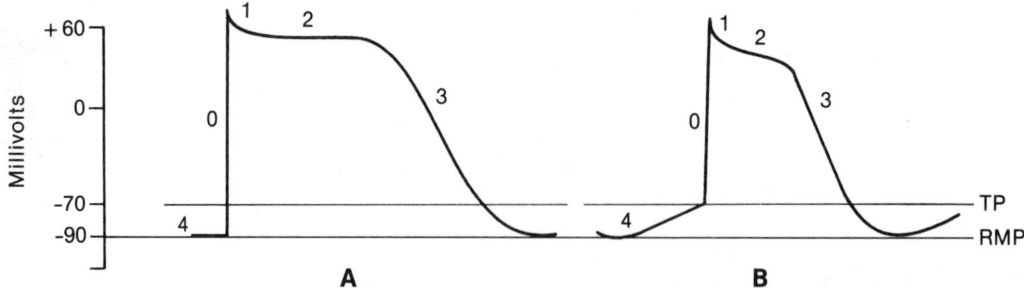

Figure 2–2. **The action potential.** *A,* The action potential of a typical atrial or ventricular cell. *B,* The action potential from the cells of the specialized conducting system, such as the sinoatrial node, the atrioventricular node or the His-Purkinje system. (TP = threshold potential; RMP = resting membrane potential.)

sequence of these processes in which the membrane rapidly changes its electrical potential is called an *action potential.*

The action potential of each muscle cell in the atria and ventricles demonstrates five phases (Fig. 2–2). *Phase 0* is the period of rapid depolarization that results from sodium ions flooding into the cell. Throughout all other phases the cell pumps sodium back out of the cell. *Phases 1, 2 and 3* are periods of variable duration in which the cell is returned to its resting potential (repolarization). During phase 1 the influx of sodium slows, and the cell begins to repolarize. The plateau period, phase 2, is caused by the slow inward movement of calcium and the outward movement of potassium. During phases 1 and 2 the cell is in the *absolute refractory period.* This means that a stimulus, no matter how strong, is unable to excite the cell to produce another action potential. Phase 3 results from the cessation of sodium and calcium inflow and, more importantly, the rapid outflow of potassium. This results in a rapid repolarization to the resting potential.

During the end of phase 3 the cell is in the *relative refractory period.* This means that the cell can be excited to produce an action potential but only by a stimulus that is much stronger than normal.

Phase 4 is the resting membrane potential. It is a stable, highly negative potential that will persist until an impulse arrives to cause excitation (Fig. 2–2*A*).

During phase 4 of the action potential, the cell membrane is largely permeable to potassium, with the net loss of intracellular potassium. In fact, it is the transmembrane

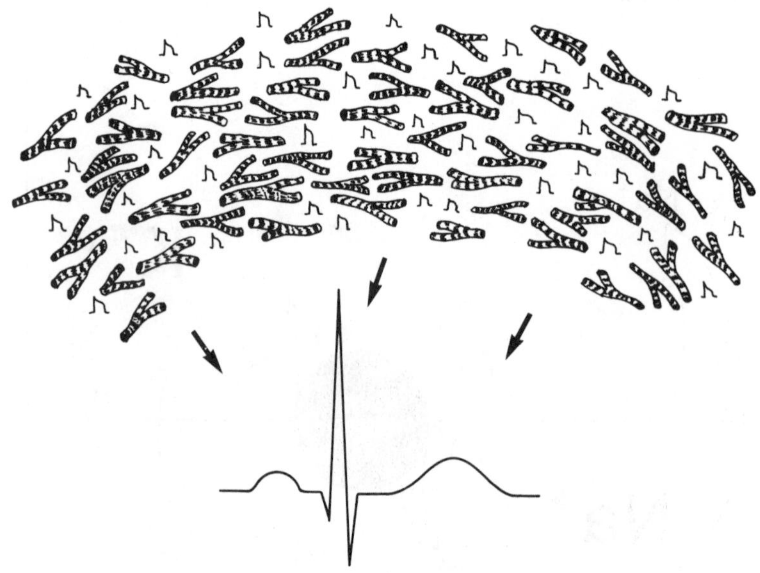

Figure 2–3. The net result of all action potentials in the heart produces the P wave, QRS complex and T wave.

concentration of potassium that largely determines the magnitude of the resting potential. This relationship is described by the *Nernst equation,* which states that an increase in extracellular potassium decreases the resting membrane potential (becomes less negative). Conversely, lowering of the extracellular potassium will result in a state of hyperpolarization or an increase in the resting membrane potential (becomes more negative).

In the cells of the specialized conducting system such as those in the sinoatrial node, atrioventricular node and the His-Purkinje system, repolarization is followed by a period during which the resting potential is not stable (Fig. 2–2*B*). Instead, immediately after the end of repolarization, the membrane potential begins to decrease slowly (resting membrane potential gets closer to 0). This slow depolarization during phase 4 lowers the resting potential toward the *threshold potential,* the potential at which activation occurs (i.e., the trigger point). If the slow depolarization reaches the threshold potential, excitation occurs, and the cell repeats an action potential. Cells that demonstrate this slow depolarization are said to be *automatic.* Normal cardiac rhythm results from this spontaneous excitation in the sinoatrial node.

There are many other groups of automatic cells in the heart, and any factor that changes the intrinsic rate of the normal sinoatrial node or increases the automaticity of these cells can result in arrhythmias.

The electrocardiogram records the sum effect of all the individual action potentials of myocardial cells (Fig. 2–3). The different complexes on the electrocardiogram correlate with activation, depolarization and repolarization. Atrial depolarization produces the *P wave.* Rapid depolarization, phase 0, of the ventricular muscle cells transmits electrical impulses that together produce the *QRS complex,* while the *ST segment* and *T wave* are produced by ventricular repolarization.

3

Vectors and Leads

What is a vector? Physical laws of nature describe a *vector* as any force that has both magnitude and direction. A simple example is provided by examining a 100-pound weight on a table (Fig. 3–1*A*). The weight has a force of 100 pounds—that is its magnitude. What about its direction? If the table were quickly removed from under the weight, the weight would fall to the ground. Thus, the action of the weight is directed downward.

Vectors are represented as arrows pointed in the direction of the force, while the size of the arrow reflects the magnitude of the force. For this example, the vector describing the weight is shown in Figure 3–1*B*.

Electricity is a force with a magnitude and direction. Thus, vectors can be used to represent electrical action. The heart's electrical actions can also be represented by vectors. These vectors are caused by the spread of waves of depolarization and repolarization throughout the myocardium.

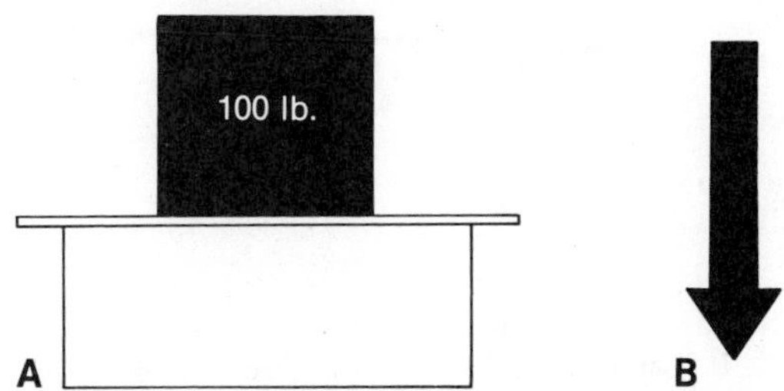

Figure 3–1. The concept of a vector, as outlined in the text.

Electrocardiographic leads are electrodes that sense the heart's electrical action. They respond to the heart's electrical actions by causing a positive deflection (above baseline) on the electrocardiographic paper when the depolarization is directed toward a lead (Fig. 3–2*A*) and a negative deflection (below baseline) when the depolarization is going away from the lead (Fig. 3–2*B*). When the depolarization is perpendicular to the lead, no net deflection results. The wave is said to be equiphasic (Fig. 3–2*C*).

There are 12 leads in the routine electrocardiogram. Leads I, II and III are standard bipolar limb leads (Fig. 3–3*A*). In a bipolar lead, a positive and a negative electrode are placed on any two limbs. Lead I is composed of two electrodes: The right arm is negative, while the left arm is positive. Lead II measures the difference in potential between the right arm, which is negative, and the left leg, which is positive. Lead III is composed of the left arm, which is negative, and the left leg, which is positive. These three leads form a triangle, shown in Figure 3–3*A*. Einthoven described the relationship between these three leads: The sum of any complex in leads I and III equals that of lead II (I + III = II). This formula is especially useful when examining the waves and complexes in the limb leads. For example, since the P wave is usually upright in the limb leads, it will be most prominent in lead II. Understanding Einthoven's formula will give the reader insight into the height and width of the P waves, QRS complexes and T waves seen in these leads.

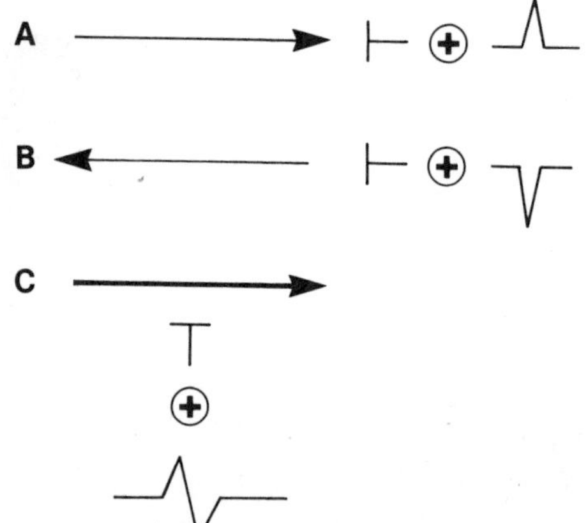

Figure 3–2. **Electrical vectors and the resultant deflections.** *A*, The generation of a positive deflection when the impulse is approaching the exploring electrode. *B*, The development of a negative deflection when the exploring electrode views an impulse going away from it. *C*, The electrode perpendicular to the impulse. An initial positive followed by a negative deflection is inscribed. Note that there is no net positive or negative deflection, and the complex is therefore called "equiphasic."

Leads AVR, AVL and AVF are unipolar augmented limb leads and provide three additional directions for viewing the wave of depolarization. The positive electrodes are measured on the right arm, left arm and the left leg, respectively. Together, the three standard limb leads and the three augmented limb leads view the heart in the frontal plane. They are termed the frontal plane hexaxial system and are shown in Figure 3–3*B*. As can be seen, the leads are evenly spaced and are 30° apart.

In addition to limb leads, there are six precordial leads (V1 to V6) that are placed on the anterior and lateral chest wall (Fig. 3–4*A*). These leads view the heart and the wave of depolarization in the horizontal plane. Leads V1 and V2 are placed in the fourth intercostal space at the right and left sternal edge, respectively. Lead V4 is placed in the fifth intercostal space in the midclavicular line. Lead V3 is placed equidistant between leads V2 and V4 in a straight line with them. Leads V5 and V6 are placed in the anterior and mid axillary lines, respectively, at the same horizontal level as lead V4 (Fig. 3–4*B* and C).

These 12 leads are useful in an electrocardiogram because a single lead cannot view all of the heart's electrical action. In fact, each lead can only view the heart's electrical activity as vector components directed toward, away from or perpendicular to itself. This is why each lead inscribes different P, QRS and T waveforms.

Figure 3–5 illustrates how myocardial depolarization vectors can be broken down into components—a method termed *vector resolution*. Although an infinite number of vectors are produced by myocardial depolarization, it is common to illustrate this process by using three representative vectors. These oc-

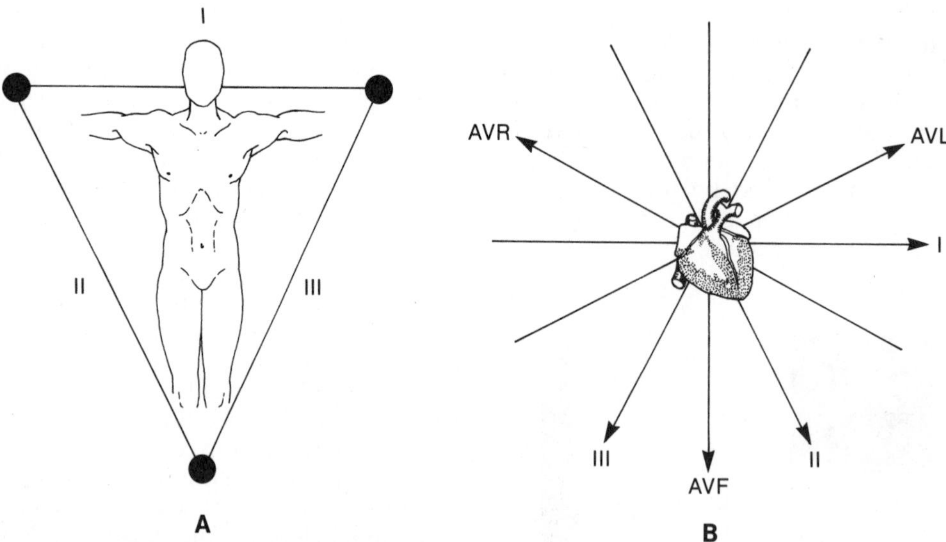

Figure 3–3. **Limb leads.** *A*, Einthoven's triangle made up of leads I, II and III. *B*, The hexaxial lead system of the limb leads as it runs through the heart. The leads are equally spaced, 30° apart. The leads are indicated at their positive poles.

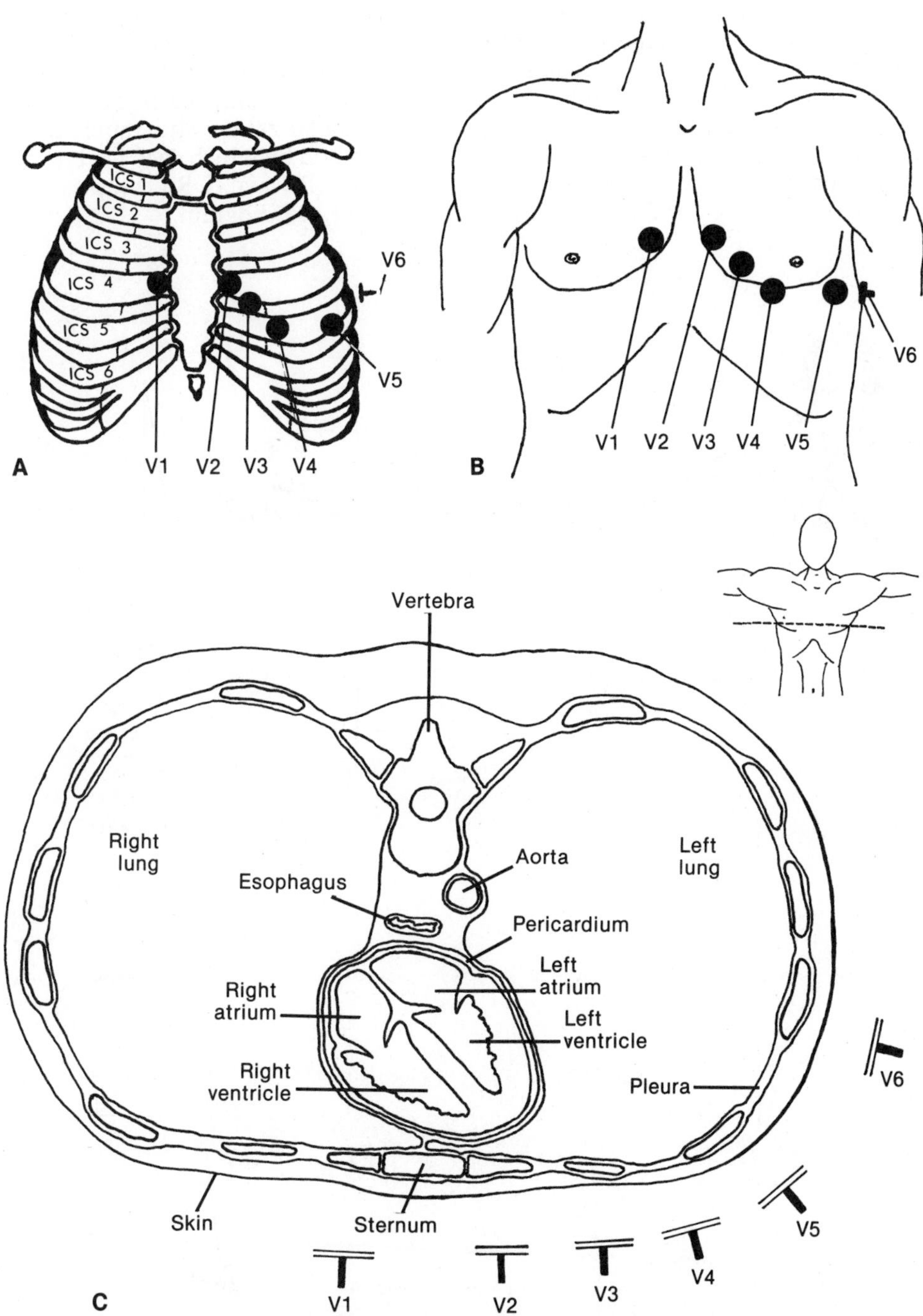

Figure 3–4. **Precordial leads.** *A,* The anatomical location of the six precordial leads. *B,* The surface anatomy for the placement of the leads. *C,* A cross-sectional cut through the chest illustrating the view that each electrode visualizes. (ICS = intercostal space.)

cur in sequence and are labeled vectors 1, 2 and 3.

Lead I will view vector 1 as a component that moves away from lead I, thus a negative deflection in this lead results. Vector 2 will be viewed as a component progressing toward lead I, so a positive deflection is produced. Vector 3 is viewed as a largely positive component approaching lead I, and again a positive deflection results.

Lead AVF views vector 1 as a vector component progressing toward it. This results in a positive deflection. Vector 2 is also viewed as progressing toward lead AVF, so a positive deflection is inscribed. Finally, lead AVF views vector 3 as a vector component directed away from it. This results in a negative deflection in this lead.

This method of resolving each vector into its basic components that are directed parallel to an electrocardiographic lead is useful for understanding how each lead views myocardial depolarization and repolarization. It is the method by which each lead inscribes each complex (P wave, QRS complex, T wave) of the electrocardiogram.

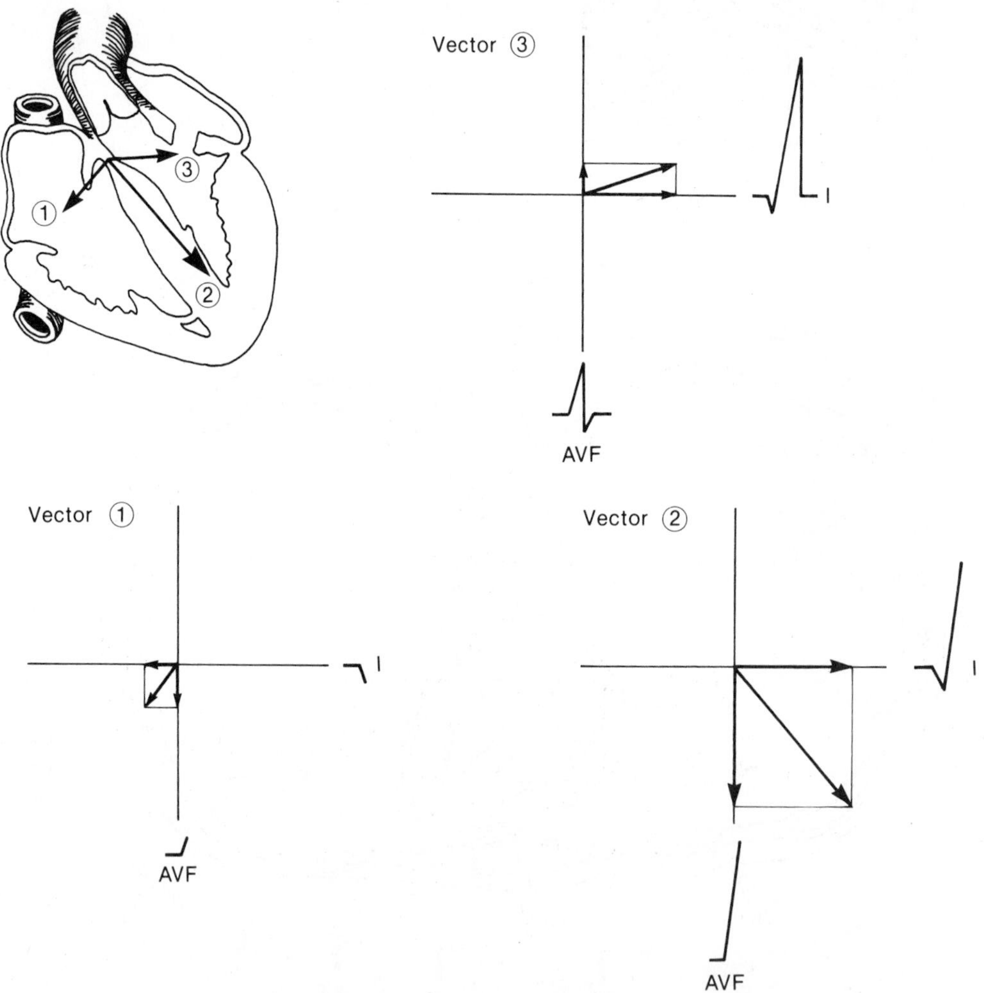

Figure 3–5. **The three main vectors of depolarization and their resolution into components in leads I and AVF.** Note that the magnitude of each vector component is equal to the amplitude of the deflection seen in that lead.

4

Review of Complexes

Figure 4–1 shows a normal electrocardiographic tracing. The morphologies of the P wave, QRS complex and T wave are shown. The following discussion includes the important characteristics for rate determination and for each of the complexes and intervals. This information is presented in a comprehensive format. The beginning student should not feel overwhelmed by trying to memorize all of this information. It is presented in outline form for easy reference.

STANDARDIZATION

The standardization of the electrocardiogram is 10 mm (10 small boxes) equals 1 millivolt. This is important and must be present on all

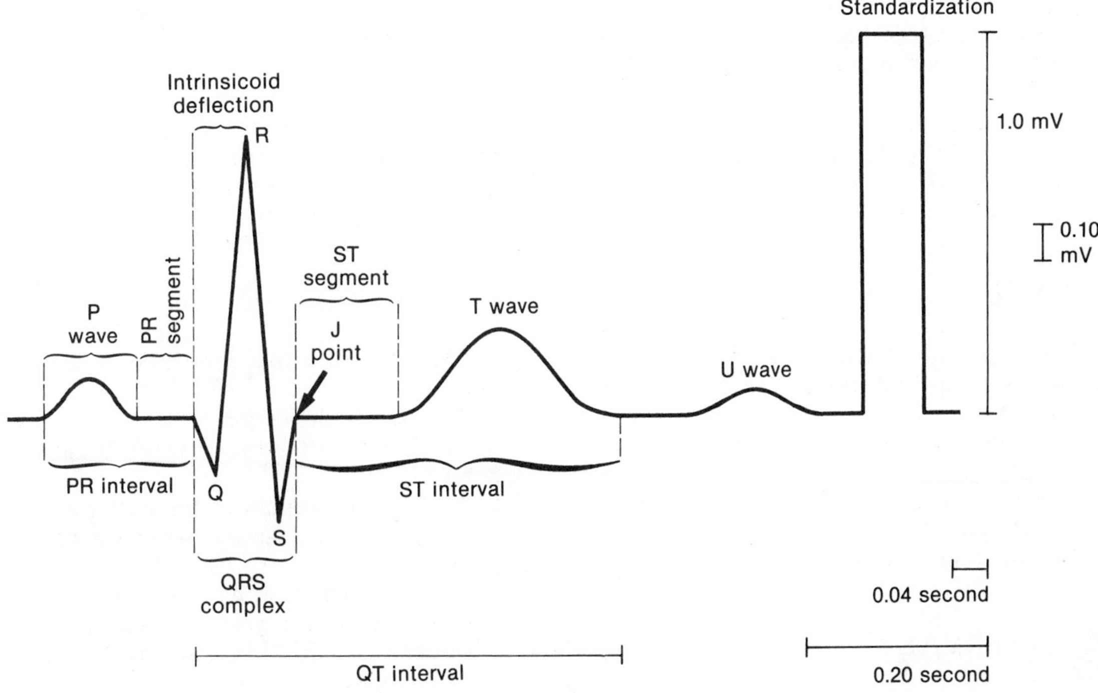

Figure 4–1. A normal electrocardiogram showing the morphologies of the P wave, QRS complex, T wave and U wave as well as the standardization.

tracings. If one sees a wave 10 mm in height, one should recognize that this is the result of 1 millivolt of electrical activity in the myocardium (Fig. 4–1).

RATE DETERMINATION

In a routine electrocardiogram, the recording speed of the paper is 25 mm per second. Therefore, the following relationships exist:

1 small box = 1 mm = 0.04 second
1 large box = 5 mm = 0.20 second
6 large boxes = 30 mm = 1.20 seconds

Four methods to determine heart rate are listed as follows:

1. Count the number of complete QRS cycles in 6 large boxes (1.2 seconds) and multiply by 50. This is very useful for fast heart rates, since the other methods described are more inaccurate at these rapid rates (Fig. 4–2*A*).
2. Since each large box equals 0.2 second (one fifth of a second), count the number of large boxes between consecutive beats and divide into 300. This is very useful for slow heart rates (300 divisions = 1 minute) (Fig. 4–2*B*).
3. Remember: *300–150–100–75–60–50.* These numbers represent the heart rate for consecutive large boxes (i.e., 1 large box gives a heart rate of 300 beats per minute, 2 give 150 beats per minute and so on (Fig. 4–2*C*).
4. One method that is accurate at all rates is to count the number of small boxes between two QRS complexes and divide the number into 1500 (Fig. 4–2*D*).

P WAVE

1. Represents atrial activation.
2. Normally upright in leads I, II, AVF and V4 to V6.
3. Normally inverted in lead AVR.
4. Variable in other leads.
5. Atrial disease increases the duration of the P wave to greater than 0.10 second (2.5 small boxes).

PR INTERVAL

1. Normally 0.12 to 0.20 second (3 to 5 small boxes).
2. Measures the time for the impulse to travel from the sinoatrial node to the atrioventricular node.
3. Used to measure atrioventricular node conduction.
4. With a shortened PR interval, consider atrioventricular nodal or low atrial rhythm; pre-excitation. May be a normal variant.
5. With a prolonged PR interval, consider atrioventricular block, hyperthyroidism or coronary artery disease. Atrial disease increases the P wave duration. This is differentiated from atrioventricular nodal disease, which increases the duration of the P wave and also the PR interval. This may also be a normal variant.

PR SEGMENT

It is part of the PR interval. This is the baseline between the end of the P wave and the beginning of the QRS complex. Although normally isoelectric, it can be displaced in atrial infarction and in acute pericarditis.

QRS COMPLEX

1. Represents ventricular activation.
2. Duration is normally 0.05 to 0.10 second (< 2.5 small boxes). Measurement is made most often from the limb leads.
3. If the amplitude is less than 10 mm in all leads (*low voltage*), heart disease, pericardial effusion, myxedema or pulmonary disease may be present.
4. QRS complex abnormalities are seen in conduction disturbances.
5. Nomenclature of QRS complexes (Fig. 4–3):
   a. The first downward deflection is called a *Q wave.*
   b. The first upward deflection is an *R wave.*
   c. A negative deflection (below baseline) that occurs after the R wave is called an *S wave.*
   d. All R waves are above the baseline.
   e. All Q and S waves are below the baseline.
   f. A low amplitude R wave may be noted by using a lower case "r" instead of an upper case "R"; likewise for "q" and "s" waves.
   g. If a second complex occurs, it is noted by using a prime (rSR′).

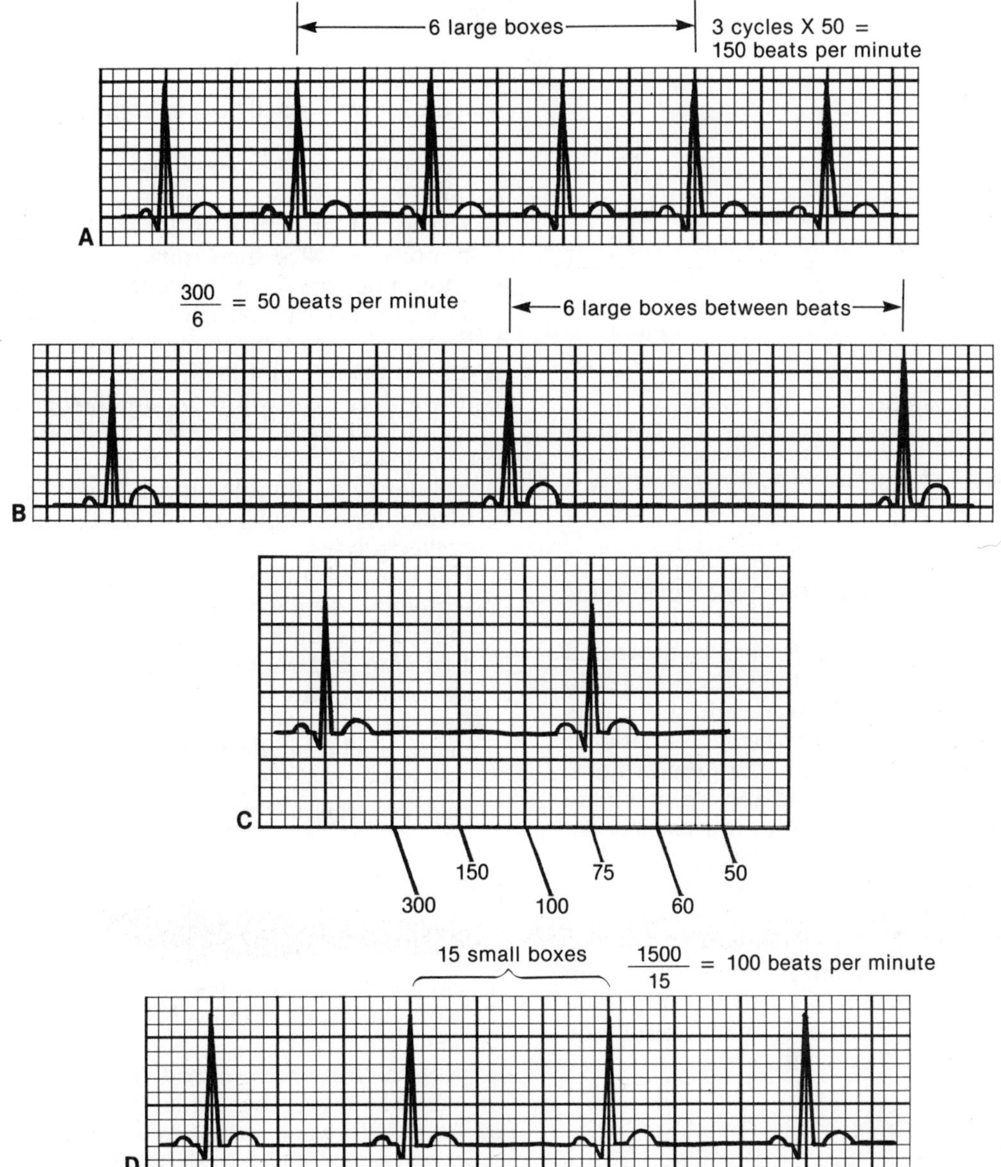

Figure 4–2. **Methods of determining heart rate (see text).** *A,* A heart rate of 150 beats per minute. *B,* A heart rate of 50 beats per minute. *C,* A heart rate of 75 beats per minute. *D,* a heart rate of 100 beats per minute.

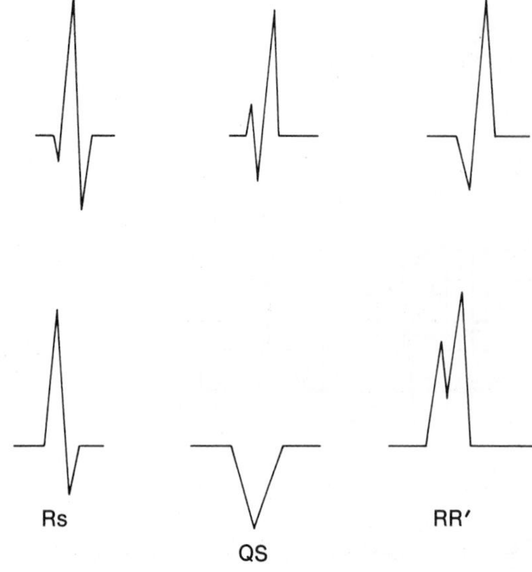

Figure 4–3. **Nomenclature of QRS complexes.** Any upward, or positive, wave is an *R wave*. The first downward, or negative, wave before an R wave is a *Q wave*. A downward, or negative, wave after an R wave is an *S wave*.

6. QRS complexes in the precordial leads (Fig. 4–4*A*):
   a. The *intrinsicoid deflection* is measured from the onset of the QRS complex to the peak of the R wave and represents the arrival of the wave of excitation from endocardium to epicardium. Only leads V1 or V2 and V5 or V6 are used. In lead V1, the intrinsicoid deflection should not be greater than 0.035 second (< 1 small box). In lead V6, it should not be greater than 0.055 second (< 1.5 small boxes).
   b. As the QRS complex progresses from leads V1 to V6, the S wave amplitude decreases as the R wave amplitude increases (Fig. 4–4*B*).

Q WAVES

1. Should not be greater than 0.03 second (less than 1 small box). Significant Q waves are greater than 0.04 second (1 small box) and/or greater than one third the height of the QRS complex.
2. Q waves can normally be found in leads I, AVL and V5 to V6. These represent normal septal activation from the left to the right.
3. It is important to take into consideration the clinical setting when deciding on the significance of Q waves.
4. A Q wave in leads V1 and V2 must be considered abnormal.

ST SEGMENT

1. Usually isoelectric but an elevation of less than 1 mm (1 small box) in limb leads may be normal.
2. Normally not depressed more than 0.5 mm (½ small box).
3. The point at which it leaves the QRS complex is called the *J point*.
4. Should not pursue a horizontal course but should curve sigmoidally into the T wave.
5. Primary ST segment changes are abnormal displacements of the ST segment either upward or downward and are associated with ischemia or inflammation. Secondary changes are related to conduction abnormalities (e.g., bundle branch block), ventricular hypertrophy or the effect of drugs or electrolytes.
6. The most common causes of primary ST segment elevation are myocardial ischemia and injury related to myocardial infarction and pericarditis.
7. Elevations of the ST segment at the J point may be a normal variant, especially in children, young adults or black men. This variant is called *early repolarization* or *juvenile ST segment abnormality*.

T WAVE

1. Represents recovery period or repolarization of the ventricles.
2. Normally upright in leads I, II and V3 to V6.
3. Normally inverted in lead AVR.
4. Variable in all other leads.
5. As the R wave increases in amplitude from leads V1 to V6, so should the amplitude of the T wave.
6. T wave shape is normally rounded; notching may be a normal variant in children but is also seen in pericarditis.
7. Amplitude is normally not greater than 5 mm (1 large box) in the limb leads or 10 mm (2 large boxes) in the precordial leads.
8. Tall T waves may suggest infarction, potassium excess ("tented T waves"),

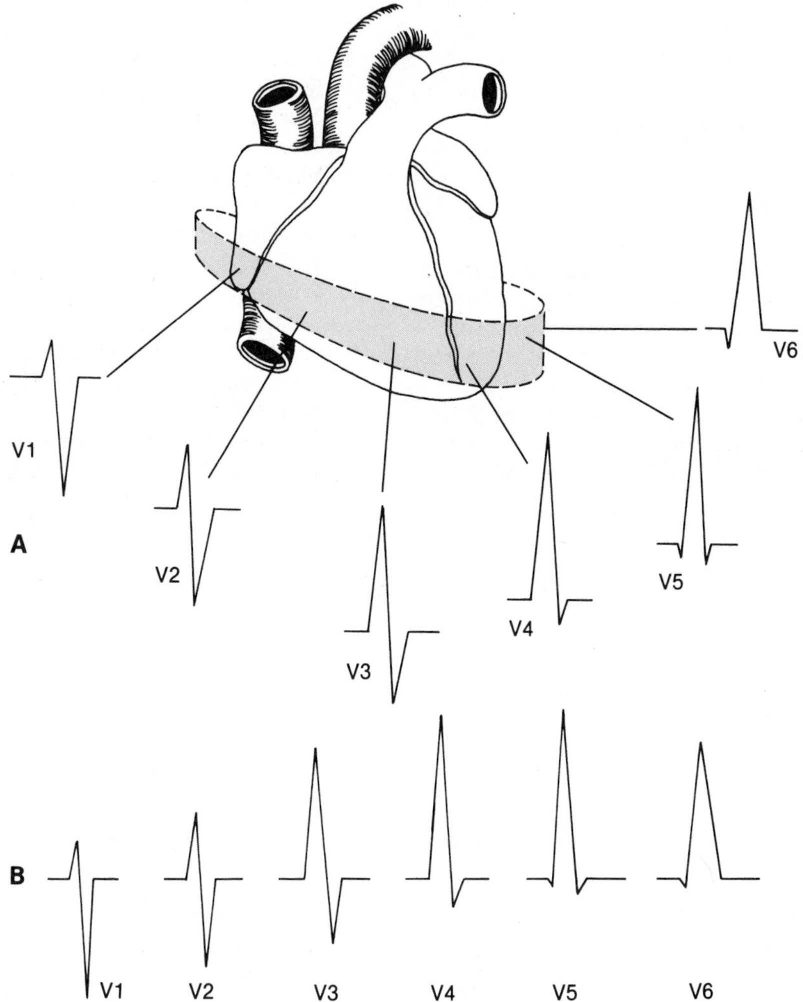

Figure 4–4. **Configuration of the precordial QRS complexes.** These figures demonstrate that as the electrode moves in position from leads V1 to V6, the S wave amplitude decreases as the R wave amplitude increases. In addition, septal depolarization is shown by the development of the Q wave in leads V5 and V6 and the R wave in leads V1 and V2.

ischemia, ventricular overload, use of antipsychotic drugs and cerebral vascular accidents. Very wide, bizarrely shaped T waves may be seen in cerebrovascular accidents or strokes.

9. Primary T wave changes are related to ischemia or inflammation. These conditions will produce T wave inversion if the T wave was originally upright. However, if the T wave was initially inverted, there may be a return of this T wave to an upright position, a state called *pseudonormalization*. Secondary T wave changes result from conduction abnormalities or ventricular hypertrophy.
10. The atria also produce a T wave during repolarization. This wave normally occurs during the QRS complex and therefore is buried within that complex and is not seen; however, when the PR interval is increased, it may occur before the QRS complex. If the PR interval is shortened, the atrial T wave may occur in the ST segment. This may be the mechanism for depressed ST segments associated with sinus tachycardia.

QT DURATION

1. Represents the total time of systole.
2. Varies with heart rate, sex and age.
3. Useful rule: QT interval should be less than one half the preceding R-R interval. This is only true for rates between 65 and 90 beats per minute.

4. To measure the QT interval more accurately, the corrected QT interval for rate (QTc) is defined as:

$$QTc = \frac{QT}{\sqrt{RR}}$$

5. Normal QTc is approximately 0.44 ± 0.02 second.
6. QTc is prolonged by congestive heart failure, infarction, hypocalcemia and quinidine and procainamide administration.
7. QTc is shortened by digitalis, hypercalcemia and hyperkalemia.
8. Prolonged QTc predisposes to the *R on T phenomenon*, which may result in ventricular tachycardia (see Ventricular Tachycardia).

U WAVE

1. A small wave of low voltage that follows the T wave.
2. Normally follows the same polarity as the T wave.
3. Most visible in the midprecordial leads (V3 to V4).
4. Is made more prominent by hypokalemia and bradycardia.
5. Polarity is reversed by ischemia and left ventricular strain.
6. Amplitude is increased by digitalis, quinidine, epinephrine, hyperthyroidism and exercise.
7. Represents a period of supernormal excitability during repolarization of the ventricles.

5

Electrical Axis

The QRS complex represents ventricular depolarization. This depolarization can be summated into a single vector that is normally directed toward the apex of the ventricles (Fig. 5–1). This summated vector is the mean electrical axis of the ventricles; it is not the anatomical axis of the heart.

Limb leads can determine the axis of the frontal plane and can provide information about the position of the electrical activity of the heart as it rotates around an anteroposterior axis. Precordial leads can determine the axis of the horizontal plane. This axis is situated in a mediolateral direction and is referred to as the rotational axis.

An electrical axis is not unique to ventricular depolarization; P and T waves also demonstrate this electrical property. Their respective axes can be determined by the same methods used to determine the frontal plane axis.

DETERMINING THE AXIS

In determining the axis it is important to remember that when the ventricular depolarization is parallel to and in the direction of a positive electrode, a large positive deflection will result (see Chapter 3, Vectors and Leads,

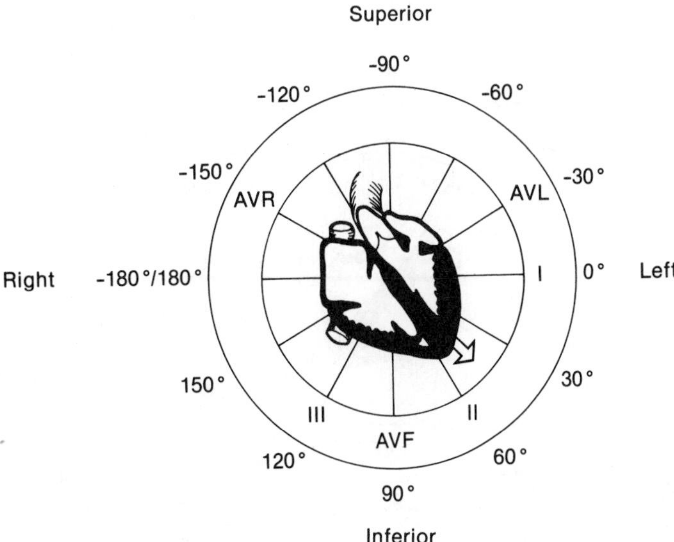

Figure 5–1. **Electrical axis.** The hexaxial limb leads are shown superimposed on the heart at its electrical center. The arrow is the mean QRS complex vector. The leads are indicated at their positive poles. Note that the leads are 30° apart.

page 13). When the depolarization is perpendicular to a positive electrode, a small, equiphasic deflection will result (see Chapter 3, Vectors and Leads, page 14 and Fig. 3–2).

Although there are numerous methods for determining the axis, a simple and easy method is outlined as follows and is shown in Figure 5–2:

1. Find the quadrant of the mean QRS vector by using leads I and AVF. When the QRS complex in lead I is above the baseline (positive), the mean QRS vector points to the left: quadrants B and D (Fig. 5–2*B*). When the QRS complex in lead AVF is above the baseline (positive), the mean QRS vector points to quadrants C and D. In this example, leads I and AVF indicate that the mean QRS vector is located in quadrant D.
2. Find either the limb lead with the smallest deflection or the lead in which the positive wave equals the negative wave (the isoelectric lead). This is the limb lead that is most nearly perpendicular to the axis. In this example, lead AVL has the smallest deflection.
3. Move 90° from the lead with the smallest deflection toward the proper quadrant. In this example, move 90° from lead AVL toward quadrant D.
4. If the lead with the smallest deflection is slightly positive, the axis is not quite a full 90° away from the lead. If the lead with the smallest deflection is slightly negative, the axis is actually slightly greater than 90°.

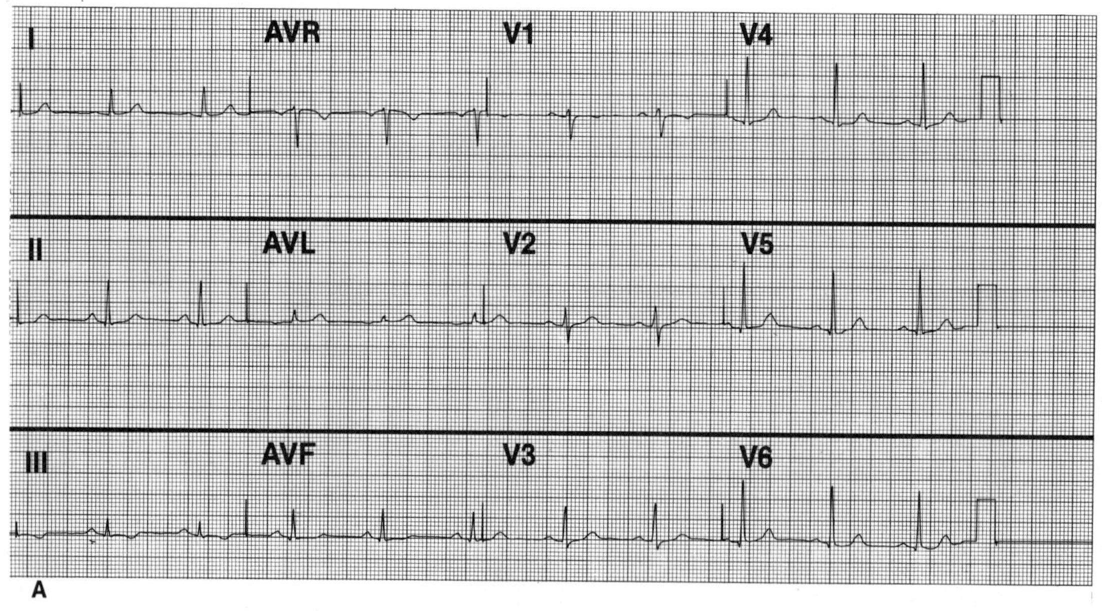

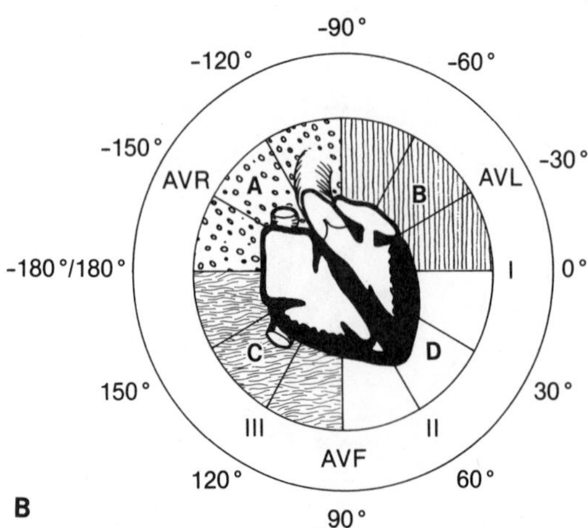

Figure 5–2. **Determination of the axis.** *A,* A representative electrocardiogram. Follow the text and use Figures 5–2*A* and *B* to determine the axis.

In the example provided, since the QRS complex is slightly positive in lead AVL, the mean QRS axis is slightly less than 90° toward quadrant D, and the axis is 50°. Most commonly, the axis is approximated to within 10 to 20°

AXIS DEVIATION

This is an important concept and is helpful in diagnosing certain electrocardiographic abnormalities. The axis of the mean QRS vector varies in individuals, depending upon age and body structure. In early life, this mean axis is deviated to the right. As the child grows, the mean QRS vector rotates leftward. By early adolescence, the QRS axis ranges between 0 and 90°.

The QRS axis may be between 0 and 90° or can be deviated to the right or left. Figure 5–3 depicts the degrees of rotation that are considered normal, left axis deviation, right axis deviation and extreme, or abnormal, left and right axis deviation. Although the QRS axis from −30 to +120° is normal, the term left axis deviation is used to denote a QRS axis from 0 to −30; right axis deviation denotes a QRS axis from +90 to +120°. Beyond these extremes, the axis is considered abnormal. In addition, a QRS axis between −90 and +180° is called indeterminant, since it is impossible to determine if it is extreme right or extreme left axis deviation.

When considering the importance of axis deviation, it is useful to know the clinical state of the patient in order to be sure that the deviation is abnormal. For instance, the QRS axis is normally deviated to the left in late pregnancy because of the gravid uterus's pushing up on the diaphragm and heart. The major causes of axis deviation are listed in Table 1.

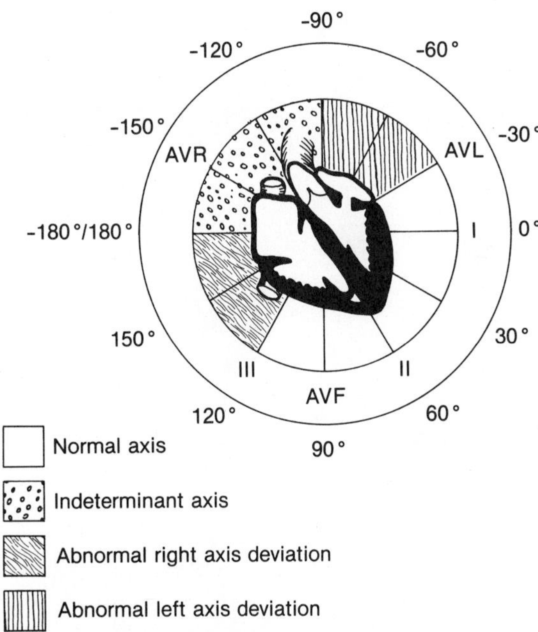

Figure 5–3. **Axis deviation.** A normal axis lies between −30° and +120°. An axis from 0 to −30° is called a left axis deviation. An axis greater than −30° is called abnormal left axis deviation. An axis between +90 and +120° is called right axis deviation. An axis greater than +120° is called abnormal right axis deviation. Since it is impossible to determine from which direction an axis has come, an axis between −90 and +180° is called an indeterminate axis.

Table 1. COMMON CAUSES OF AXIS DEVIATIONS

LEFT AXIS DEVIATION	RIGHT AXIS DEVIATION
Left ventricular hypertrophy*	Right ventricular hypertrophy†
Left bundle branch block	Right bundle branch block
Wolff-Parkinson-White syndrome	Left posterior hemiblock
	Left ventricular ectopic beats
High diaphragm, pregnancy, ascites, abdominal tumor	Emphysema (causes flat diaphragm)
	Pulmonary infarcts and emboli
Normal variants, especially elderly and obese patients	Normal variants, especially young and thin patients

*Left ventricular hypertrophy causes left axis deviation in only about 50 per cent of cases.

†Right axis deviation is seen in almost 100 per cent of cases.

6

Fundamentals of Rhythms

Normal cardiac rhythm results from the spontaneous depolarization of pacemaker cells within the sinoatrial node and conduction of these impulses to the atrioventricular node, bundle of His and bundle branches to the Purkinje system. An abnormality in the rate or site of origin of the impulse is termed an arrhythmia. Disturbances in rhythm are usually related to abnormalities in excitability, automaticity, conductivity or a combination of these properties. In order to better understand rhythm disorders, a brief review of some basic electrophysiological properties of heart tissue will be helpful (see Chapter 2, The Action Potential).

EXCITABILITY

Excitability is the capacity of the cell to depolarize and to form an action potential when exposed to a sufficiently strong stimulus. This property is common to all myocardial cells. However, the depolarization threshold potentials of the different cells vary.

AUTOMATICITY

Automaticity is the capability of a cell to initiate an impulse without extrinsic stimulation. Cells such as those in the sinoatrial node, atrioventricular node, bundle of His and Purkinje system demonstrate automaticity by allowing a slow influx of ions, which reduces their resting membrane potentials (see Fig. 2–2*B*, phase 4). When the changing resting membrane potential reaches the threshold, the cell will rapidly depolarize (phase 0).

It is apparent that the automaticity of a cell is dependent upon the slope of phase 4, the magnitude of the resting potential and the threshold potential. Sinus node cells have the steepest phase 4, so that they reach threshold at a faster rate than other cells of the conducting system. However, if the sinus node fails to fire, other tissues of the conducting system can take over as secondary pacemakers. Myocardial cells do not normally possess the property of automaticity because they do not allow an influx of ions in phase 4 (see Fig. 2–2*A*, phase 4).

In summary, the rate of automaticity can be changed by three mechanisms:

1. Changing the slope of the phase 4 depolarization.
2. Changing the threshold.
3. Changing the resting potential.

For example, if the slope of phase 4 is increased, the threshold will be reached sooner, and consequently the automatic rate will increase (Fig. 6–1*B*). If the threshold is increased (the threshold potential is made less negative), the automatic rate will slow, since it will take longer for phase 4 depolarization to reach the threshold level (Fig. 6–1*C*). If the resting membrane potential is increased (made more negative), the rate of automaticity will decrease because it will take longer for phase 4 to reach the threshold (Fig. 6–1*D*).

Changes in automaticity can be induced by

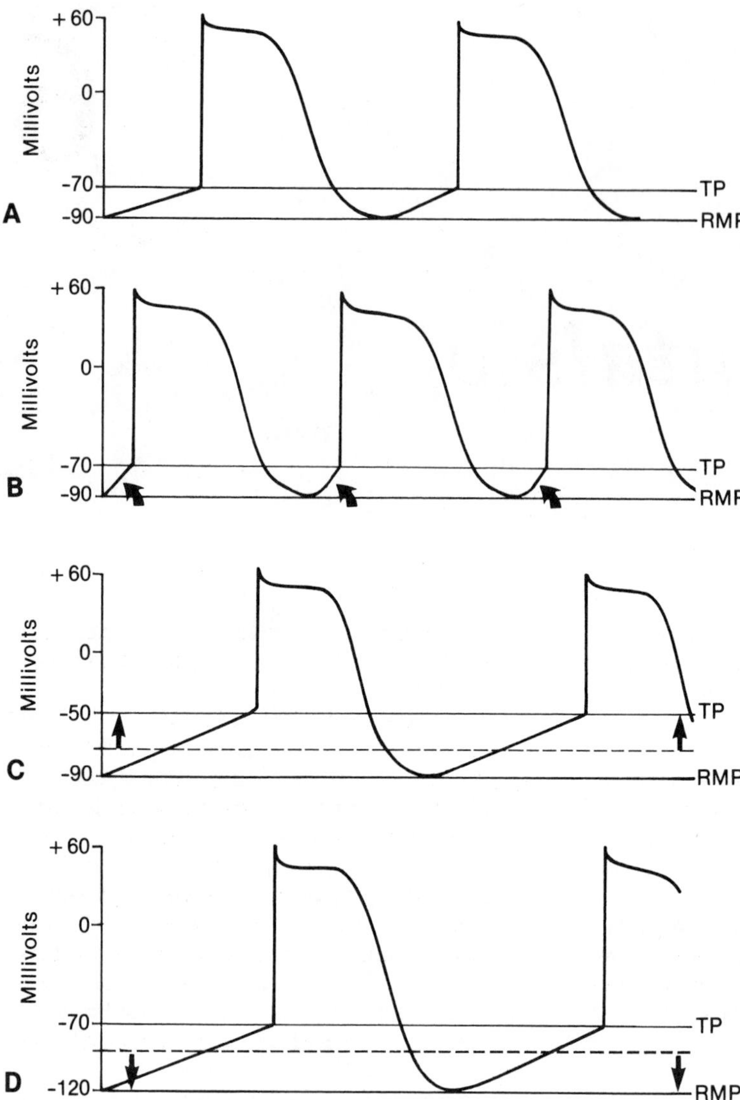

Figure 6–1. **Mechanisms for changing automaticity.** *A,* The normal action potentials at a rate used for reference in this figure. *B,* By increasing the slope of phase 4 (arrows), the automaticity can be increased, thereby increasing the rate. *C,* By making the threshold potential less negative (arrows), it will take longer to reach this potential; thus, the rate will slow. *D,* By making the resting membrane potential more negative (arrows), it will also take longer to reach the threshold potential, and the rate will again slow. Notice also that the height of the action potential is greater than normal. This is a result of the more negative position of the resting membrane potential. (TP = threshold potential; RMP = resting membrane potential.)

various factors. Vagal stimulation slows the heart rate by decreasing the slope of phase 4 and by increasing the resting membrane potential in the sinoatrial node. In contrast, increasing sympathetic tone will increase automaticity in all heart tissue by increasing the slope of phase 4. Hypoxia also increases the slope of phase 4 and leads to increased automaticity. In addition, any type of injury to the myocardium may increase the irritability and automaticity of cells in the conducting system and myocardium and may even induce the property of automaticity in cells that do not normally possess it.

A variety of arrhythmias result from changes in automaticity. For example, when the automaticity of the sinus node is increased, *sinus tachycardia* will result. If the automaticity of the sinus node is slowed, *sinus bradycardia* will result. If the sinus rhythm is too slow, other cells that possess automaticity may fire. This produces *escape beats,* which prevent long pauses in rhythm. If other automatic cells completely take over the sinus node's function, they are referred to as *secondary* or *latent pacemakers* (Fig. 6–2). In addition, premature contractions and ectopic tachycardias are often caused by an increase in the automaticity of the offending cells.

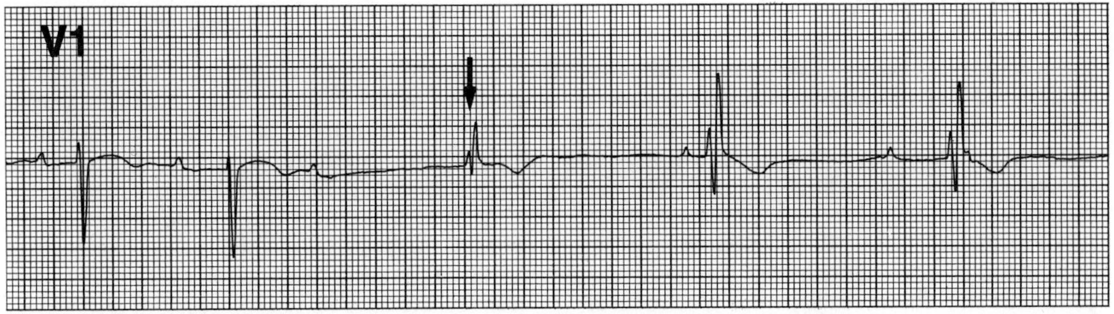

Figure 6–2. **Latent (secondary) pacemaker.** This tracing shows the sudden development of complete heart block after a P wave fails to capture the ventricles. A ventricular, or secondary, pacemaker then takes over. The arrow points to a ventricular escape beat, after which a ventricular rhythm at a rate of 36 beats per minute serves as the pacemaker.

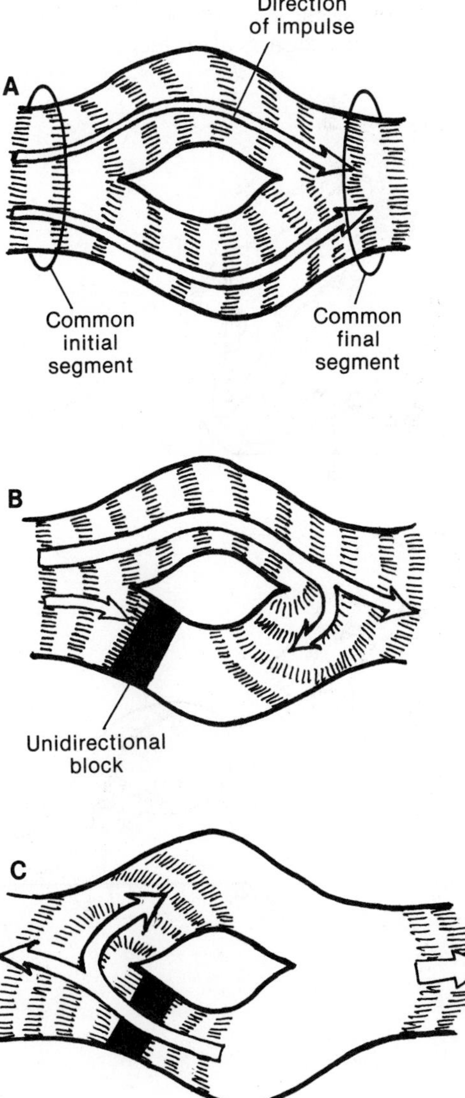

Figure 6–3. **Requirements for re-entry.** *A,* The presence of two pathways with a common initial and final segment. *B,* A unidirectional block, represented by the black bar, in one of these pathways. *C,* A slowing of the impulse in the unblocked pathway caused by the passing of the earlier impulse.

CONDUCTIVITY

Conductivity, which is a property of all myocardial cells, is the ability of a cell to propagate an electrical impulse. The rate of propagating the impulse varies with the type of myocardial cell. The rate is fastest in the His-Purkinje system, while it is slowest in the atrioventricular node. It is the slow conduction through the atrioventricular node that produces the PR interval in the electrocardiogram.

The physiological factors affecting conductivity are the following:

1. Rate of phase 0 depolarization.
2. Amplitude of the action potential.

There is a direct relationship between these factors and conductivity. Simply stated, as the rate of phase 0 or the amplitude is decreased, conduction is also decreased.

Changing both the resting membrane potential and the threshold potential are the two common mechanisms that produce changes in the rate of phase 0 and in amplitude. For example, hypokalemia increases the resting membrane potential (makes it more negative). This increases the rate of rise of phase 0 and speeds conduction. Conversely, hyperkalemia decreases the resting potential (makes it more positive). This decreases the rate of rise of phase 0 and slows conduction. These mechanisms are also utilized by the autonomic nervous system and by digitalis in controlling conduction through the atrioventricular node. They are also the mechanisms by which cardiac disease and electrolyte disturbances produce changes in conduction.

There are few arrhythmias caused by increased conductivity; therefore, it is more useful to understand the effects of decreased

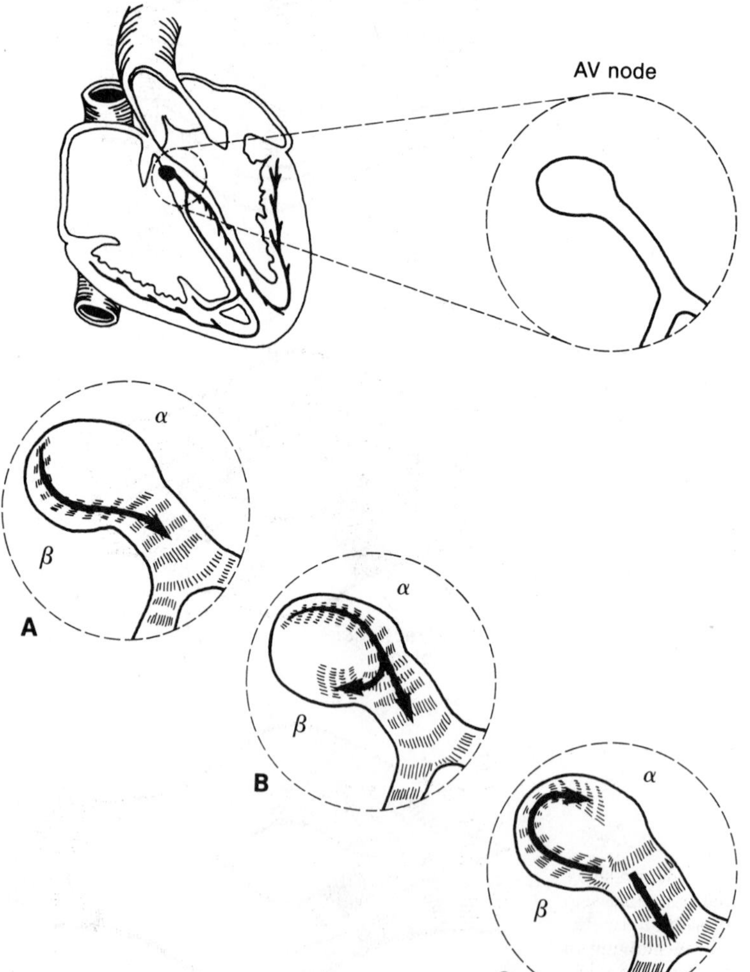

Figure 6–4. Atrioventricular nodal re-entry. *A, B,* and *C,* Enlargements of the area of the atrio-ventricular node, which is circled. These enlargements show the two pathways, "alpha" and "beta," and the development of re-entry (see text for discussion).

conductivity. In general, decreased conductivity can range from a simple slowing of conduction to a complete block in impulse transmission; thus, decreased conductivity can lead to serious arrhythmias.

Decreased conductivity in the sinus node or atria may impair sinus impulses from spreading throughout the heart. This may produce long pauses in rhythm that encourage *escape beats* and *secondary pacemaker* formations. Decreased conduction through the atrioventricular node impairs the relationship between atrial and ventricular contractions. This can result in very slow rhythms that inhibit cardiac output. Ventricular conduction disturbances may impair ventricular contraction. They may also result in a decrease in cardiac output.

In addition to these arrhythmias, changes in conductivity are significant because they can lead to the formation of arrhythmias caused by re-entry.

RE-ENTRY

A common method by which decreased conduction produces arrhythmias is termed *re-entry*. Re-entry is the phenomenon in which a stimulus re-excites a conduction pathway through which it has already passed. Once started, this impulse may circulate repeatedly.

The re-entry phenomenon has three requirements (Fig. 6–3). The *first* is that two different pathways for conduction have the same initial and final segments (Fig. 6–3*A*). The *second* requirement is that conduction is slowed to such an extent in one of the pathways that there is a failure of conduction in one direction. This is termed *unidirectional block* (Fig. 6–3*B*). The *third* requirement for re-entry is that conduction be slower than normal in the unblocked pathway. Essentially, these three requirements produce a circuit that once activated may be able to re-excite itself, thus producing a tachyarrhythmic focus (Fig. 6–3C).

Re-entry can occur anywhere in the heart. Re-entry in the sinus node can produce premature atrial contractions and atrial tachycardias. Paroxysmal supraventricular tachycardia results from re-entry in the atrioventricular node; and ventricular tachycardia results from re-entry at the ventricular level.

A good example of re-entry is atrioventricular nodal re-entry. This is the most common cause of supraventricular tachycardia. Most patients with this condition have two pathways within the atrioventricular node (Fig. 6–4). These pathways are called "alpha" and "beta." "Alpha" has a slower conduction; therefore, the impulse is propagated down the "beta" pathway (Fig. 6–4*A*). However, a premature atrial impulse may reach the atrioventricular node during the refractory period of the "beta" pathway. Since the refractory period will act as a block to conduction, the impulse will proceed down the "alpha" pathway (Fig. 6–4*B*). This impulse will then enter the "beta" pathway in a retrograde fashion and create a circuit rhythm that may result in a supraventricular tachycardia (Fig. 6–4C).

7

Supraventricular Rhythms

Cardiac rhythms can be classified in a variety of ways. We have chosen to use an anatomical approach, since this seems to be the easiest to conceptualize. Essentially, a rhythm is classified according to the location of its origin. For example, *supraventricular* rhythms include those originating in the sinoatrial node, atria or atrioventricular node. *Ventricular* arrhythmias arise anywhere within the ventricular conducting system or myocardium. *Conduction disturbances* constitute a separate division of arrhythmias and refer to blocks of electrical conduction within the heart. Finally, *pre-excitation syndromes* are characterized by cardiac conduction through aberrant pathways.

SINUS RHYTHM

Normally, cells in the sinoatrial node depolarize spontaneously at a rate of 60 to 100 beats per minute. This depolarization spreads throughout the atria and produces P waves; it then spreads to the atrioventricular node where it is delayed before continuing down to the bundle of His and then to the Purkinje fibers in the ventricles (Fig. 7–1).

Normal sinus rhythm produces P waves that occur at regular intervals and precede each QRS complex by a fixed interval. The P waves should be upright in leads I, II and AVF, since these leads are parallel to the wave of atrial depolarization. In addition, the rate is between 60 and 100 beats per minute (Fig. 7–2*A*). A sinus rate below 60 beats per minute is considered sinus bradycardia (Fig. 7–2*B*), whereas a sinus rate greater than 100 beats per minute is termed sinus tachycardia (Fig. 7–2*C*).

Sinus bradycardia is common in athletes and may be a normal variant. It may also result from drug therapy, which may increase vagal tone or decrease sympathetic tone. Hypothy-

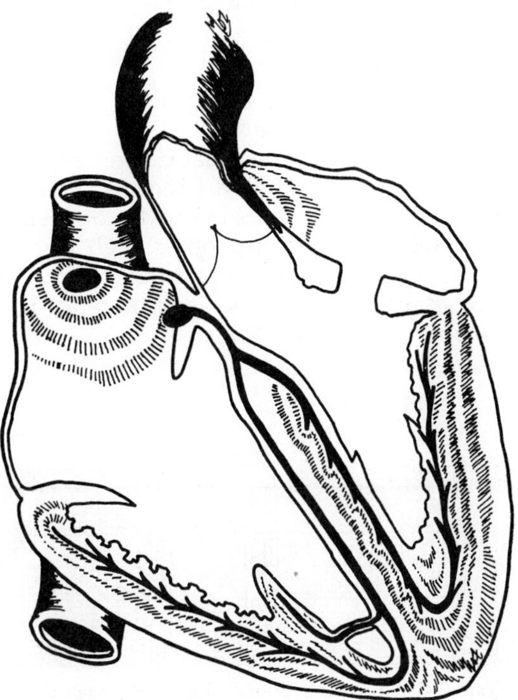

Figure 7–1. The normal conduction pathway.

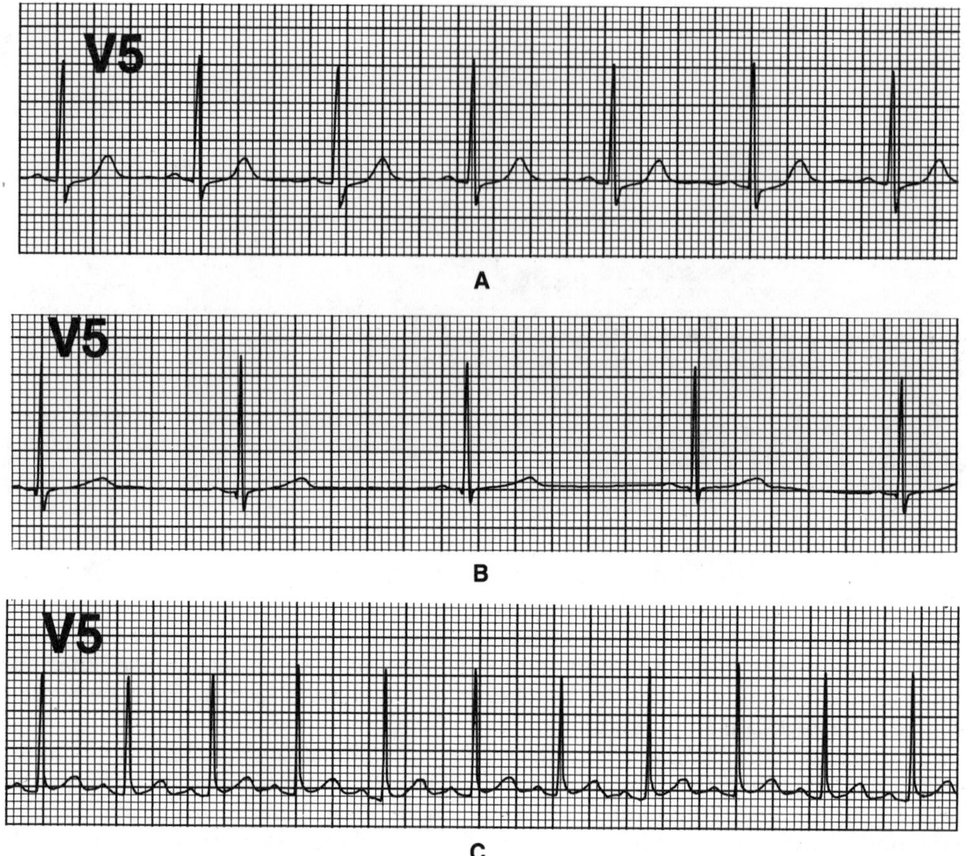

Figure 7–2. **Sinus rhythms.** *A,* Normal sinus rhythm at a rate of 79 beats per minute. *B,* Sinus bradycardia at a rate of 50 beats per minute. *C,* Sinus tachycardia at a rate of 125 beats per minute. Notice that all of these tracings show sinus P waves that precede the QRS complexes and have fixed PR intervals.

roidism, by slowing metabolism, can also produce sinus bradycardia.

Sinus tachycardia is normal during exercise but can be produced by the increase in sympathetic tone that occurs in shock, congestive heart failure, fever and other high output states, such as anemia. Sympathomimetics such as epinephrine and isoproterenol will likewise increase heart rate.

Sinus arrhythmia, a speeding up of the heart rate with inspiration and slowing with expiration, is caused in part by inhibition by the vagus nerve. Like all other sinus rhythms, each QRS complex is preceded by a P wave with a fixed PR interval. The QRS complexes are normal in configuration and duration. However, the R-R intervals are irregular (Fig. 7–3). Sinus arrhythmia is frequently found in

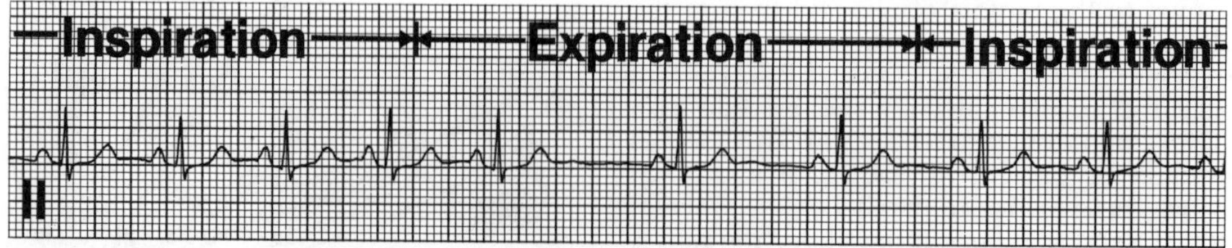

Figure 7–3. **Sinus arrhythmia.** Notice that each QRS complex is preceded by a fixed PR interval. However, upon inspiration, there is an increase in the rate of the sinus node firing, which slows with expiration.

healthy young persons without heart disease; however, in older patients it may be associated with degeneration of the sinoatrial node (see Sick Sinus Syndrome, Chapter 9, page 61) or chronic lung disease.

Pauses in sinus rhythm result from *sinus blocks* or *sinus exit blocks.* If the sinus node fails to resume pacemaker function, *sinus arrest* is present. These rhythms are characterized by the absence of sinus P waves, pauses in rhythm and escape beats. An *escape beat* is simply the firing of an ectopic focus to preserve cardiac function. It can originate in any tissue that possesses automaticity. If sinus arrest is present, the ectopic focus may take over as a *secondary pacemaker.* This pacemaker will fire at its inherent rate of automaticity. For example, an atrioventricular node pacemaker will fire at 40 to 60 beats per minute, and a Purkinje pacemaker will fire at 30 beats per minute. In some patients, an escape beat rhythm may be too slow to maintain sufficient cardiac output; an electronic pacemaker is therefore required.

ATRIAL ARRHYTHMIAS

Any impulse that does not originate in the sinus node is termed an *ectopic focus,* and any rhythm that is not normal sinus rhythm can be termed an *arrhythmia.* Atrial arrhythmias are ectopic foci of activity that may originate in any part of the atria. The electrical activity from an atrial pacemaker will produce P waves, but these waves will have a different configuration from the P waves produced by the sinus node (Fig. 7–4). In fact, different ectopic foci in the atria will produce P waves with different configurations.

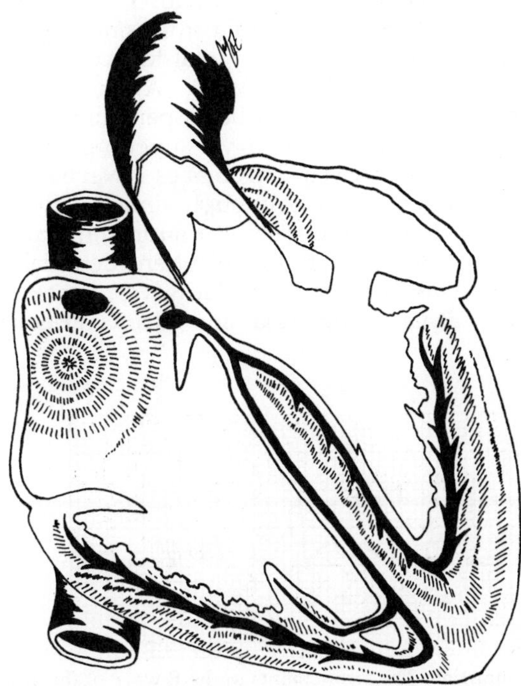

Figure 7–4. This diagram shows the generation of an ectopic atrial arrhythmia.

Most atrial arrhythmias are tachyarrhythmias and include atrial premature contractions, atrial tachycardia, atrial flutter and atrial fibrillation. In the evaluation of a tachyarrhythmia, the atrial rate is helpful in determining the arrhythmia. The so-called "rule of hundreds" is quite helpful. If the atrial rate is 200 ± 50 beats per minute, atrial tachycardia may be present. If the atrial rate is 300 ± 50 beats per minute, atrial flutter is usually present. Finally, if the atrial rate is 400 ± 50 beats per minute, the rhythm is said to be atrial fibrillation.

ATRIAL PREMATURE CONTRACTIONS

Atrial premature contractions are ectopic atrial beats that originate in any part of the atria. The terms atrial premature contraction, premature atrial contraction, atrial premature beat and atrial extrasystole are synonymous. These beats are characterized by P waves that come before the next normal sinus beat is due and have a different configuration from the P waves of sinus origin. The morphology of the P waves depends on the site of the ectopic atrial focus. When the site is high in the atrium, the P wave axis is generally normal (upright P wave in Lead II). When the ectopic focus is low in the atrium, the P wave axis tends to be directed superiorly, with upright P waves in lead AVR and negative P waves in leads II, III and AVF (Fig. 7–5).

Interestingly, the atrial activation also depolarizes the sinus node. The "reset" sinus node will continue to fire at its inherent rate, so the interval between an atrial premature beat and the next sinus beat is equal to the interval between any two normal sinus beats. In other words, the duration of two cycles, including the premature beat, is less than the sum of two normal cycles. This situation, caused by the reset sinus node, is referred to as an *incomplete compensatory pause.*

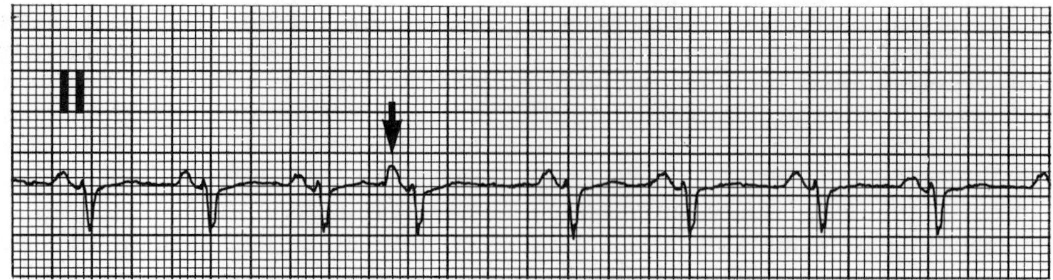

Figure 7–5. **An atrial premature contraction.** The arrow points to the P wave of the atrial premature contraction. Notice that the configuration of the P wave is different from the sinus P waves and that it is early with respect to where the next sinus P wave should occur.

Usually, each atrial beat is conducted through the atrioventricular junction to the ventricles, so the PR intervals are normal as well as the duration of the QRS complexes. In some instances, an atrial premature contraction may reach the atrioventricular junction while all or part of the conducting system is still refractory. This will result in an atrial premature contraction that is either not conducted to the ventricles (Fig. 7–6) or aberrantly conducted. An RSR′ complex (see Right Bundle Branch Block, Chapter 10, page 68) usually results from an aberrantly conducted atrial premature contraction. Aberrant conduction is discussed further under Atrial Fibrillation.

Atrial premature contractions are common in healthy individuals and often are associated with the intake of stimulants such as caffeine or tobacco. They may, however, be associated with structural heart disease. Treatment for atrial premature beats is usually not necessary. Patients should refrain from the ingestion of stimulants.

ATRIAL TACHYCARDIA

Runs of consecutive atrial premature contractions are termed *atrial tachycardia.* In atrial tachycardia, an atrial pacemaker fires regularly at 200 ± 50 beats per minute. This ectopic focus produces true P waves, but their configuration is different from the P waves produced by normal sinus rhythm. Because the arrhythmia has a sudden onset and termination, it is often called *paroxysmal atrial tachycardia.* Since the atrioventricular node is able to conduct each atrial impulse to the ventricles, the rhythm is regular, with a ventricular rate of 150 to 250 beats per minute. The QRS complex is not widened (Fig. 7–7). Occasionally, one will find paroxysmal atrial tachycardia with varying degrees of atrioventricular block. The ventricular rhythm is, therefore, irregular. Paroxysmal atrial tachycardia with block is frequently seen in patients with digitalis toxicity.

It is frequently difficult to differentiate paroxysmal atrial tachycardia from sinus tachycardia, atrioventricular nodal tachycardia or atrial flutter with 2:1 block. At ventricular rates greater than 150 beats per minute, all these rhythms may have superimposed P waves on T waves. This makes P wave identification difficult. Although sinus tachycardia and atrial flutter are of a supraventricular origin, these rhythms are often identifiable based on other criteria. However, paroxysmal atrial tachycardia and atrioventricular

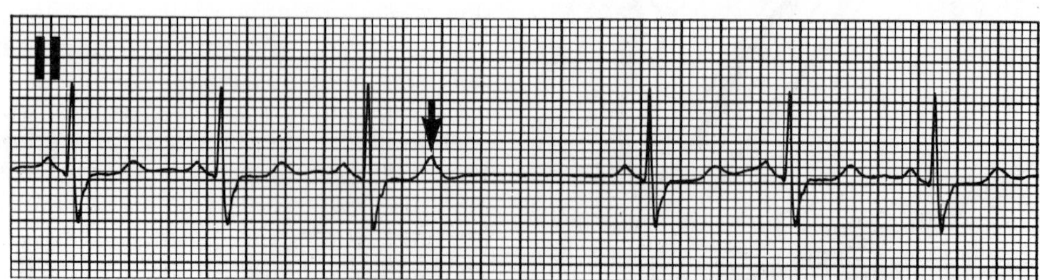

Figure 7–6. **A blocked, or nonconducted, atrial premature contraction.** The arrow points to the P wave of the atrial premature contraction, which has occurred so early that the ventricles are still in the absolute refractory period. The ectopic P wave has made the T wave, on which it has fallen, much more peaked than any other.

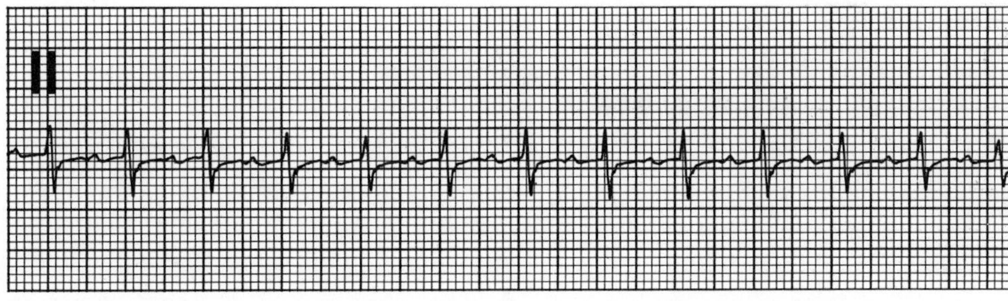

Figure 7–7. **Supraventricular tachycardia.** The atrial and ventricular rates are 150 beats per minute. The term supraventricular tachycardia is used to denote a tachycardia with a focus above the ventricles. This term therefore includes both atrial and junctional tachycardias.

nodal tachycardia are often indistinguishable and are grouped together under the term *supraventricular tachycardia.*

In most cases supraventricular tachycardias are caused by re-entrant or circus rhythm phenomena (see Re-entry, page 31). They are characterized by regular ventricular rates of 150 to 250 beats per minute and are common in young, healthy individuals as well as in patients with atherosclerotic or hypertensive heart disease. Their onset is abrupt, and episodes are usually transient, lasting a few seconds to minutes. These paroxysms may be related to emotional stress, consumption of caffeine, tobacco or alcoholic beverages as well as mental or physical fatigue. During these episodes, patients may experience palpitations. Following a paroxysm, patients frequently experience acute polyuria. Supraventricular tachycardias are usually benign arrhythmias; however, patients with pre-existing heart disease may suffer hemodynamic compromise.

Vagal maneuvers such as gagging, carotid massage and the Valsalva maneuver are often helpful in determining the underlying rhythm and in converting a supraventricular tachycardia to normal sinus rhythm. By increasing vagal tone, these maneuvers slow sinus tachycardia. In paroxysmal atrial tachycardia, the rhythm will either remain unchanged or abruptly revert to normal sinus rhythm. In atrial flutter, vagal maneuvers will increase the atrioventricular block (e.g., 2:1 to 3:1 to 4:1; see the following discussion on Atrial Flutter). This will make flutter waves more prominent on the electrocardiogram and will decrease the heart rate.

If vagal maneuvers are unable to convert a supraventricular tachycardia back to normal sinus rhythm, pharmacological treatment with propranolol, a beta blocker, or verapamil is useful. Rapid atrial pacing and electrical cardioversion can also be employed to convert supraventricular tachycardia to normal sinus rhythm.

ATRIAL FLUTTER

Atrial flutter is a common abnormality of rhythm in which the atria beat regularly at a rapid rate, usually 300 ± 50 beats per minute. These atrial beats do not produce true P waves. Rather a "saw-toothed" or "picket-fenced" baseline is apparent, which is best seen in leads II, III and AVF. Each saw-toothed wave is referred to as an "F" wave; these may superimpose on the QRS complexes, T or U waves and distort their configurations (Fig. 7–8*A*).

As in atrial fibrillation, the atrioventricular node is unable to conduct all the atrial impulses to the ventricles. The relationship between the atrial rate and the ventricular rate can be expressed as a ratio. Many patients with atrial flutter have 2:1 atrioventricular block. This means that for every two atrial impulses (two F waves reach the atrioventricular node), one will get through and stimulate the ventricles. As the degree of atrioventricular block increases, the ventricular response will decrease. If the atrial rate is 300 beats per minute in atrial flutter with a 2:1 atrioventricular block, the ventricular rate is 150 beats per minute; with 3:1 block, 100 beats per minute and with 4:1 block, 75 beats per minute. Not uncommonly, patients will have varying degrees of atrioventricular block on the same tracing. This will result in an irregular rhythm (Fig. 7–8*B*). However, one should notice that the atrial flutter waves are regular at 300 beats per minute. This should provide a clue that it is the degree of atrioventricular block that is varying.

Although rare, atrial flutter with 1:1 con-

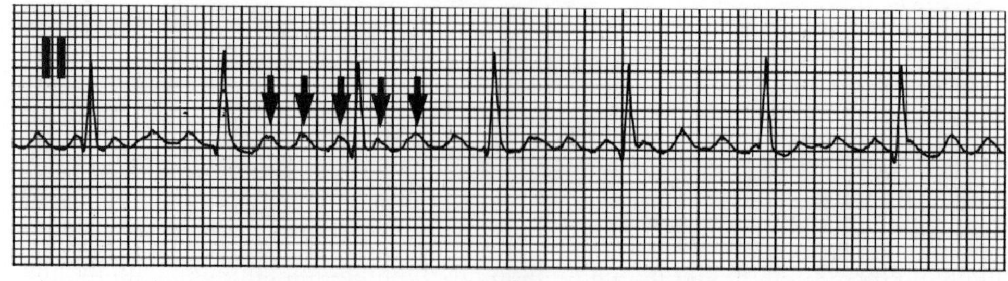

A

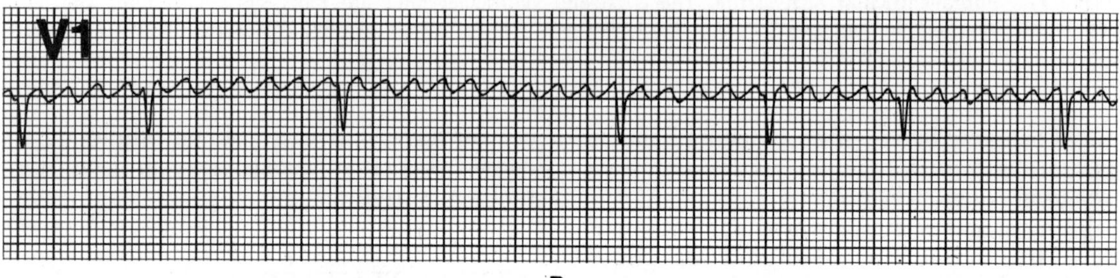

B

Figure 7–8. **Atrial flutter.** *A,* The saw-toothed pattern of the F waves, as indicated by the arrows. The F wave rate is approximately 300 beats per minute, and there are four F waves for every QRS complex; the ventricular rate is 88 beats per minute. The rhythm is atrial flutter with 4:1 atrioventricular block. The fourth F wave is not clearly seen, as it tends to be buried in each QRS complex. *B,* Atrial flutter with varying atrioventricular block, which produces irregular R-R intervals.

duction can occur. This is usually incompatible with adequate cardiac output and frequently occurs in patients who have been medicated with vagolytic drugs, such as quinidine. By decreasing vagal tone, quinidine will allow more impulse to pass through the atrioventricular node, so the block will decrease, resulting in an increase in the ventricular response.

Clinical Significance

Atrial flutter is rare in healthy individuals. It is often found in patients with thyrotoxicosis, mitral valve disease, atrial septal defects and chronic lung disease. It is an unstable rhythm caused by re-entry or circus rhythm phenomenon. It often reverts spontaneously to normal sinus rhythm or degenerates to atrial fibrillation. The danger to patients with atrial flutter is the rapid ventricular response that can lead to a decrease in cardiac output.

Treatment of atrial flutter is directed toward slowing the ventricular rate and converting the rhythm to normal sinus rhythm or atrial fibrillation. Digitalis will increase the atrioventricular block (change 2:1 to 3:1 to 4:1) and will produce a slower ventricular rate. It also can increase the atrial rate and change the rhythm to atrial fibrillation. Verapamil or propranolol can also be used to control the ventricular rate by decreasing conduction through the atrioventricular node.

When the ventricular response is controlled, conversion of atrial flutter to normal sinus rhythm can be attempted using quinidine, verapamil or propranolol. If pharmacological treatment fails, rapid atrial pacing or electrical conversion is often used to convert atrial flutter to normal sinus rhythm.

ATRIAL FIBRILLATION

In *atrial fibrillation* the atria contract approximately 400 to 500 times per minute. Because most of these contractions are weak and incomplete, P waves are not produced. Instead, a wavy undulating baseline is seen. These atrial contractions bombard the atrioventricular node with impulses, but because of the inherent delay at the atrioventricular node, many of these impulses are "blocked" from reaching the ventricles. This atrioventricular nodal block results in a ventricular rate that is usually between 120 and 200 beats per minute; the ventricular response is grossly irregular with irregular R-R intervals and QRS complex amplitudes. This is probably caused by waves of atrial depolarizations

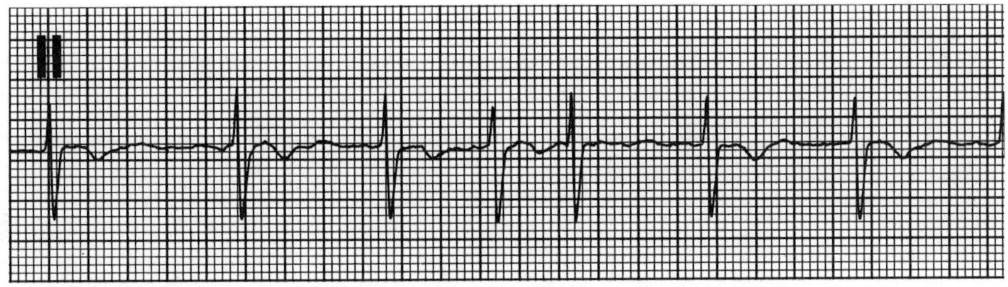

Figure 7–9. **Atrial fibrillation.** Notice the absence of P waves and the undulating baseline. The R-R intervals are irregularly irregular, which means that there is no regularity to the irregularity.

of various strengths reaching the atrioventricular node in an unorganized fashion.

The fibrillatory atrial waves, sometimes referred to as "F" waves, are best seen in lead V1 because it is closest to the fibrillating atria. Since it is almost impossible to discern the "F wave" rate, one must learn to recognize the pattern of fibrillation. Besides producing the undulating baseline and absence of P waves, "F waves" may superimpose on the QRS complexes or T or U waves, thereby distorting their configurations (Fig. 7–9).

The major characteristics of atrial fibrillation include the following:

1. Undulating baseline; absence of P waves.
2. Irregular ventricular response, including irregular R-R intervals and QRS complex amplitudes.

In addition to these criteria, widened QRS complexes are often seen in patients with atrial fibrillation. This is called *aberrant ventricular conduction.* Aberrant conduction is a form of transient abnormal intraventricular conduction and results from unequal refractoriness of the bundle branches. To understand the concept of aberrancy, it is important to remember that the ventricles are capable of firing at about 200 beats per minute. Secondly, that the atrioventricular node, bundle of His and fascicles are being stimulated at 400 to 500 beats per minute, but only 120 to 200 beats get through these sections of the conducting system to reach the ventricles. Thus, the ventricular rate (R-R interval) reflects the refractory period for the conducting system. For example, a longer R-R interval is associated with a longer refractory period of the conducting system. Likewise, a shorter R-R interval represents a shorter refractory period of the conducting system. Now, if a long R-R interval is followed by a shorter R-R interval, part of the conducting system may still be refractory when the QRS complex fires, and aberrant conduction will occur. This aberrant conduction caused by the changing R-R intervals is called *Ashman's phenomenon* (Fig. 7–10).

Since the right bundle branch has the longest refractory time of the conducting system, an RSR′ complex in lead V1 of right bundle branch block is the aberrancy pattern usually found in association with atrial fibrillation. It is very important to differentiate aberrant conduction from premature ventricular complexes, which look similar. Although, certainly open to exception, the premature ventricular contraction is more likely to have a slurred or notched R-wave in lead V1 rather than an RS or RSR′ complex, which is associated with aberrancy. If one looks in lead V6, a deep S wave is usually associated with

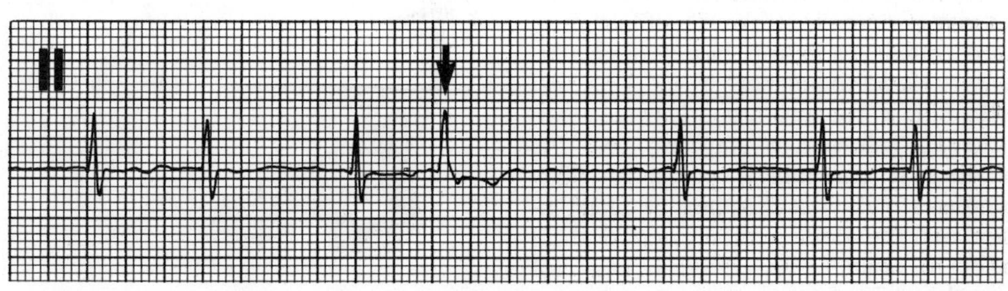

Figure 7–10. **Ashman's phenomenon.** The rhythm is atrial fibrillation. The arrow points to the beat conducted aberrantly, which occurs at a shorter R-R interval compared with the previous longer R-R interval (see text).

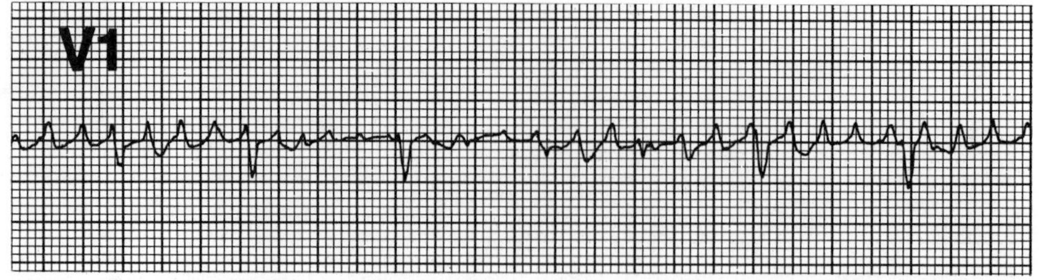

Figure 7–11. **"Atrial fibrillation-flutter."** Although flutter waves appear to be present, the baseline has periods without these waves, and the rhythm is irregular. This rhythm is best called coarse atrial fibrillation.

a premature ventricular contraction, whereas a wide *slurred* S wave is associated with the right bundle branch pattern frequently associated with aberrancy. The presence of the Ashman's phenomenon leads to the conclusion that aberrancy is present.

Fibrillatory waves may be fine or coarse. The term *"fibrillation-flutter"* is a poor term, indicating that the rhythm is irregular but has evidence of a saw-toothed pattern (flutter). The rhythm is actually a coarse atrial fibrillation (Fig. 7–11).

Clinical Significance

The clinical consequences of atrial fibrillation include a decrease in cardiac output and a tendency to form thrombi due to stasis of blood in the enlarged fibrillating atria. The decreased cardiac output is in part a result of the inability of the fibrillating atria to pump blood into the ventricles. The loss of this "atrial kick" results in decreased ventricular filling and, hence, a decrease in cardiac output. More importantly, the rapid ventricular rate shortens the ventricular filling time. This also results in a decrease in the amount of blood filling the ventricles during diastole and reduces cardiac output.

Because of the stasis of blood in the atria, patients with atrial fibrillation have an increased risk of embolic stroke. The fibrillating atria are unable to pump blood normally. This allows blood to stagnate in the atria and form thrombi. If the atria are enlarged, even more blood is allowed to stagnate, and the risk of forming thrombi is increased. This risk increases with the duration of atrial fibrillation and the sudden conversion of atrial fibrillation to normal sinus rhythm. If a clot exists in the atria, the onset of normal atrial contraction caused by the conversion of atrial fibrillation to normal sinus rhythm may propel the clot into the circulation (Fig. 7–12).

The mainstay of treatment for patients with atrial fibrillation is to decrease the heart rate. This is important because the rapid ventricular rate poses the most immediate threat to the patient's cardiovascular stability. Digitalis is useful because it slows conduction through the atrioventricular node. This will prevent many of the atrial impulses from passing through the atrioventricular node to stimulate the ventricles, resulting in a slower ventricular response.

When the ventricular rate is under control (less than 100 beats per minute), conversion of atrial fibrillation to normal sinus rhythm is often attempted. Some patients convert to normal sinus rhythm with digitalis alone.

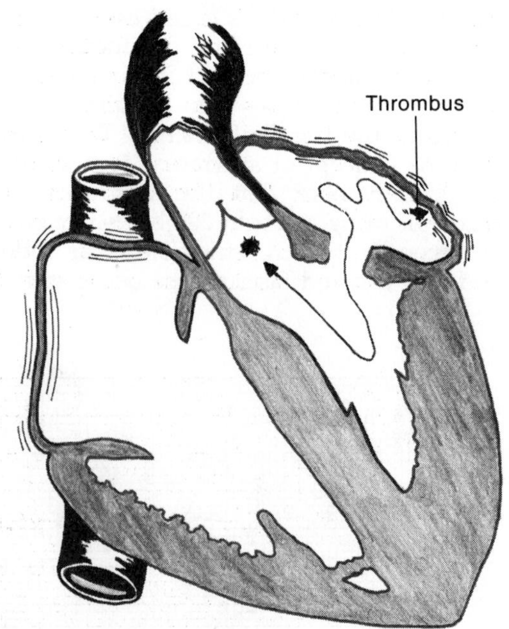

Figure 7–12. This diagram shows the development of emboli from fibrillating atria.

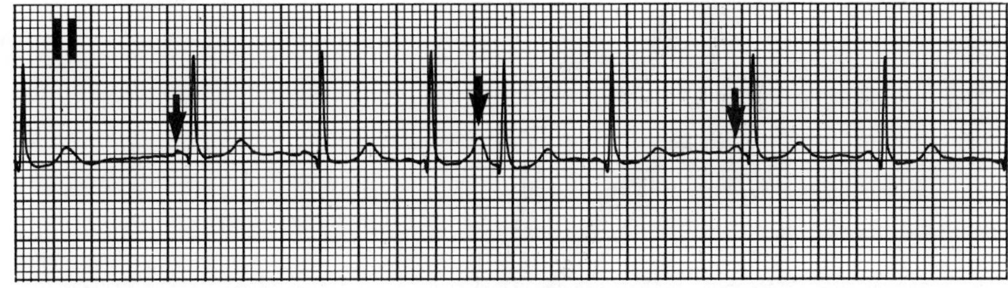

Figure 7–13. **Wandering atrial pacemaker.** The arrows point to three differently shaped P waves, indicating three different atrial foci.

Others may require quinidine or calcium channel blockers. And still others may require electrical cardioversion. Prior to any attempted conversion, patients with atrial fibrillation and atrial enlargement should be treated with anticoagulants as prophylaxis against emboli.

WANDERING ATRIAL PACEMAKER

Wandering atrial pacemaker is a disturbance of rhythm in which the atria are stimulated from different sites in the atrium. The PR intervals and the R-R intervals are therefore likely to change as well as the configuration of the P waves (Fig. 7–13). When the wandering atrial pacemaker exceeds the rate of 100 beats per minute, the term *multifocal atrial tachycardia,* or *chaotic atrial tachycardia,* is used. Multifocal atrial tachycardia is characterized by P waves with at least three different shapes and PR intervals (Fig. 7–14). This rhythm, frequently seen in elderly patients, is commonly associated with pulmonary disease, cor pulmonale and diabetes.

JUNCTIONAL RHYTHMS

There has been much confusion regarding the terms junctional and nodal as they relate to etiologies of rhythm. The atrioventricular node is a discrete anatomical structure, and the area surrounding the atrioventricular node is termed *junctional tissue.* Subjunctional refers to the His-Purkinje system. By using new techniques such as His bundle electrocardiography, it has been found that ectopic rhythms formerly attributed to the atrioventricular node actually arise in the His bundle and junctional tissue. In addition, ectopic rhythms that arise low in the atria cannot be distinguished from true junctional beats. Thus, the term *junctional* is frequently used in place of atrioventricular nodal to indicate a degree of vagueness regarding the site of origin of the ectopic rhythm or the site of delay in atrioventricular conduction. Many cardiologists continue to use the terms atrio-

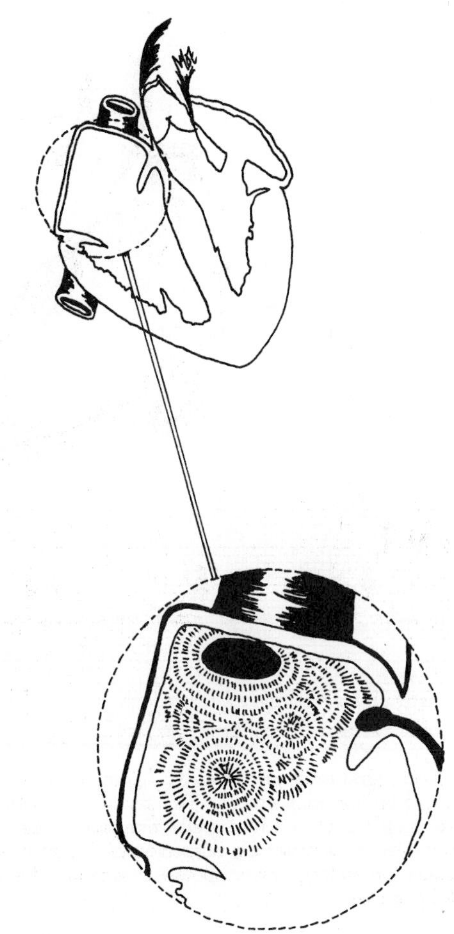

Figure 7–14. This diagram shows many foci discharging in the atria, producing a multifocal atrial tachycardia.

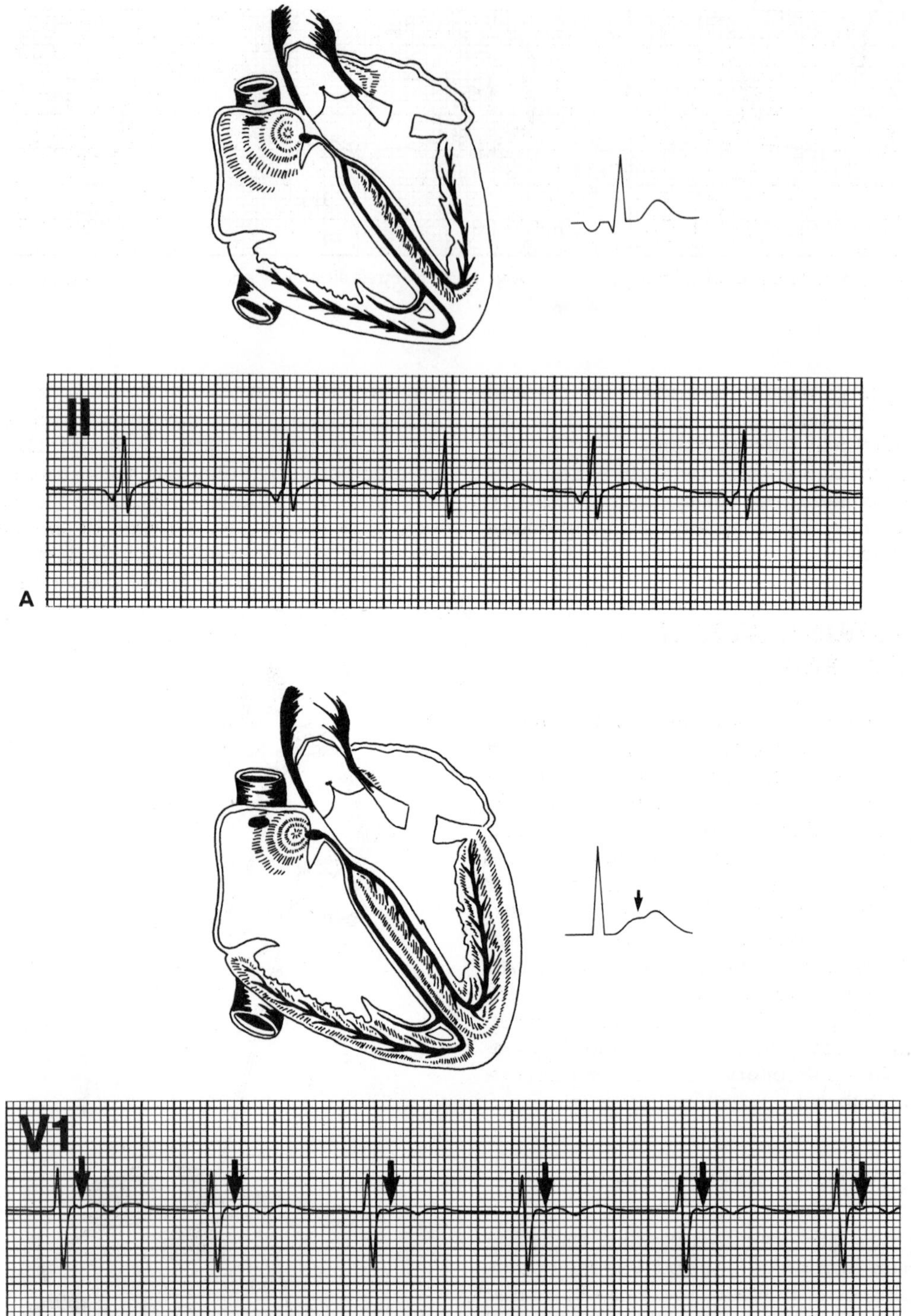

Figure 7–15. **Junctional rhythms.** *A,* A junctional rhythm in which the impulse originates closer to the ventricular conducting system than normal. This produces a shorter than normal PR interval. In order to stimulate the atria, the impulse must travel in a retrograde direction. Thus, it produces inverted (retrograde) P waves, which precede the QRS complex. *B,* Retrograde activation of the atria after the ventricles. In this example, the impulse reaches the ventricular conducting system before it activates the atria. The arrow points to the retrograde P wave that follows the QRS complex.

Illustration continued on opposite page

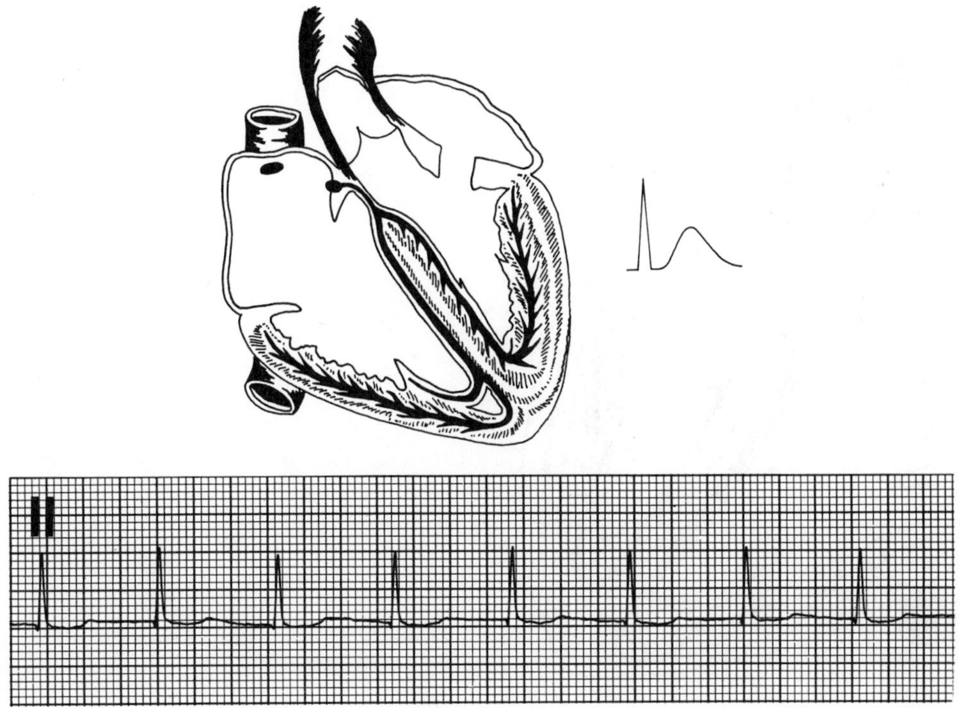

Figure 7–15. Continued. *C,* Another pattern of junctional rhythm. In this example, the impulse originates in the junctional tissue and conducts normally to the ventricles. However, either retrograde conduction to the atria does not occur, and the P waves are absent, or the P wave is buried in the QRS complex.

ventricular nodal, nodal and atrioventricular junctional interchangeably, and we have chosen to continue this tradition.

Common junctional rhythms include junctional escape beats, junctional pacemakers and accelerated junctional rhythms. These rhythms are characterized by the following:

1. Absent or retrograde inverted P waves, which precede or follow the QRS complex.
2. QRS complex of normal duration.

When an impulse arises in junctional tissue, it will be conducted normally to the ventricles and sometimes retrogradely to the atria. This results in several different P wave-QRS complex relationships. For example, Figure 7–15*A* illustrates that when the impulse originates close to the atrioventricular node and conducts retrogradely, inverted (retrograde) P waves result. These *retrograde P waves* have the exact opposite characteristics of normal sinus P waves: The P waves are inverted in leads I, II and III but are upright in lead AVR. Because the impulse is close to the ventricular conducting system, the PR interval is shorter than normal: less than 0.10 second (2.5 small boxes). Figure 7–15*B* illustrates the circumstance in which the junctional impulse activates the ventricles before the retrograde conduction can stimulate the atria to produce P waves. This usually occurs when the ectopic impulse actually arises in the junction. Again, retrograde (inverted) P waves result, but these follow the QRS complex. The most common and most easily recognizable characteristics of a junctional impulse is the absence of P waves with a normal QRS complex. This occurs when there is no retrograde conduction and when no P waves are produced (Fig. 7–15C). Alternately, the P waves may be masked by the QRS complex.

A junctional impulse will also conduct to the ventricles. Since it will follow the normal route to the conducting system (i.e., atrioventricular node to bundle of His to bundle branches to Purkinje fibers), the QRS complex will not be widened and will have the same configuration as the QRS complex in normal sinus rhythm (Fig. 7–16).

An *atrioventricular junctional escape beat* is a beat that interrupts a pause in rhythm caused

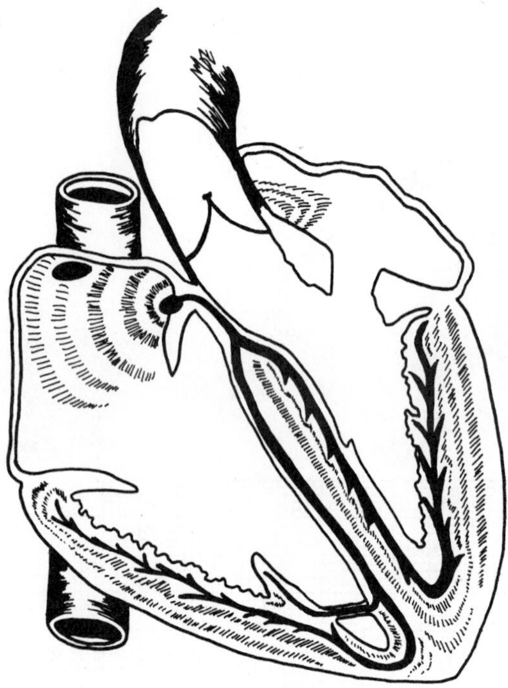

Figure 7–16. This diagram shows the propagation of a junctional arrhythmia.

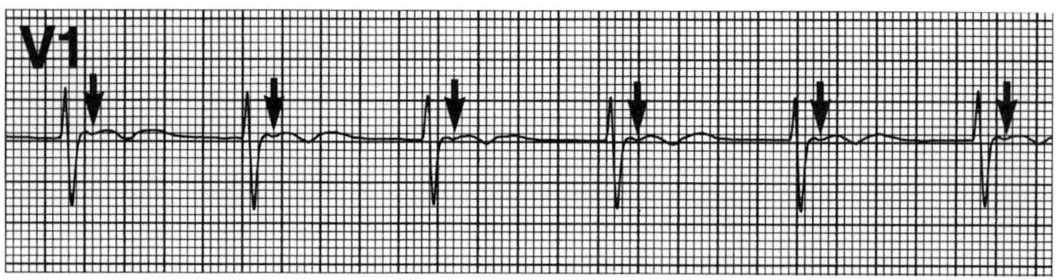

Figure 7–17. **Junctional rhythm.** The rate is 62 beats per minute. The arrows point to the retrograde (inverted) P waves deforming the ST segment.

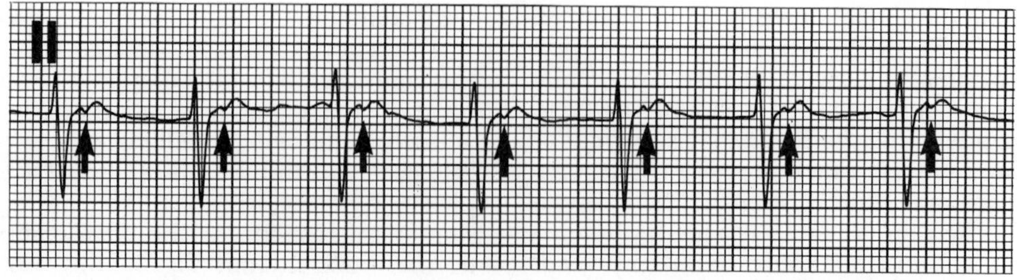

Figure 7–18. **Nonparoxysmal junctional tachycardia.** The junctional and ventricular rates are 83 beats per minute. The arrows point to the retrograde P waves that have deformed the upstroke of the T waves.

by the failure of the sinus node to pace. Essentially, escape beats are safety mechanisms that prevent long pauses in the rhythm of the heart. If the sinus node does not resume its pacemaker function, the atrioventricular junction may continue to fire escape beats and a *junctional pacemaker* may take over the function for the failing sinus node. Junctional pacemakers fire at an inherent rate of 40 to 60 beats per minute.

Junctional escape beats and junctional pacemakers are common in patients with hypoxia, hyperkalemia, myocardial infarction and other clinical settings that may cause the sinus node to fail. Sometimes the junctional rhythm is too slow to maintain adequate cardiac output. In these cases, atropine and isoproterenol are used to enhance the automaticity of the atrioventricular junction.

Since the normal rate of a junctional pacemaker is 40 to 60 beats per minute (Fig. 7–17), a junctional rhythm at a rate greater than 75 beats per minute is termed an *accelerated junctional rhythm* (e.g., junctional tachycardia). *Paroxysmal junctional tachycardia* is similar to atrial tachycardia in that the QRS complex duration is generally normal, the rhythm is regular, between 140 and 200 beats per minute, and the onset and termination are abrupt (see Atrial Tachycardia, Chapter 7, page 36). However, paroxysmal junctional tachycardia differs from atrial tachycardia in that the P waves tend to be inverted, indicative of retrograde activation of the atria. The P waves may come shortly before or after the QRS complex or may even be buried within the QRS complex. Paroxysmal junctional tachycardia has the same significance as paroxysmal atrial tachycardia. It is frequently seen in healthy individuals without heart disease, although it may be seen in patients with coronary artery disease, hypertension and rheumatic heart disease. It is occasionally seen in patients with digitalis intoxication. Paroxysmal junctional tachycardia also occurs in patients who have two pathways in the atrioventricular node. These pathways are conducive to the formation of a re-entry circuitry as described in Chapter 6, Fundamentals of Rhythms.

Another accelerated junctional rhythm is *non–paroxysmal junctional tachycardia.* In this arrhythmia, the P wave, QRS complex and T wave are similar to the paroxysmal variety, but the heart rate is only increased to 70 to 130 beats per minute (Fig. 7–18). This rhythm, however, lacks the abrupt onset and termination that is so characteristic of paroxysmal arrhythmias. The clinical significance of non–paroxysmal junctional tachycardia is its association with digitalis toxicity. This is related to the capacity of digitalis to increase the excitability of the myocardium (see Digitalis, Chapter 14, page 107). It is also associated with acute myocardial infarction and is generally a poor prognostic sign.

8

Ventricular Rhythms

Ventricular arrhythmias are caused by ectopic impulses that may originate in any part of the ventricles. Since these impulses originate in the ventricle, the normal route of depolarization is bypassed (Fig. 8–1). This prevents the simultaneous depolarization of the right and left ventricles that normally occurs. Instead, the impulse must travel a longer, circuitous route in order to stimulate the ventricles. This results in a widened, bizarrely shaped QRS complex that is greater than 0.12 second (3 small boxes) in duration.

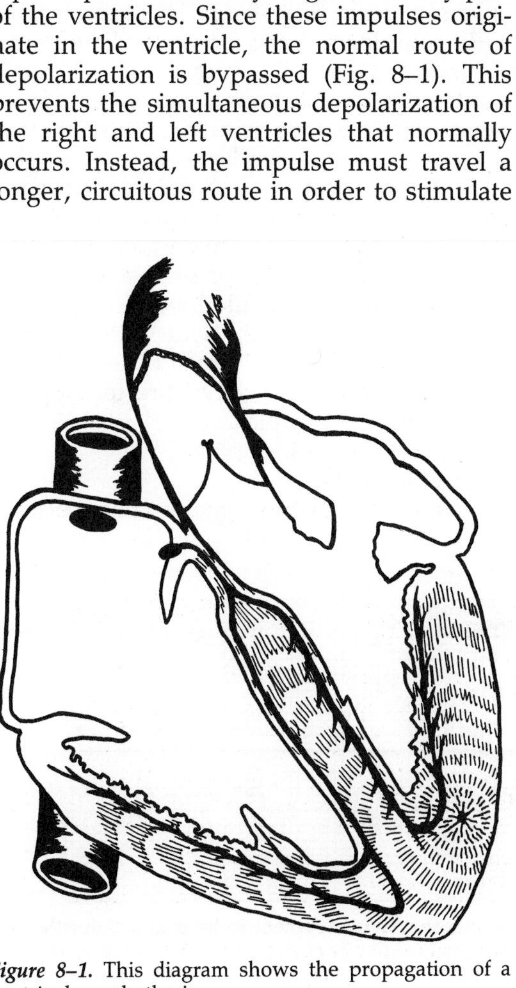

The configuration of the QRS complex is influenced by the site of origin. For example, a QRS complex that originates in the right ventricle will have a left bundle branch block pattern: primarily negative complexes in the right precordial leads (V1 to V3) and positive complexes in the left precordial leads (V4 to V6). In contrast, a QRS complex that originates in the left ventricle will have just the opposite pattern. If the ventricular septum is the site of the ectopic focus, the QRS complex is usually positive in all the precordial leads.

Ventricular arrhythmias of major importance include ventricular premature contraction, ventricular tachycardia, ventricular flutter and ventricular fibrillation.

Figure 8–1. This diagram shows the propagation of a ventricular arrhythmia.

VENTRICULAR PREMATURE CONTRACTION

A *ventricular premature contraction* is an ectopic ventricular impulse that stimulates the myocardium prematurely. The terms ventricular premature contraction, premature ventricular contraction, ventricular premature beat and ventricular extrasystole are all synonymous.

Premature ventricular contractions are characterized by bizarre, widened QRS complexes. This abnormal depolarization also results in an abnormality of repolarization. This produces T waves that are directed opposite to those of the QRS complex. The abnormal

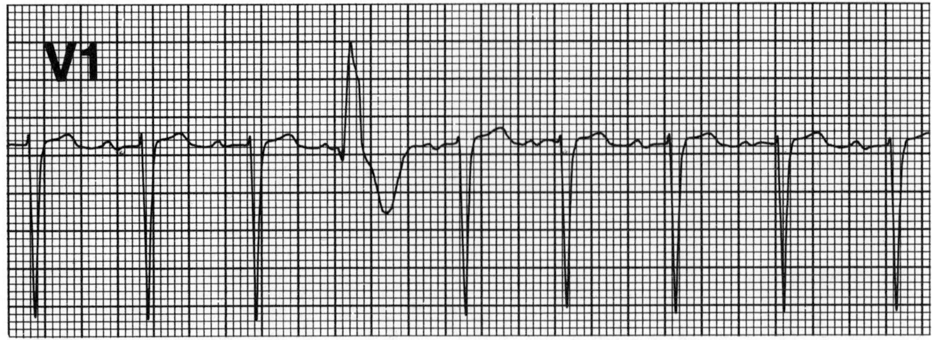

Figure 8–2. **Ventricular premature contraction.** Notice that this wide complex comes prematurely when compared with the next sinus P wave.

QRS complexes and T waves may also obscure the ST segments (Fig. 8–2).

In some instances, the ectopic impulse will be conducted retrogradely to the atrioventricular node, and then to the atria. This will result in inverted (retrograde) P waves that follow the QRS complexes; however, it is more common for the retrograde impulse to be blocked at the atrioventricular node so that P waves are not produced. More importantly, the sinus node is not depolarized or "reset" in this situation. Consequently, the sinus node is unaffected by the premature ventricular contraction, and it will continue to fire on schedule during and after the premature ventricular contraction. Therefore, premature ventricular contractions usually have a *full compensatory pause.* This means that the duration of two cycles, including the premature ventricular contraction, is the same as the duration of two normal cycles. On an electrocardiogram tracing, a compensatory pause appears as a pause between the premature ventricular contraction and the next normal sinus beat (Fig. 8–3).

Although the sinus node continues to fire during a premature ventricular contraction, most of the time its impulses arrive during the refractory period of the conducting system. Sometimes, the sinus beat will conduct to the ventricles at the same time that the ventricular ectopic focus is firing. This results in *fusion beats* (Fig. 8–4). These beats have QRS complexes that are intermediate in configuration between a premature ventricular contraction and a normal sinus beat. In essence, the two depolarizations "fuse" to form a complex that is similar to both beats (Fig. 8–5). Fusion beats are reliable indicators that the rhythm is from a ventricular origin.

In summary, the major electrocardiographic characteristics of premature ventricular contractions include the following:

1. Premature, bizarre, wide QRS complex (0.12 second, i.e., 3 small boxes).
2. ST segment and T wave directed opposite of the QRS complex.
3. Full compensatory pause.
4. Fusion beats.

In addition to these major characteristics,

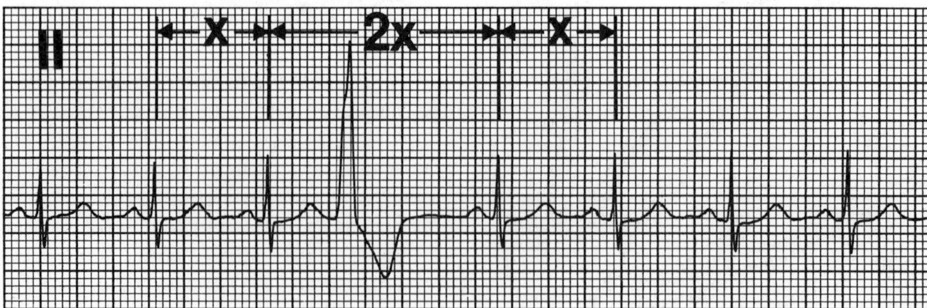

Figure 8–3. **Full compensatory pause.** The interval before and after the premature ventricular contraction is labelled "x." Notice that the interval containing the premature ventricular contraction is exactly "2 ×" or twice the normal R-R interval.

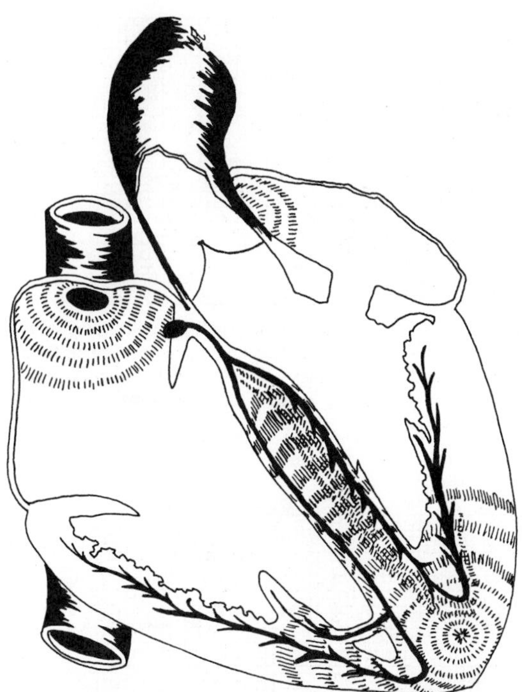

Figure 8–4. This diagram shows the generation of a fusion beat. Notice that there are two foci: the sinoatrial node and a ventricular focus. If the timing is correct, the beat produced will be a "fusion" of these two impulses.

there are many minor findings that help identify ventricular beats. These include *concealed retrograde conduction,* abnormalities of the *postectopic beat* and the *R on T phenomenon.*

Concealed retrograde conduction occurs when the retrograde impulse is blocked in the atrioventricular node but leaves the node refractory to the next descending sinus beat. This increases the delay at the atrioventricular node and results in a prolonged PR interval for this next sinus beat. Since the retrograde impulse is not conducted to the atria and does not produce P waves, the only way to recognize retrograde conduction is by the presence of a prolonged PR interval (Fig. 8–6).

The *postectopic beat* is the normal beat that follows an ectopic beat. This beat may have abnormalities of the T wave or the QRS complex, referred to as *postectopic T wave changes* and *postectopic aberrancy,* respectively. T waves in postectopic beats may show changes in amplitude, configuration or direction. They are caused by an abnormality in repolarization that persists after a premature ventricular contraction and usually indicate underlying heart disease. Postectopic aberrancy is generally thought to be caused by a sinus impulse that activates a partially refractory ventricle. As a result, the QRS complex is often disfigured.

Another important consideration in recognizing ventricular beats is the *R on T phenomenon.* This refers to the occurrence of a premature ventricular contraction near the peak of the T wave. The T wave represents a vulnerable period for the ventricles. During this period, part of the conducting system is refractory, and all of the requirements for reentry are present (see Chapter 6, Fundamentals of Rhythms). If a ventricular premature contraction occurs near the peak of this vulnerable period, a circus rhythm may be generated, leading to ventricular tachycardia or ventricular fibrillation.

The terminology used in describing ventricular beats is simple but important. A premature ventricular contraction that originates in a single ventricular location is called a *unifocal* premature ventricular contraction (Fig. 8–7*A*). In any single lead, each unifocal premature ventricular contraction will be identical. *Multifocal* premature ventricular contractions have different sites of origin,

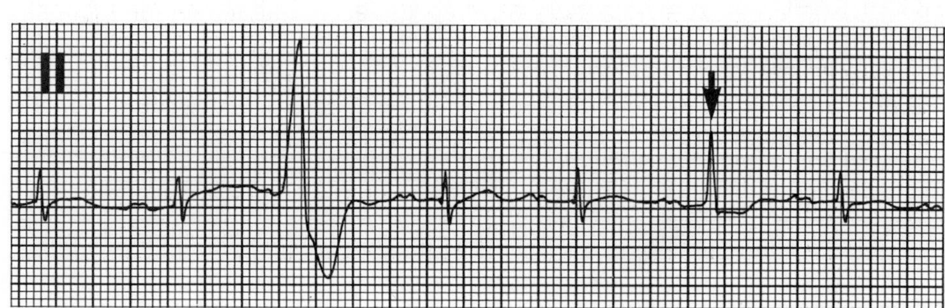

Figure 8–5. **Fusion beat.** The third beat is a premature ventricular contraction. The arrow points to a fusion beat. This beat is preceded by a sinus P wave, which is on time, but the beat is slightly wider than the sinus-generated QRS complex; it looks somewhat similar to the premature ventricular contraction.

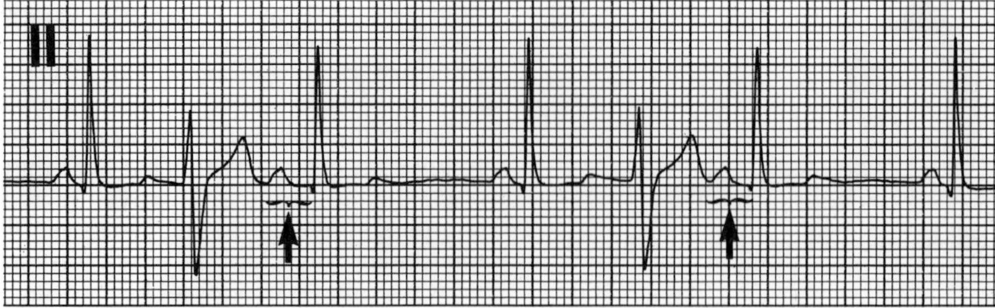

Figure 8–6. **Concealed retrograde conduction.** Occasionally, a premature ventricular contraction will fall exactly between two sinus beats. This will not produce any change in the regularity of the sinus mechanism. These beats are called *interpolated*. Notice that the arrows point to the PR intervals of the next sinus beats, which are prolonged compared with the PR intervals of the beats that are not preceded by an ectopic beat. This represents concealed retrograde conduction (see text).

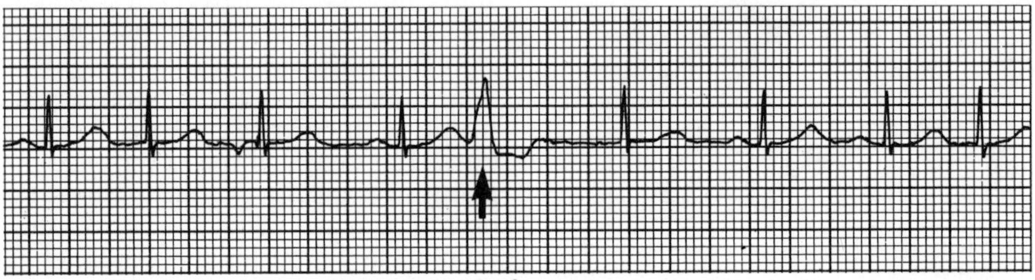

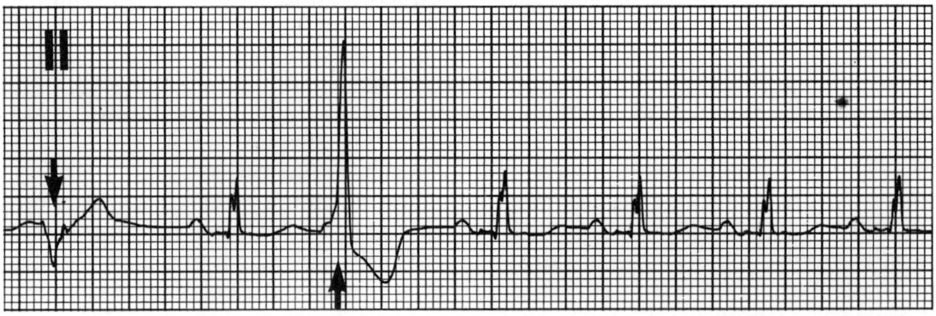

Figure 8–7. Terminology of ventricular premature contractions. *A*, A premature ventricular contraction, which is indicated by the arrow. *B*, Two arrows pointing to two different premature ventricular contractions in the same lead. These are called *multifocal* premature ventricular contractions. *C*, A pair of premature ventricular contractions, called a *couplet*.

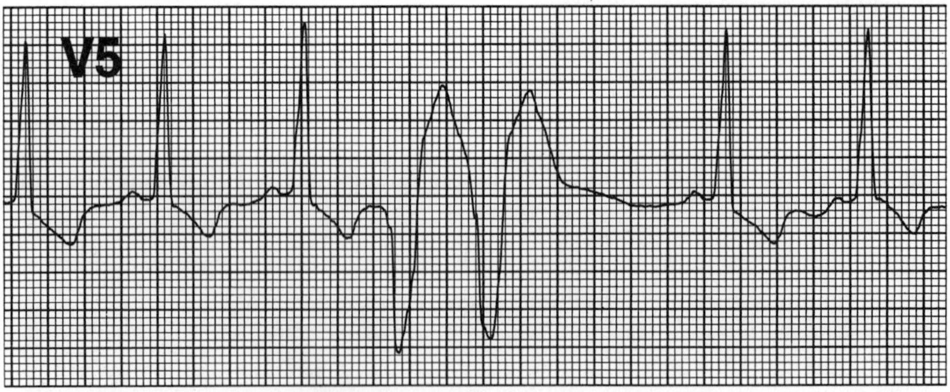

Illustration continued on opposite page

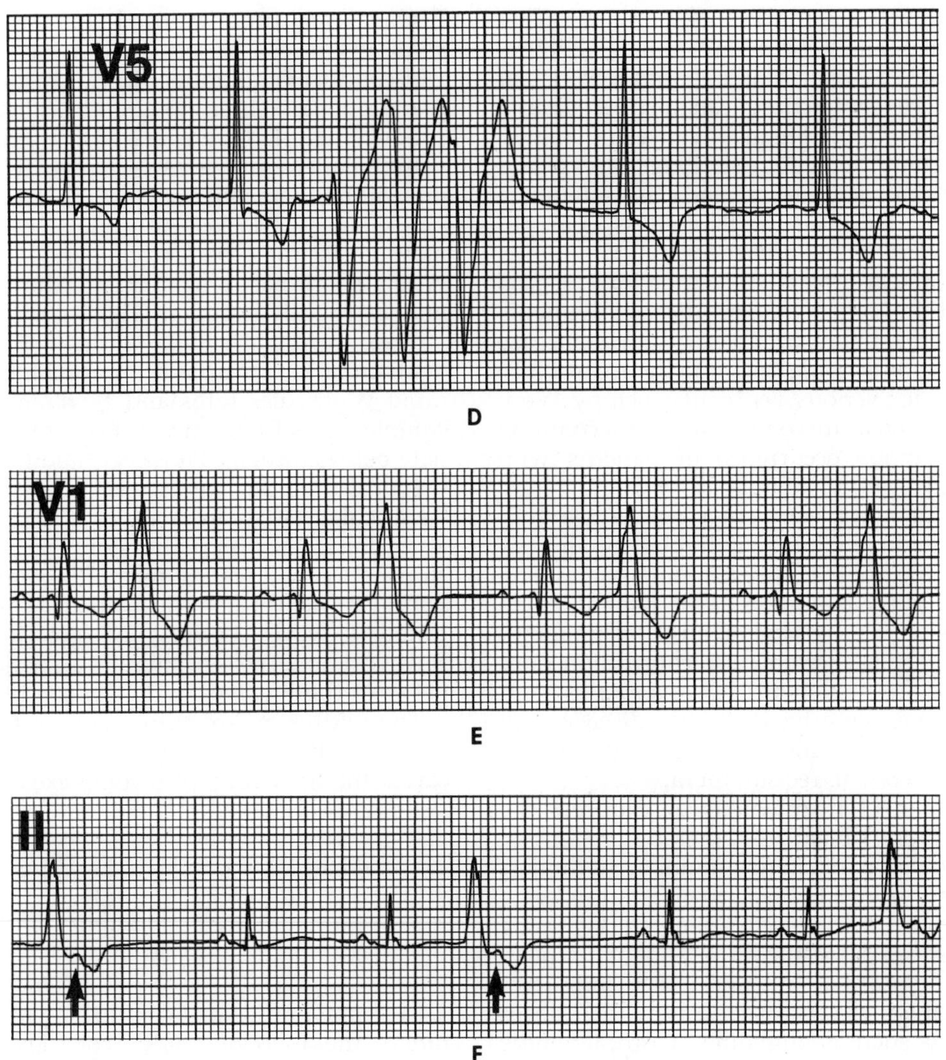

Figure 8–7. Continued. *D,* Three consecutive ventricular premature contractions. Three or more such beats are called *ventricular tachycardia. E,.* The alternation of a sinus beat with a ventricular premature contraction is called *bigeminy. F,* Illustration of *trigeminy,* which is one ventricular beat alternating with two sinus beats. The arrows point to retrograde P waves from the ventricular focus.

and their QRS complexes have different configurations in the same lead (Fig. 8–7*B*). Premature ventricular contractions can occur singly or in pairs called *couplets* (Fig. 8–7*C*). Three or more consecutive premature ventricular contractions are by definition called *ventricular tachycardia* (Fig. 8–7*D*). The repetitive sequence of one ventricular beat coupled to one normal beat is called *ventricular bigeminy* (Fig. 8–7*E*). *Ventricular trigeminy* is the sequence of one ventricular beat alternating with two normal beats (Fig. 8–7*F*). In these arrhythmias, the interval between the premature ventricular contraction and its preceding normal beat is called the *coupling interval.* Although the coupling interval can vary, it is usually fixed. Sometimes a ventricular premature contraction will occur exactly between two normal beats. In this case, the ventricular premature contraction is referred to as an *interpolated beat* (Fig. 8–6). There is no compensatory pause associated with an interpolated beat.

Clinical Significance

Clinically, premature ventricular contractions are the single most common arrhythmias. An occasional unifocal ventricular premature contraction occurs in virtually all normal individuals. These beats are usually benign. However, multifocal or frequent ventricular premature contractions can also occur and are more serious. Frequent causes of ventricular ectopy include emotional stress and ingestion of stimulants, such as caffeine or tobacco, as well as drugs such as epinephrine, isoproterenol and theophylline.

Ventricular premature contractions are also caused by organic heart disease. Patients with ischemic heart disease, lung disease with hypoxia or digitalis toxicity are at highest risk for serious ventricular ectopy. Ventricular premature contractions are a common and ominous occurrence in patients with acute myocardial infarction.

Treatment of ventricular premature contractions depends on the frequency and nature of the ventricular premature contraction as well as the condition of the patient. In an otherwise healthy person, an occasional unifocal ventricular premature contraction does not require treatment; however, a patient with pre-existing heart or lung disease with frequent or multifocal ventricular premature contractions will require therapy.

The aim of treatment is to suppress the ectopic ventricular focus, thereby preventing the formation of more serious arrhythmias. This can be effected simply by administering oxygen to a hypoxic patient or by using intravenous lidocaine in a patient with an acute myocardial infarction. For long-term suppression of ventricular ectopy, oral doses of drugs such as quinidine or procainamide may be required.

VENTRICULAR TACHYCARDIA

Ventricular tachycardia is, by definition, three or more consecutive premature ventricular contractions. Like ventricular premature contractions, the QRS complexes in ventricular tachycardia are bizarre and widened with a duration greater than 0.12 second (three small boxes). In addition, the ventricles and atria beat independently. The term used is *atrioventricular dissociation.* This dissociated rhythm that occurs in 50 per cent of all patients with ventricular tachycardia produces P waves that have no relationship to the QRS complexes. P waves can be found preceding, following or buried within the QRS complex. In fact, the QRS complexes may demonstrate varying morphologies as P waves are superimposed upon them. In some instances, the ectopic ventricular beat will conduct retrogradely to the atrioventricular node and then to the atria. This will produce inverted (retrograde) P waves. The ventricular rhythm is usually regular, with a rate of 140 beats per minute. It may occur paroxysmally and last only transiently, or it may persist for a prolonged period of time. When short paroxysms occur, the rhythm may be slightly irregular (Fig. 8–8).

Since ventricular tachycardia and supraventricular tachycardia with aberrancy have rapid ventricular rates and a widened QRS complex, it is frequently difficult to differentiate between them. However, a few clues to the origin of the rhythm may be present. Ventricular tachycardia often demonstrates atrioventricular dissociation with no relationship between P waves and QRS complexes. Supraventricular tachycardia usually has distorted T waves because of superimposed P waves; nonetheless, there is a relationship between the P waves and QRS complexes.

The QRS complex morphology often provides additional clues. In ventricular tachycardia the following QRS complexes may be seen:

Lead V1	Lead V6
RR′ (R′ > R)	qR
qR	QS
Rs	

In supraventricular tachycardia with aberrancy, the following QRS complexes may result:

Lead V1	Lead V6
RSR′	qRs
RR′ (R > R′)	

In addition, 75 per cent of patients with ventricular tachycardia have a QRS complex with a left axis deviation. Finally, most patients (60 per cent) with ventricular tachycardia have QRS complexes that are 0.14 second or greater in duration, while most patients with aberrancy have complexes less than 0.14 second in duration.

One reliable sign of ventricular tachycardia is the *fusion beat* (Fig. 8–9). This beat is a composite of a normal sinus beat that simultaneously fires with the ectopic ventricular beat. The resultant QRS complex configuration is intermediate between a normal sinus QRS complex and the ventricular QRS com-

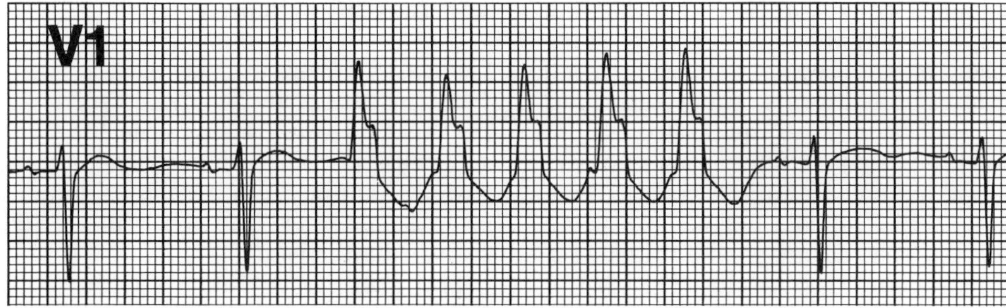

Figure 8–8. **Ventricular tachycardia.** This five-beat run of ventricular tachycardia occurs at a rate of 150 beats per minute.

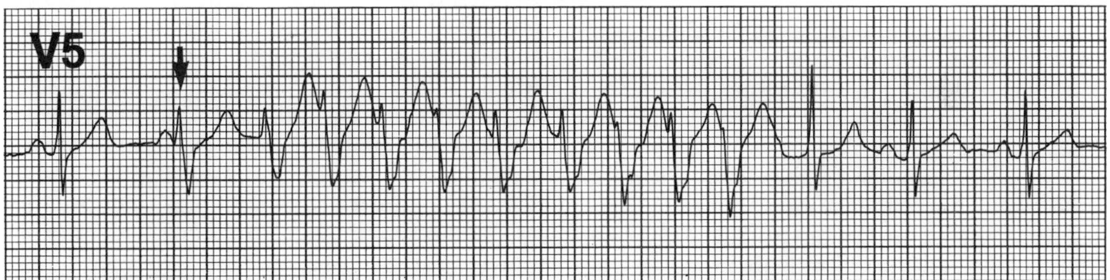

Figure 8–9. **Fusion beat.** The arrow points to a fusion beat that starts this run of ventricular tachycardia. A fusion beat is a reliable sign that a rhythm is from a ventricular focus and not from a supraventricular focus with aberrancy.

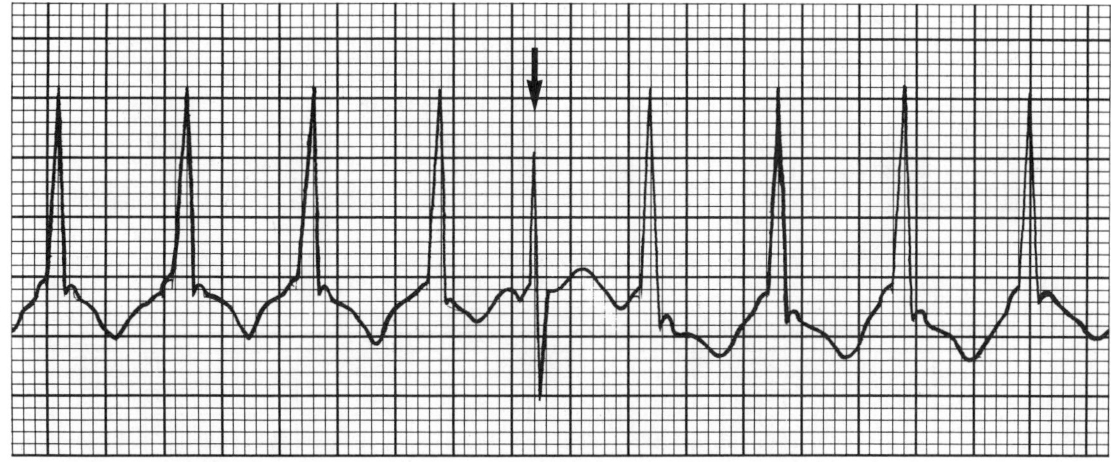

Figure 8–10. **Dressler, or capture, beat.** During a run of ventricular tachycardia, occasionally a sinus impulse will be able to conduct normally to the ventricles. The resultant QRS complex produced is narrower, since it conducts normally from the sino-atrial node through the atrioventricular node to the Purkinje fibers. This is called a *capture beat* and is the most reliable sign of a ventricular rhythm. The arrow points to the capture beat in the diagram.

plex. This beat comes on time or is slightly early and indicates that the ventricles were depolarized by two separate but simultaneous impulses: one from a supraventricular origin and one from a ventricular focus.

The most reliable sign of ventricular tachycardia is the *capture beat,* which is also called the *Dressler beat.* This is a normal-appearing QRS complex that occurs in the midst of a run of ventricular tachycardia (Fig. 8–10). During atrioventricular dissociation, a rare sinus impulse may be able to depolarize the atrioventricular node and conduct through the normal pathways; this beat will capture the ventricles, and the QRS complex will be narrower than a ventricular or fusion beat.

In summary, the major electrocardiographic characteristics of ventricular tachycardia include the following:

1. Bizarre wide QRS complexes (0.12 second, i.e., 3 small boxes).
2. Atrioventricular dissociation, with the P waves distorting the QRS complex or retrograde P waves.
3. Regular ventricular rhythm with a rate of 140 to 200 beats per minute.
4. QRS complex morphology: RR′ (R′ > R) in lead V1, qR or QS in lead V6.
5. Fusion beats.
6. Capture beats.

Clinical Significance

Clinically, ventricular tachycardia can have dire consequences. The rapid ventricular rate prevents adequate filling time for the heart, so cardiac output is drastically reduced, and patients suffer from hypotension. Also, it often degenerates into ventricular fibrillation and cardiac arrest.

The majority of patients with ventricular tachycardia have underlying cardiac disease, especially ischemic heart disease. Ventricular tachycardia has also been associated with cardiomyopathies and with mitral valve prolapse.

Treatment of patients with ventricular tachycardia depends on their hemodynamic status. Some patients tolerate bouts of ventricular tachycardia well and are able to maintain adequate cardiac output. These patients should be treated with intravenous lidocaine to suppress the ectopic ventricular focus. Most patients with ventricular tachycardia experience precipitous falls in blood pressure. If the patient is conscious and hemodynamically stable, intravenous lidocaine should be given. If the patient is unconscious or hemodynamically unstable, electrocardioversion is used to convert ventricular tachycardia back to normal sinus rhythm.

Another form of ventricular tachycardia is

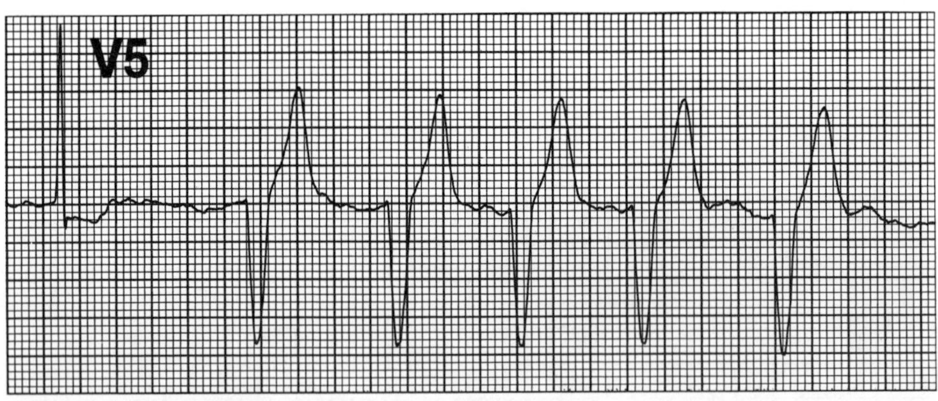

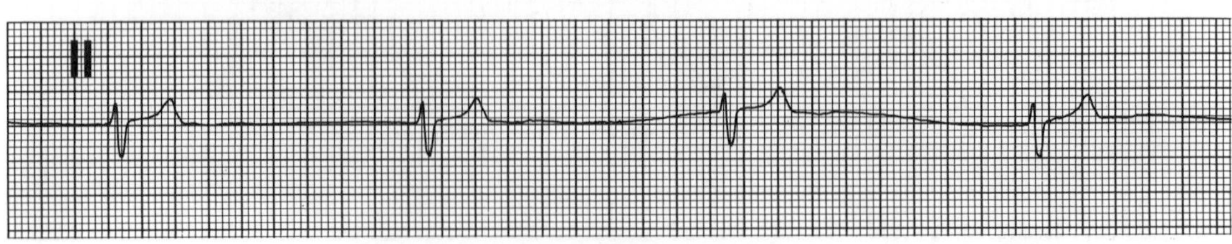

Figure 8–11. **Idioventricular rhythms.** *A,* An *accelerated* idioventricular rhythm at a rate of 88 beats per minute. *B,* An idioventricular rhythm at a rate of 32 beats per minute. This rhythm can also be called a *ventricular escape rhythm.* Notice that the QRS complex is widened to 0.12 second.

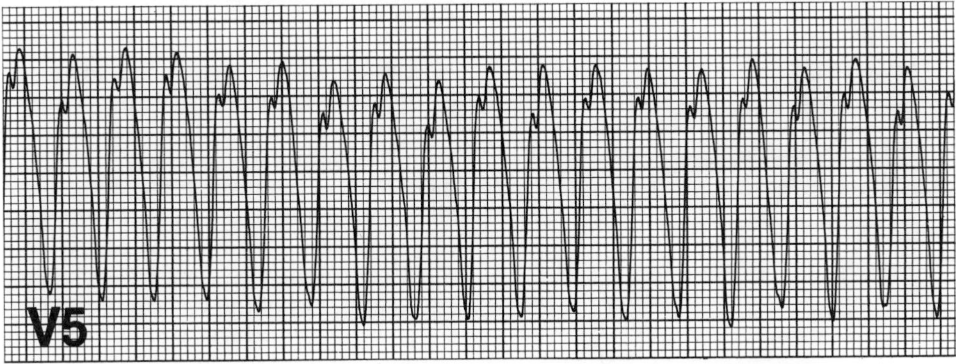

Figure 8–12. **Ventricular flutter.** The rate is 214 beats per minute.

called *accelerated idioventricular rhythm.* This rhythm is regular and has a rate between 60 and 100 beats per minute, and the QRS complexes are wide (Fig. 8–11*A*). It is apparent that idioventricular rhythm has most of the characteristics of ventricular tachycardia except that the ventricular rate is slower. However, it is an accelerated rhythm, since the normal idioventricular rhythm is 20 to 40 beats per minute (Fig. 8–11*B*).

Most episodes of accelerated idioventricular rhythm are short, lasting only seconds or minutes. It is seen in myocardial infarction and generally occurs during sinus bradycardia. Since the rate is within the range of normal sinus rhythm, little hemodynamic compromise occurs. Therefore, therapy is generally not indicated. It may also occasionally be seen in digitalis toxicity.

VENTRICULAR FLUTTER

Ventricular flutter is a rapid ventricular tachycardia. It is characterized by widened QRS complexes and a regular rate of 200 ± 50 beats per minute (Fig. 8–12). In contrast to ventricular tachycardia, there are no obvious ST segments or T waves. This is because the rapid ventricular rate in ventricular flutter precludes their visualization. The clinical presentation and therapy are discussed under the preceding section, Ventricular Tachycardia.

VENTRICULAR FIBRILLATION

Ventricular fibrillation is a ventricular arrhythmia that is recognized on the electrocardiogram by irregular, chaotic undulations of the baseline. No recognizable P waves, QRS complexes or T waves are seen (Fig. 8–13). Physiologically, the ventricle is said to look like a "bag of worms" without obvious mechanical contraction (Fig. 8–14).

Patients with existing heart disease, arrhythmias and those with an accessory pathway are at risk for developing ventricular fibrillation (see Pre-Excitation Syndrome, page 80). If a patient with an accessory pathway develops atrial fibrillation, many of the 400 or more atrial impulses may be transmitted to the ventricle via the accessory pathway. This will result in a rapid ventricular rate. Ventricular fibrillation is a serious ar-

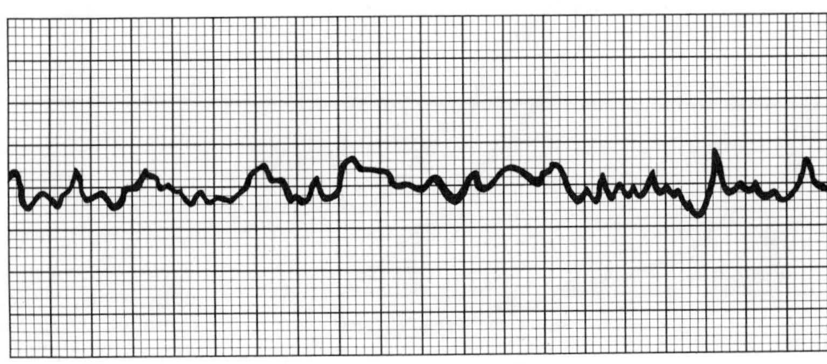

Figure 8–13. **Ventricular fibrillation.** No recognizable P, QRS or T complexes are seen.

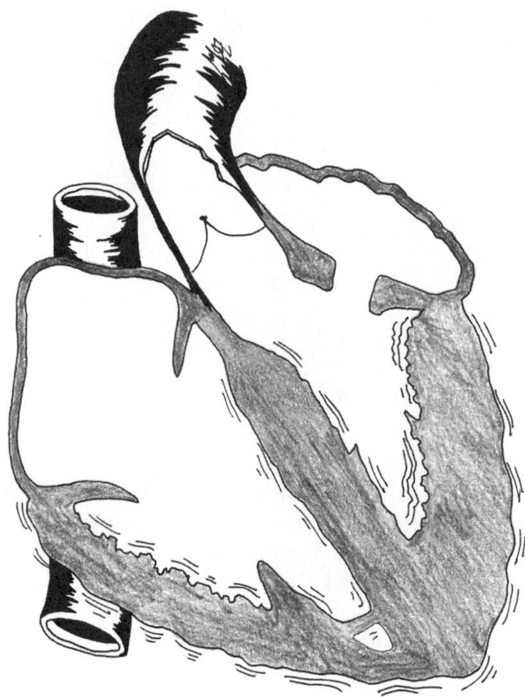

Figure 8–14. Diagram showing the disordered mechanical contraction associated with ventricular fibrillation. The ventricle looks like a "bag of worms."

rhythmia that severely compromises cardiac output and can lead to sudden death. Therapy is electrocardioversion.

PARASYSTOLE

Parasystole is the term used to describe an ectopic, unextinguishable focus that fires at a regular, uninterrupted rate and co-exists with the dominant pacemaker. This focus is protected by *entrance block,* which does not allow other impulses to enter the focus and to depolarize it. Ventricular parasystole is the most common type, but parasystole can occur in any part of the conduction system (Fig. 8–15). It can produce a pattern that may be hard to differentiate from frequent premature ventricular contractions. However, since the firing of the parasystolic focus is independent of the sinus node rate, there is no coupling of the ectopic beat to the sinus beat, as one sees with frequent unifocal premature ventricular contractions. If a ventricular parasystolic focus fires at exactly the same time as the sinus node is firing, a fusion beat may result. If the sinus rate is fast, the conduction pathways may be refractory and will not allow the parasystolic focus beat to produce a QRS complex. If the sinus rate is slow, many of the parasystolic beats will find the ventricle repolarized, and many premature ventricular contractions will occur. Since the parasystole focus is unextinguishable and therefore fires regularly, the interval between the extrasystoles will be constant, with the exception of blocked parasystolic impulses

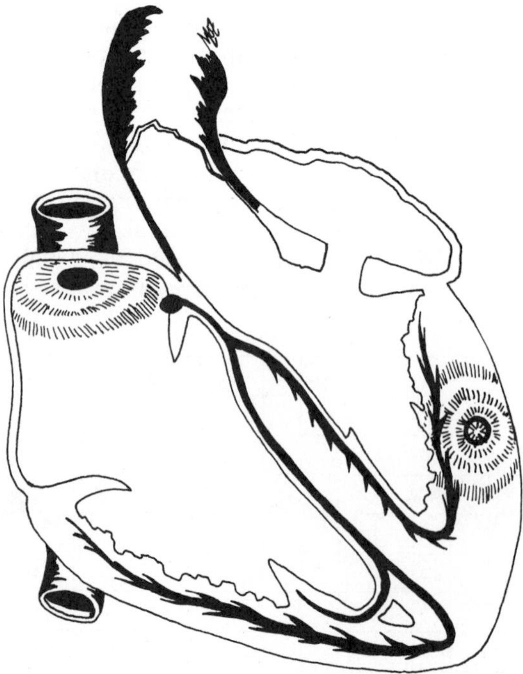

Figure 8–15. **A diagram showing a ventricular parasystolic focus.** Notice that the ventricular focus is surrounded by an area of unidirectional entrance block, producing a physiological "zone of protection."

because of the normal sinus depolarizations. Therefore, the intervals between parasystolic beats appear irregular but are always multiples of the R-R interval of the parasystolic focus.

The major characteristics of ventricular parasystole are the following:

1. R-R intervals of the ectopic beats at multiples of the shortest interectopic interval.
2. Variable coupling.
3. Fusion beats.

Clinical Significance

Parasystole is most common in elderly individuals, although it also occurs in young persons. Most individuals with parasystole are asymptomatic or complain of palpitations. The symptoms are similar to those produced by other extrasystoles. The parasystolic rhythm may be transient or longstanding. Unless the patient is symptomatic, treatment is not indicated.

9

Supraventricular Conduction Disturbances

A conduction disturbance is an abnormality in the propagation of an electrical impulse through the normal conduction pathways. Impaired conduction can range from a delay in conduction to a complete halt of impulse transmission. Conduction disturbances can occur in any part of the conducting system and are commonly found in the sinoatrial node, atrioventricular node or ventricular conducting system.

The normal conducting pathway is illustrated in Figure 9–1. An impulse is generated by the automatic cells of the sinus node. This impulse is conducted out of the sinus node to the atria. The atria depolarize, producing the P wave, and conduct the impulse to the atrioventricular node. The atrioventricular node normally delays the transition of this impulse, thus producing the PR interval. From the atrioventricular node, this impulse propagates to the bundle of His, and then simultaneously down each bundle branch and fascicle to stimulate the ventricles.

Abnormal conduction in the sinus node or in the atria will affect the characteristics of the P waves. Abnormal conduction in the atrioventricular node will affect the PR interval and the relationship between atrial and ventricular activity (that is, the relationship between P waves and QRS complexes).

When conduction abnormalities occur lower than the bundle branch fascicles, *intraventricular conduction disturbances* result. These abnormalities may prevent the simultaneous depolarization of the ventricles, and a widened QRS complex is produced.

DISTURBANCES OF SINOATRIAL CONDUCTION

The sinoatrial node is the heart's main pacemaker. However, in order for an impulse generated at the sinoatrial node to initiate a cardiac cycle, it must first exit the node before being conducted throughout the surrounding nodal tissue to the rest of the heart. Some

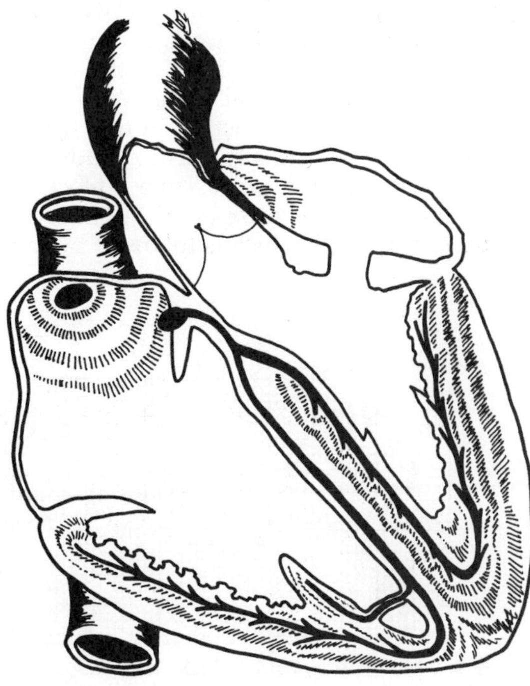

Figure 9–1. Diagram demonstrating the normal conduction pathway.

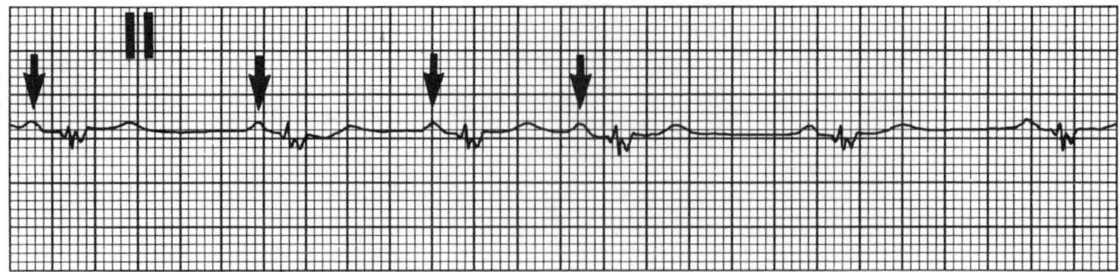

Figure 9–2. **Sinoatrial Wenckebach block.** The arrows point to the P waves. Note that the P-P interval shortens until a dropped P wave occurs.

patients have abnormalities in the sinoatrial node or its surrounding tissue that delay or block the conduction of sinus impulses. These abnormalities are termed *sinoatrial blocks.*

In first degree sinoatrial block, the conduction time in the sinoatrial node is prolonged. In second degree sinoatrial block, some of the impulses fail to be conducted out of the sinoatrial node. In third degree or complete sinoatrial block, there is complete failure of sinoatrial conduction. Since the impulse within the sinus node cannot be recorded by the surface electrocardiogram, the existence of most sinoatrial conduction defects can only be inferred from the P wave activity. Only second degree sinoatrial block can be seen in the surface electrocardiogram.

There are two types of second degree sinoatrial block. *Type I sinoatrial block,* also called *sinoatrial Wenckebach block,* is caused by a progressive conduction delay in the tissue surrounding the sinoatrial node. With each sinus impulse, the conduction in this tissue worsens, and it eventually fails to conduct a sinus impulse to the atria. Type I block is characterized by a decrease in the P-P interval of successive beats, which is followed by the loss of P wave activity. In other words, the P-P interval is progressively shortened until a dropped P wave occurs; the sequence may then begin again (Fig. 9–2).

The second kind of second degree sinoatrial block, called *Mobitz's type II sinoatrial block,* is caused by the failure of an impulse to conduct out of the sinus node (i.e., the impulse is "trapped" within the node). Type II sinoatrial block is characterized by a regular P-P interval with the occasional abrupt loss of a P wave (Fig. 9–3). This produces a pause that is a multiple of the basic P-P interval.

Clinical Significance

All types of sinoatrial block can be associated with advanced sinoatrial disease, such as the sick sinus syndrome. Sinoatrial block is also associated with digitalis toxicity. Sinoatrial block results in pauses in rhythm that can lead to escape beats or the formation of secondary pacemakers. These rhythms are often severe bradyarrhythmias, which may produce hypotension and decreased cardiac output. Treatment of patients with sinoatrial block is directed toward preventing the pro-

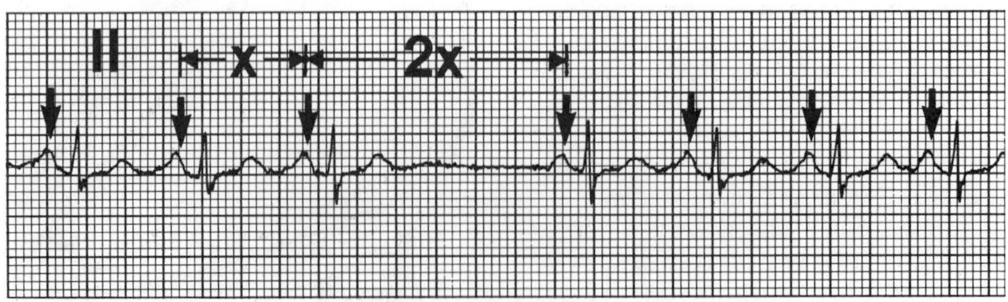

Figure 9–3. **Mobitz II sinoatrial block.** The interval marked "x" is the basic P-P interval. Notice that this interval is constant. However, after the third P wave, there is a dropped P wave. The interval surrounding this dropped beat is "2×," exactly twice the basic P-P interval.

longed pauses and bradycardias. This is usually accomplished by the insertion of an electronic pacemaker (see Electronic Pacemakers, page 82).

SICK SINUS SYNDROME

The *sick sinus syndrome* is caused by dysfunction in the heart's electrical conducting system. It is frequently associated with periods of long pauses in electrical activity followed by runs of rapid ectopic impulses. For this reason it has frequently been termed the *bradycardia-tachycardia syndrome.*

The syndrome results from either disordered impulse formation in the sinoatrial node or impaired conduction in the more distal pathways. Supraventricular tachycardia, atrial flutter and atrial fibrillation frequently act as escape rhythms after the long pauses. Both the long pauses and the rapid heart rates tend to reduce cardiac output, and syncope may result.

The etiology of the sick sinus syndrome is multiple and includes: coronary artery disease, cardiomyopathy, hypertension, rheumatic heart disease, myocarditis and surgical trauma to the sinoatrial node. Therapy for symptomatic patients is the insertion of a permanent electronic pacemaker.

DISTURBANCES OF ATRIOVENTRICULAR CONDUCTION

Atrioventricular block is a disturbance in the conduction of atrial impulses to the ventricles. Atrioventricular block is classified into three types: (1) first degree atrioventricular block, which is only a prolongation in the time for each atrial impulse to reach the ventricles; (2) second degree atrioventricular block, in which some of the atrial impulses are not conducted to the ventricles; (3) third degree atrioventricular block or complete heart block, in which none of the atrial impulses are conducted to the ventricles.

First Degree Atrioventricular Block

In *first degree atrioventricular block* it takes longer for each atrial impulse to reach the ventricles. This is caused by an increase in the delay at the atrioventricular node. Since the PR interval represents the time between atrial and ventricular activation, it is prolonged in first degree atrioventricular block (Fig. 9–4). First degree block is characterized by (1) a regular rhythm, normal P waves and normal QRS complexes and (2) a fixed, prolonged PR interval that exceeds 0.2 second (1 large box).

Clinical Significance. First degree block does not by itself produce symptoms, and it is frequently found in normal individuals with a high degree of vagal tone. This is because vagal stimulation increases the delay (i.e., impairs conduction) at the atrioventricular node. Digitalis also impairs conduction through the atrioventricular node, so patients using this medication will have a prolonged PR interval.

Other conditions that may produce first degree block include collagen vascular disease, cardiomyopathies and ischemic heart disease. In particular, patients with an inferior wall myocardial infarction often have a transient first degree block. This is because the inferior myocardial wall and the atrioventricular node are both supplied by the right coronary artery in most individuals. Occlusion of this artery produces an inferior myo-

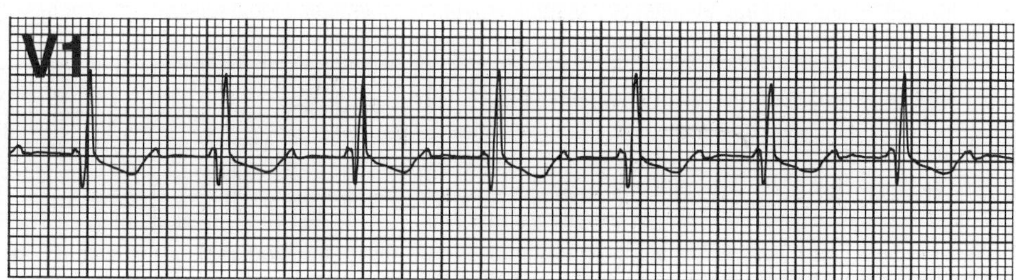

Figure 9–4. **First degree atrioventricular block.** The PR interval is 0.32 second.

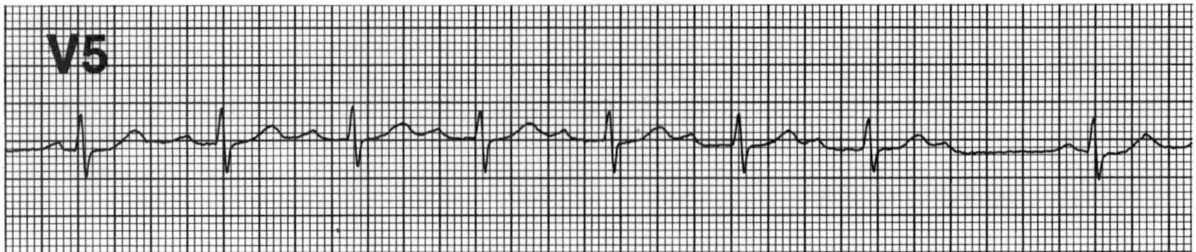

Figure 9–5. **Second degree (Wenckebach) atrioventricular block (Mobitz I).** Notice that there is a progressive lengthening of the PR interval until a dropped beat occurs. This is associated with a progressive shortening of the R-R intervals.

cardial infarction, but often ischemia of the atrioventricular node also results. This ischemia is, however, transient, since redistribution of coronary blood flow will soon result. Patients with first degree atrioventricular block do not require treatment.

Second Degree Atrioventricular Block

In *second degree atrioventricular block* some of the atrial impulses are not conducted to the ventricles. This results in "dropped" QRS complexes and an irregular rhythm. A "dropped" QRS complex refers to the absence of a QRS complex on the electrocardiogram. These are also called *dropped beats.* There are two types of second degree atrioventricular block. *Mobitz type I,* also called the *Wenckebach phenomenon,* is caused by a progressive impairment of conduction through the atrioventricular node. In this condition, successive atrial impulses find it increasingly difficult to penetrate the atrioventricular node to stimulate the ventricles. Eventually, the atrioventricular node completely blocks the transmission of the atrial impulse; this results in a "dropped" QRS complex. The electrocardiogram in Mobitz type I block is characterized by the following:

1. A progressive lengthening of the PR interval until a QRS complex is dropped.
2. A shortening of the R-R interval.
3. A regularly irregular rhythm caused by the changing PR interval and dropped QRS beats.
4. Normal configurations of P waves and QRS complexes.

After the dropped beat, the atrioventricular node recovers its ability to conduct impulses, and the entire sequence of changing PR and R-R intervals, dropped beat and recovery, repeats (Fig. 9–5). The presence of pairs or groups of beats should be a clue to alert one of a possible underlying Wenckebach phenomenon.

Clinical Significance. Mobitz type I atrioventricular block can be caused by digitalis toxicity, cardiomyopathies, intense vagal stimulation and ischemic heart disease. Patients with acute inferior wall myocardial infarction are especially prone to developing Mobitz type I block (see the preceding discussion on First Degree Atrioventricular Block, page 61). Most patients can maintain

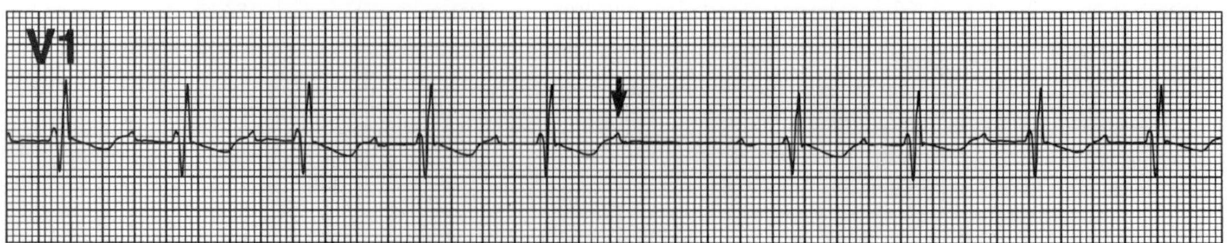

Figure 9–6. **Second degree atrioventricular block (Mobitz II).** Notice that the PR intervals are constant. The arrow points to a P wave without a QRS complex following it. Also in this example, the PR interval is prolonged to 0.30 second and there is first degree atrioventricular block.

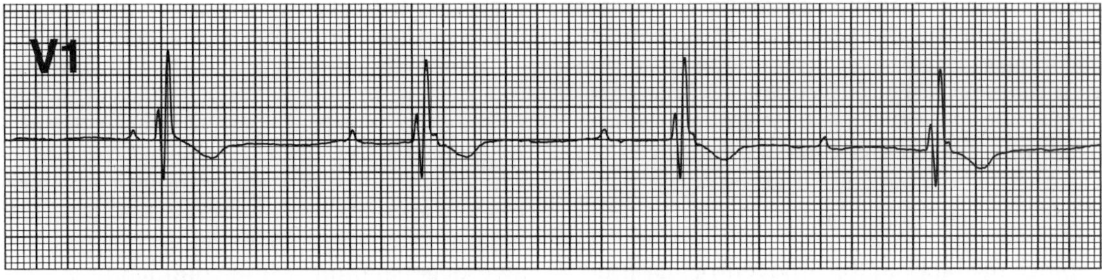

Figure 9–7. **Third degree atrioventricular block.** Notice that there is atrioventricular dissociation present. The P waves have no fixed relationship to the QRS complexes. This is an idioventricular escape rhythm at a rate of 38 beats per minute in the presence of complete heart block.

adequate cardiac output and do not require electronic pacemakers. However, some patients do experience a decrease in cardiac output because of the bradyarrhythmia and require insertion of an electronic pacemaker.

The second type of second degree atrioventricular block, *Mobitz type II second degree atrioventricular block,* is less common than type I. This condition is caused by the occasional total block of an atrial impulse in the bundle of His or in the bundle branches, resulting in a dropped QRS beat. Because the block is further down the conducting system than the atrioventricular node, the ventricles do not depolarize simultaneously; hence the QRS complex may be prolonged and widened. Since the conduction block is occasional, the PR intervals of the beats preceding and following the dropped beat are the same (Fig. 9–6).

In summary, the major electrocardiographic characteristics of Mobitz type II block include the following:

1. A regular rhythm with rare periods of irregularity caused by the abrupt, intermittently dropped QRS beats.
2. Widened QRS complexes caused by the intraventricular conduction delay.
3. Constant PR intervals.

Clinical Significance. Clinically, Mobitz type II atrioventricular block reflects progressive disease of the conduction system, and it often proceeds to third degree heart block. Unlike the Wenckebach block, Mobitz type II is usually not associated with an inferior wall myocardial infarction. Instead it is more commonly found in patients with an anterior wall myocardial infarction. Since the presence of Mobitz type II forebodes a progression to third degree heart block, an electronic pacemaker should be inserted in patients with this condition.

Third Degree Atrioventricular Block

In *third degree atrioventricular block,* also called *complete heart block,* no atrial impulses are conducted to the ventricles. This "complete block" at the atrioventricular junction prevents atrial impulses from pacing the ventricles. As discussed previously, whenever the primary pacemaker fails to pace the ventricles, a secondary pacemaker will arise in the automatic cells of the atrioventricular junction or Purkinje system. The rate at which these ectopic pacemakers will fire is dependent upon their inherent automaticities. For example, a junctional pacemaker will fire at 40 to 60 beats per minute, while a Purkinje pacemaker will fire at about 30 beats per minute. Thus, the ventricular rhythm in third

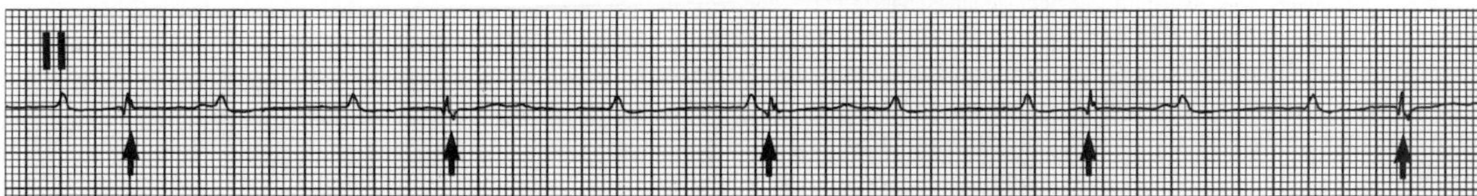

Figure 9–8. **Complete heart block.** The arrows point to the ventricular complexes, which occur at a rate of 30 beats per minute. The P waves are seen marching independently of the atrial rhythm. Therefore, there is atrioventricular dissociation present as well as sinus node disease, which is the cause of the slightly irregular P-P intervals.

degree block usually produces a severe bradycardia. In addition, the location of the secondary pacemaker will determine the morphology of the QRS complex. If the pacemaker is high in the atrioventricular junction, a normal QRS complex may be produced. In contrast, a low junctional or Purkinje pacemaker will produce bizarre, widened QRS complexes (Fig. 9–7).

Since the block at the atrioventricular junction is bidirectional in third degree block, the secondary pacemaker only regulates the ventricular rate; it has no effect on the atrial rate. Likewise, the sinus node regulates only the atrial rate. In essence, the atria and ventricles beat totally independently; this is called *atrioventricular dissociation*. Because of the independent rhythms, the P waves have no relationship to the QRS complexes, and the PR intervals are totally variable (Fig. 9–8).

In summary, the main electrocardiographic characteristics of third degree atrioventricular block include the following:

1. A regular atrial rate.
2. Atrioventricular dissociation (no relationship between P waves and QRS complexes).
3. A regular ventricular rate, which is frequently a bradycardia.

Clinical Significance. The causes of third degree block are many and include all the conditions that produce first and second degree blocks, albeit more advanced forms of these conditions. In elderly individuals it most commonly results from a chronic degeneration of the conduction system.

Regardless of the course, third degree block is a serious conduction abnormality because it leads to the formation of secondary pacemakers that produce severe bradycardias. With such slow ventricular rates, cardiac output is decreased and blood flow to the vital organs may be inadequate. In particular, cerebral ischemia may develop, causing patients to transiently lose consciousness. This is called the *Stokes-Adams syndrome*.

In managing patients with third degree block, it is important to recognize that the block can occur transiently or become a permanent abnormality (Fig. 9–9). Drug intoxication with digitalis, propranolol or electrolyte disorders usually produce transient blocks. In contrast, patients with a progressive degeneration of the conducting system or an anterior myocardial infarction may develop a permanent block.

Treatment of third degree block is directed toward maintaining cardiac output by controlling the ventricular rate. In patients with a transient block who are symptomatic, a temporary electronic pacemaker is employed, whereas patients with chronic third degree block require permanent artificial pacing.

HIGH-GRADE, OR ADVANCED, ATRIOVENTRICULAR BLOCK

In this type of atrioventricular block, a ventricular complex follows every second or third or greater atrial complex, resulting in a 2:1 or 3:1 or greater atrioventricular block. The atrial P-P interval and PR interval of the conducted beats are normal (Fig. 9–10). In order to maintain the ventricular rate, a junctional pacemaker usually arises distal to the site of the atrioventricular block to stimulate the ventricles.

The clinical consequences and therapy for advanced atrioventricular block are similar to those of third degree block. Depending upon the ventricular rate and the clinical situation, insertion of an electronic pacemaker may be indicated.

Some cardiologists consider *high-grade atrioventricular block* a form of Mobitz type II second degree block. The distinction in terminology is not universally accepted, and

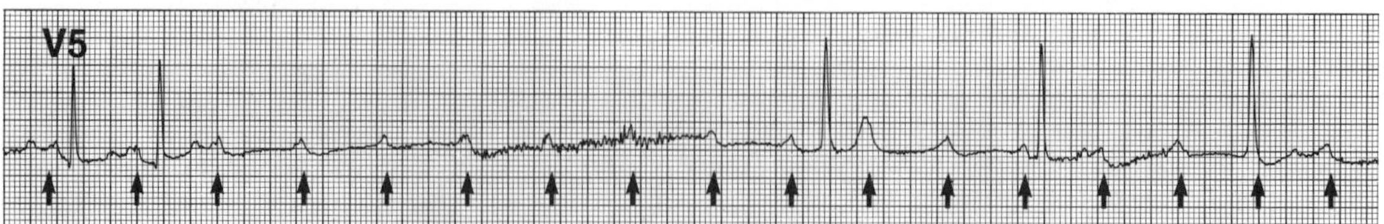

Figure 9–9. **Complete heart block.** This figure shows the sudden onset of complete heart block in a 60 year old woman during an episode of vomiting. The vomiting affected a strong cholinergic (vagal) surge that produced the over 5-second pause in ventricular rhythm. The arrows point to the P waves.

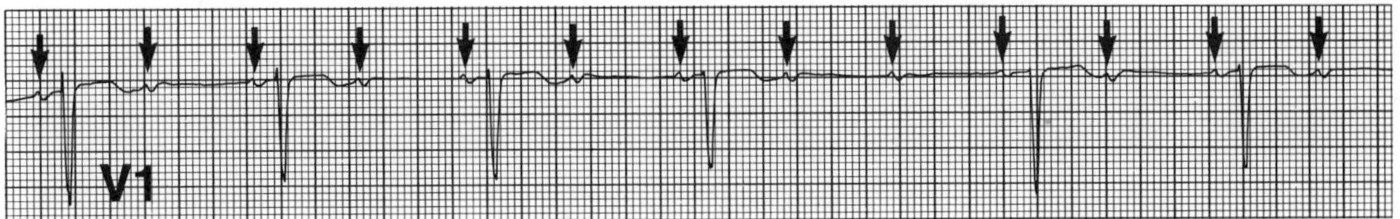

Figure 9–10. **High grade atrioventricular block.** The arrows point to the P waves. The P-P intervals are constant. Notice that there is more than one P wave for every QRS complex; there are conducted and nonconducted P waves.

there are several differences between these conduction disturbances. In Mobitz type II, a single dropped beat occurs intermittently. In comparison, high-grade block demonstrates a regular constant absence of QRS complexes. It takes several atrial impulses to the atrioventricular node to finally stimulate the ventricles. In addition, advanced block may cause the formation of an ectopic secondary pacemaker.

10

Ventricular Conduction Disturbances

The intraventricular conducting system is shown in Figure 10–1. The purpose of this system is to propagate the impulse to the ventricles and to allow it to stimulate both ventricles almost simultaneously.

Normally, as the impulse is conducted down each bundle branch, the surrounding myocardium is stimulated. The function of the *right bundle branch* is mainly to stimulate the right ventricle. The *left bundle branch* stimulates the intraventricular septum; then it divides into two fascicles, the *left anterior fascicle* and the *left posterior fascicle*, before stimulating the more massive left ventricle. Each segment of the intraventricular conducting system is connected to Purkinje cells. These cells are insinuated throughout the myocardium and form a network for the rapid conduction of the impulse.

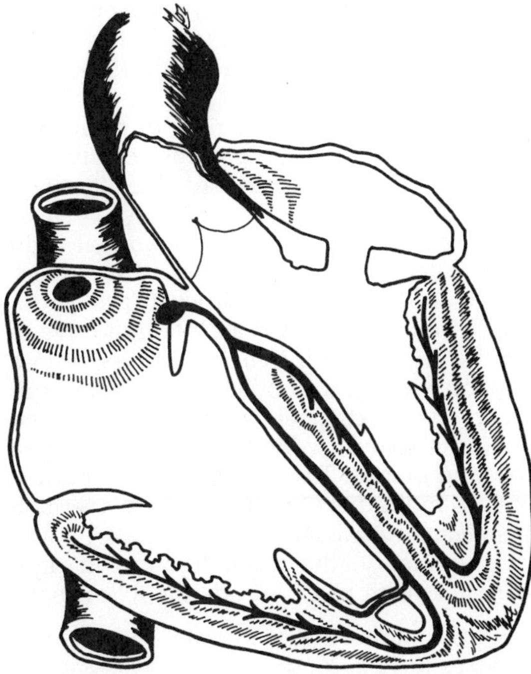

Figure 10–1. This diagram demonstrates the intraventricular conduction system.

Since each segment of the intraventricular conducting system demonstrates very rapid conduction, the whole process of ventricular activation takes less than 0.10 second. This is viewed on an electrocardiogram as the QRS complex, which is less than 2½ small boxes in duration. Abnormalities in conduction will disrupt the normal route of depolarization. This will increase the time of ventricular activation and will prolong the QRS complex. In addition, characteristic changes in the QRS complex morphology will be effected. This exact situation occurs in conduction abnormalities of the bundle branches, referred to as *bundle branch blocks*.

Abnormal conductions through the left anterior or left posterior fascicles are referred to as *hemiblocks*. These conditions generally do not prolong the QRS complex but do disrupt the normal route of left ventricular activation. This results in characteristic changes in the QRS complex morphology. In addition, since the left ventricle is largely responsible for the heart's electrical axis, hemiblocks produce abnormal axis deviations.

In some instances in which the QRS complex is prolonged, the nature of the conduction disturbance cannot be identified. These abnormalities are placed in a vague category termed *intraventricular conduction disturbances*.

BUNDLE BRANCH BLOCKS

The term bundle branch block is applied to either a physiological (see Aberrancy, Chapter 7, page 39) or pathological lesion involving the right or left bundle branch. The hallmark of a bundle branch block is a prolonged QRS complex duration of greater than 2½ small boxes (0.10 second). More specific terms are used to describe the QRS complex prolongation: An *incomplete bundle branch block* refers to a QRS complex duration of 2½ to 3 small boxes (0.10 to 0.11 second). A *complete bundle branch block* is said to be present when the QRS complex duration is equal to or greater than 0.12 second (3 small boxes).

In addition to the prolonged QRS complex duration, bundle branch blocks are characterized by specific QRS morphologies. These changes in the QRS complex result from the abnormal route of ventricular depolarization. Leads V1 and V6 best demonstrate the QRS complex configurations. This is because these two leads have the best view of the right and left ventricles, respectively.

Rather than list the QRS complex morphologies associated with bundle branch blocks, it is more helpful to understand how the abnormal ventricular depolarization produces these changes. The mechanisms for these changes are discussed as follows.

RIGHT BUNDLE BRANCH BLOCK

The characteristic QRS complex morphology of right bundle branch block is caused by a delay in the activation of the right ventricle. In fact, the right ventricle is actually stimulated following the completion of left ventricular activation.

The process of ventricular activation in right bundle branch block is illustrated in Figure 10–2. Although this process is continuous, it can be divided into three steps for easy understanding. The *first step* is septal activation by the left bundle branch. Since the left bundle is unaffected by a right bundle branch block, septal depolarization proceeds normally. This produces normal septal "r" waves in lead V1 and septal "q" waves in lead V6. Because of the right bundle branch block, the ventricles do not depolarize simultaneously. This leads to *step 2*, which is the depolarization of the left ventricle. This occurs at the normal time and produces the S wave in lead V1 and the R wave in lead V6. *Step 3* is the stimulation of the right ventricle; however, in order for this to occur, the impulse must travel from the left ventricle across the muscular septum and then spread throughout the right ventricle. This prolongs the duration of right ventricular activation and produces a slow wave of electrical activity that is directed toward the right. The result is a wide positive terminal deflection in lead V1, referred to as an R′ (R prime), and produces right axis deviation. It also causes the deep, slurred S wave in lead V6. The rSR′ complex in lead V1 is often referred to as an "M" pattern. The RSR′ complex in lead V1 together with the deep, slurred S waves in lead V6 are the characteristic QRS complex findings in right bundle branch block (Fig. 10–3). Recognize, however, that other leads can demonstrate these patterns. For instance, the right precordial leads (V1 to V3) may show the RSR′ complex, while the left precordial leads (V3 to V6) as well as leads I and AVL may display the deep slurred S waves of right bundle branch block. This is because these leads have views of the heart that are similar to the views of leads V1 and V6, respectively.

Another major characteristic of right bundle branch block is the presence of inverted T waves in the right precordial leads; these are called *secondary T-wave changes*. These changes are a result of the abnormal right ventricular repolarization that is secondary to the abnormal right ventricular activation. These inverted T waves are not indicative of disease; however, if ischemia is present in a patient with right bundle branch block, primary T-wave changes will be superimposed on the already inverted T waves. This will result in upright T waves that appear normal but are indicative of ischemia. This is termed *"pseudonormalization."*

In summary, the major findings in right bundle branch block include the following:

1. QRS complex interval greater than 3 small boxes (0.12 second).
2. RSR′ complex or "M" pattern in lead V1.

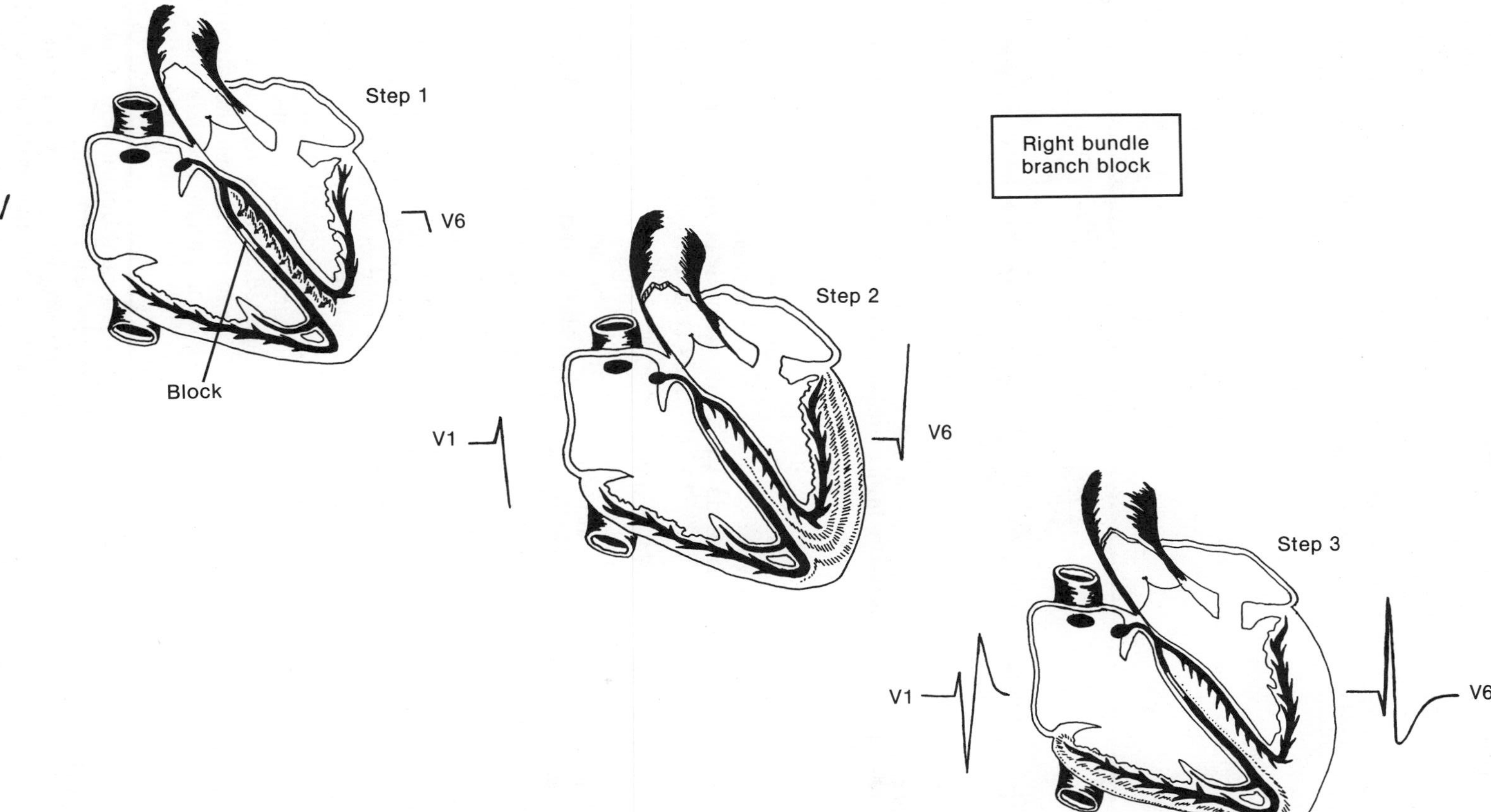

Figure 10–2. This diagram shows the process of ventricular activation in right bundle branch block (see text).

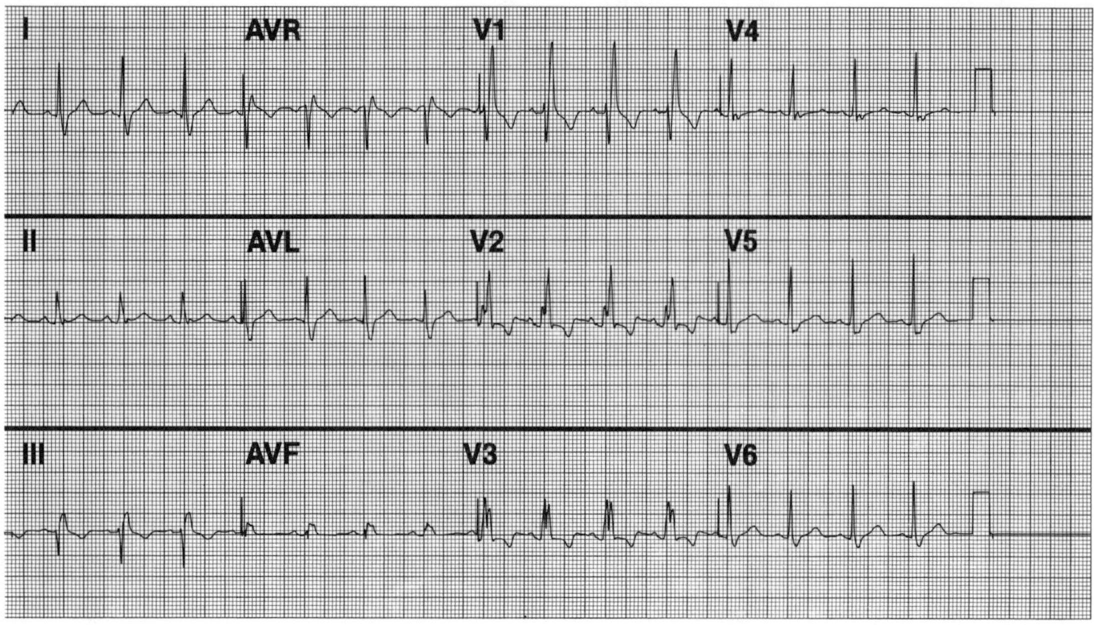

Figure 10–3. **Right bundle branch block.** Notice the rSR′ complex in lead V1 and the slurred S waves in leads I, AVL, V5 and V6, indicating an abnormality in the terminal QRS complex vector. The QRS complex is wide, measuring 0.14 second.

3. Right axis deviation.
4. Deep slurred S waves in lead V6.
5. Secondary T wave inversion in leads V1 to V3.

Another finding in right bundle branch block is an increase in the intrinsicoid deflection. The *intrinsicoid deflection* is the interval measured from the start of the QRS complex to the peak of the initial QRS complex (see Chapter 4, Review of Complexes). This interval represents the time of myocardial activation. The intrinsicoid deflection in lead V1 measures the activation time of the right ventricle, and in lead V6, it measures the time of left ventricular activation. In right bundle branch block, the right ventricular activation time is increased. This results in an increase in the intrinsicoid deflection in lead V1. Activation of the left ventricle is normal, so the intrinsicoid deflection is normal in lead V6.

Associated Findings

Right bundle branch block is usually a fixed, permanent abnormality; however, it may occur intermittently. *Intermittent block* is usually related to rapid ventricular rates. Essentially, at rapid rates the impulses from the atrioventricular junction may arrive at the right bundle while it is still in the refractory period. This results in a physiological block of the right bundle and produces the characteristic RSR′ complex in lead V1. Intermittent right bundle branch block is common in atrial fibrillation, atrial flutter and other supraventricular tachycardias.

In diagnosing right bundle branch block on an electrocardiogram, one should be aware that several conditions such as right ventricular hypertrophy, a posterior myocardial infarction and the Wolff-Parkinson-White syndrome can produce the RSR′ complex in lead V1 seen with right bundle branch block. Since there is no block of the right bundle in these conditions, the RSR′ complex is referred to as a *right bundle branch block pattern*. In most cases the differential diagnosis is apparent because these conditions do not usually prolong the QRS complex.

It is also important to note that the presence of a right bundle branch block does not interfere with the diagnosis of a myocardial infarction. This is obvious when one recognizes that a right bundle branch block affects only the terminal segment of the QRS complex, while a myocardial infarction affects the initial segment by producing Q waves (see Myocardial Infarction, Chapter 12).

Clinical Significance

Clinically, right bundle branch block does not necessarily imply organic heart disease. In fact, it is not uncommon in healthy individuals; however, it may be associated with almost any type of heart disease, especially those diseases involving the right side of the heart. For example, congenital lesions of the septum that produce left to right shunting, pulmonary hypertension and myocardial infarction often cause a right bundle branch block. In addition, patients with valvular anomalies or degenerative changes in the conducting system may demonstrate a block in the right bundle branch.

Pulmonary embolism frequently causes a right bundle branch block because the embolism produces acute right ventricular strain. Thus, in any patient with chest pain and the sudden onset of a right bundle branch block, one should always consider a pulmonary embolism as the cause.

Since a right bundle branch block does not cause hemodynamic instability, nor does it usually lead to more serious arrhythmias, treatment is generally not indicated. However, in patients with an acute anterior myocardial infarction who develop a right bundle branch block, a temporary pacemaker is indicated, as these patients often progress to complete heart block (see Third Degree Atrioventricular Block and Supraventricular Conduction Disturbance, page 63).

LEFT BUNDLE BRANCH BLOCK

The characteristic QRS complex morphology of left bundle branch block is caused by an abnormal activation of the septum and a delay in the activation of the left ventricle.

Figure 10–4 illustrates the process of ventricular activation in left bundle branch block. This process can again be divided into three steps. The *first step* is septal activation. Since the left bundle is blocked, normal septal depolarization does not occur. This results in the loss of both septal R waves in the right precordial leads (V1 to V3) and septal q waves in the left precordial leads (V4 to V6). Instead, the septum is activated from right to left by impulses from the right bundle branch. This results in the QRS complex having an initial negative deflection in lead V1 and an initial positive deflection in lead V6. After septal activation, the impulse continues toward the left ventricle. *Step 2* is the combined effect of right ventricular and left ventricular activations. Although the right ventricle is activated normally, its electrical vector is negated by the slow conduction in the septum, which is progressing in an abnormal leftward direction. *Step 3* is simply the prolongation of left ventricular activation. This produces a broad, monophasic QRS complex. Thus, the QRS complex in left bundle branch block demonstrates a loss of the normal septal "q" waves in lead V6, a broad QS complex in lead V1 and a broad, notched R wave in lead V6 (Fig. 10–5).

Other leads may demonstrate these patterns. For instance, right precordial leads that have a similar view of the heart as lead V1 may show a broad monophasic QS complex. Leads V4, V5, AVL and in particular lead I may demonstrate the loss of septal "q" waves and the broad, notched R wave found in lead V6. This is because leads V4, V5, AVL, and lead I have views of the left ventricle that are similar to the view of lead V6.

Another major characteristic of left bundle branch block is secondary T wave inversions in the left precordial leads. Analogous to the T wave changes in right bundle branch block, these T wave inversions are produced by an abnormality in left ventricular repolarization. They are not indicative of disease. Ischemic states may superimpose primary T wave inversions upon these secondary changes. The result may be upright "pseudonormal" T waves (see preceding discussion on Right Bundle Branch Block).

In summary, the major findings in left bundle branch block include the following:

1. QRS complex greater than 3 small boxes (0.12 second).
2. Absence of septal q waves in leads I and V6.
3. Broad, monophasic QS complex in lead V1 and wide notched R wave in leads I and V6.
4. Secondary T wave inversion in leads I and V6.

Associated Findings

Additional findings in left bundle branch block include an increase in the *intrinsicoid deflection* in lead V6 to greater than 0.045 second and occasionally a *left axis deviation*.

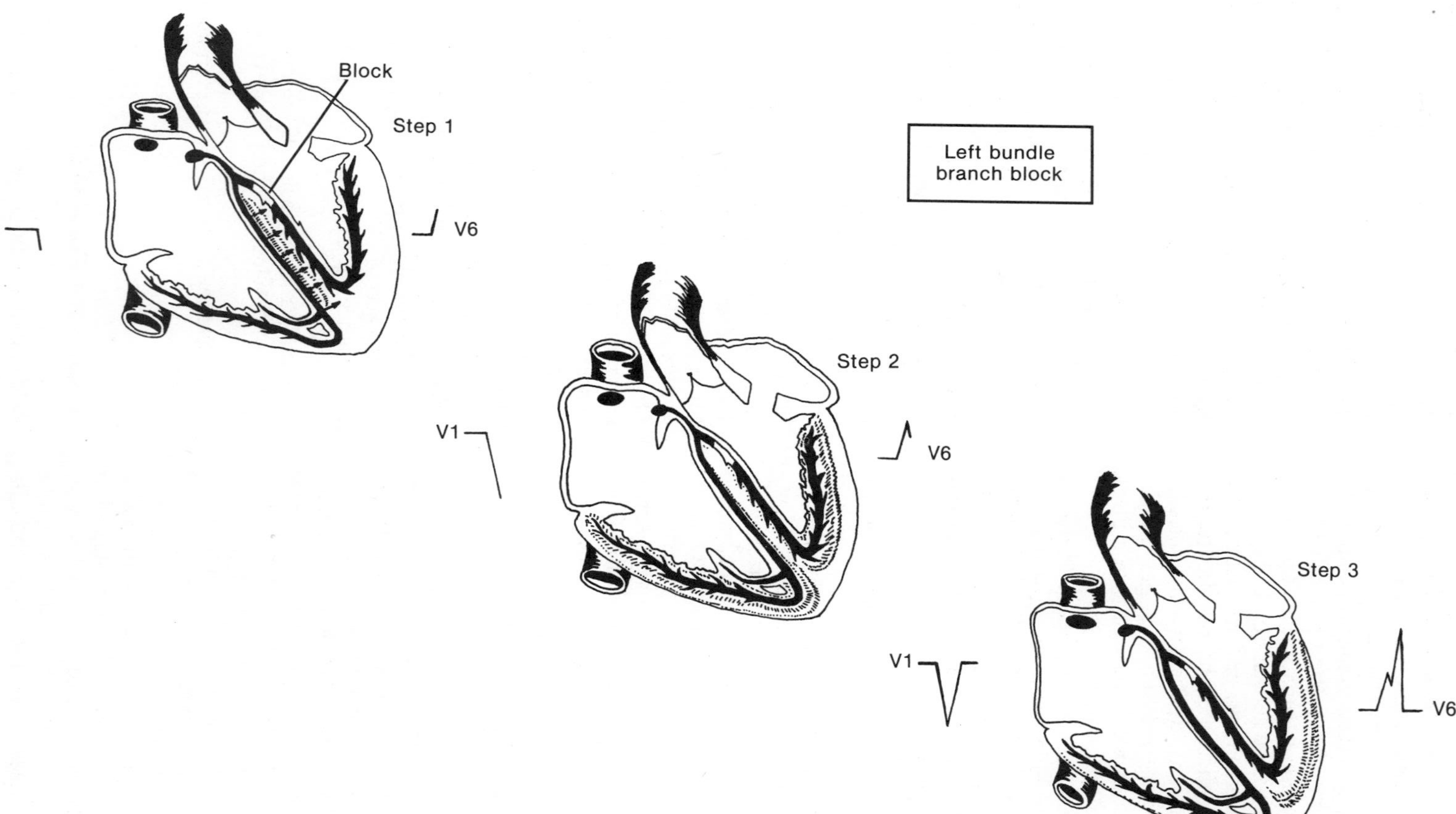

Figure 10–4. This diagram shows the process of ventricular activation in left bundle branch block (see text).

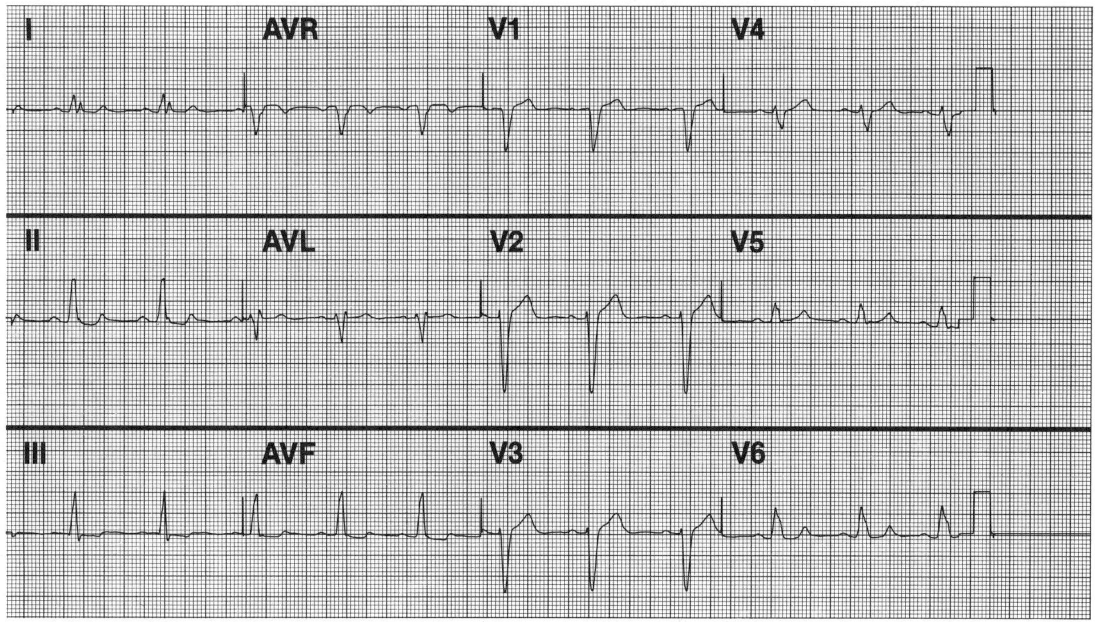

Figure 10–5. **Left bundle branch block.** Notice the absence of septal Q waves in leads I, AVL, V5 and V6 as well as the notching of the R waves in these leads. This indicates an abnormality in the initial QRS vector. The QRS complex is widened and measures 0.14 second.

As previously stated for right bundle branch block, the *intrinsicoid deflection* represents the actual time of myocardial depolarization. In left bundle branch block, the time of left ventricular depolarization is increased, and so the intrinsicoid deflection in lead V6 is also prolonged.

Unlike the right axis deviation found in right bundle branch block, left axis deviation is not a frequent finding in left bundle branch block. This is because the left ventricle is normally electrically predominant, and a left bundle branch block does nothing to change the main electrical vector; it simply changes the path by which the main vector is reached (i.e., it changes the route of depolarization, not the resultant). Occasionally a patient with left bundle branch block will demonstrate a left axis deviation. In these cases, one should suspect that an additional myocardial abnormality is producing the leftward axis.

Finally, there is an interesting and important association between left bundle branch block and acute anterior myocardial infarction. Simply stated: A pre-existing diagnosis of left bundle branch block may preclude the electrocardiographic diagnosis of an acute anterior myocardial infarction. Why? Remember, a left bundle branch block affects the initial vector or segment of the QRS complex in the precordial leads. Thus, the initial Q wave of an anterior myocardial infarction may not be recognizable in a patient with left bundle branch block. One must use clinical judgment and laboratory studies to make the diagnosis of infarction in such patients. A more ominous association between left bundle branch block and myocardial infarction occurs in a patient who suffers an acute infarction and then develops a sudden onset of left bundle branch block. This is discussed in the following section.

Clinical Significance

Unlike right bundle branch block, which occasionally occurs in normal healthy individuals, left bundle branch block is usually found in patients with organic heart disease. Left bundle branch block may be transient or permanent. Transient left bundle branch block may develop in the course of a myocardial infarction, heart failure, myocarditis or antiarrhythmic therapy. Permanent left bundle branch block is practically always the result of structural heart disease, chronic degeneration of the conducting system or an illness that produces long-standing left ventricular strain, such as valvular anomalies or hypertension.

Left bundle branch block usually does not require any specific treatment, and management of the underlying heart disease is all that is necessary. A notable exception to this occurs in patients with an acute myocardial infarction and the new onset of a left bundle branch block. These patients are at risk for developing complete heart block. Consequently, the insertion of a temporary pacemaker is indicated.

HEMIBLOCKS

As previously mentioned, the left bundle branch consists of two divisions: an *anterior fascicle* and a *posterior fascicle*. Abnormalities of conduction in the fascicles are referred to as *hemiblocks*. In general, hemiblocks do not prolong the QRS complex because each fascicle is in contact with the rapidly conducting Purkinje network. Purkinje fibers, once stimulated, will rapidly conduct the impulse throughout the myocardium. Although hemiblocks do not appreciably increase the time of myocardial activation, they do change the route of left ventricular depolarization. This results in axis deviations and changes in the QRS complex morphology. These effects are best demonstrated in the limb leads.

The topic of hemiblocks is a complex one. Understanding the anatomy of the fascicles will prove invaluable in learning this difficult subject. Figure 10–6 illustrates the anatomy of the fascicles. The anterior fascicle is located in the superior, anterior portion of the left ventricle near the base of the anterior papillary muscle. It is also lateral to the posterior fascicle. The posterior fascicle is found in the inferior, posterior portion of the left ventricle. It is near the posterior papillary muscle and is medial to the anterior fascicle.

Left Anterior Hemiblock

In *left anterior hemiblock,* left ventricular activation can only be initiated by impulses from the posterior fascicle (Fig. 10–7). Consequently, the impulse will spread from the region of the posterior fascicle to the anterior wall in an upward, anterior and leftward direction.

The initial depolarization of the posterior wall and the early spread of the impulse along the medial wall of the left ventricle produces a small q wave in lead I and a small r wave in lead III. As already described, however, the bulk of the depolarization proceeds in an upward, anterior and leftward direction. This inscribes an R wave in lead I and an S wave in leads III and AVF. This resultant depolarization produces left axis deviation. This should be apparent by recognizing that the major wave of depolarization is directed toward the left. Evidence of the

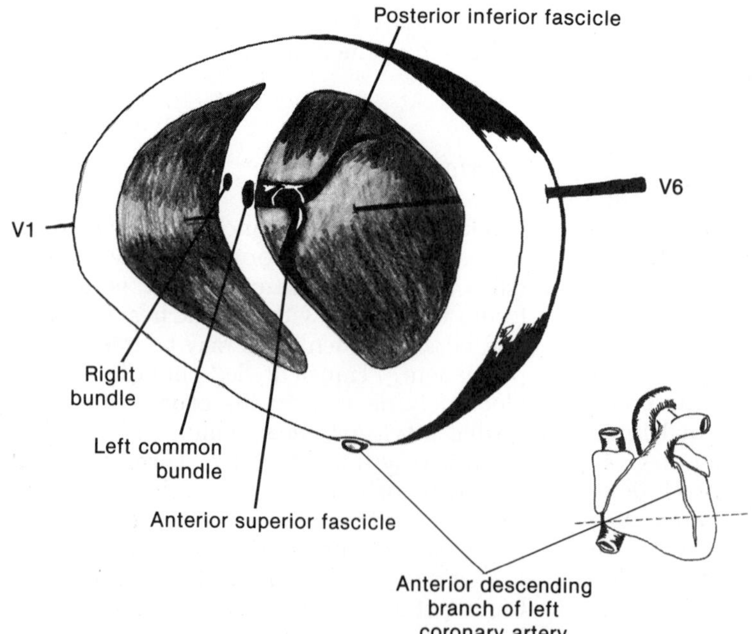

Figure 10–6. This diagram demonstrates the anatomy of the left bundle branch fascicles. The level of the cross section is shown by the dotted line.

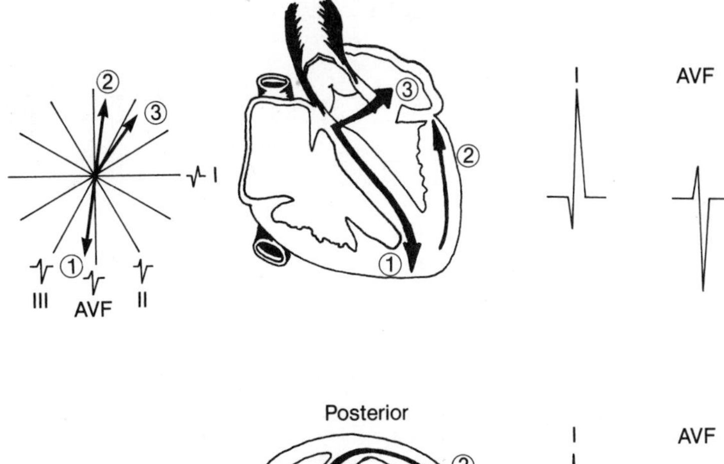

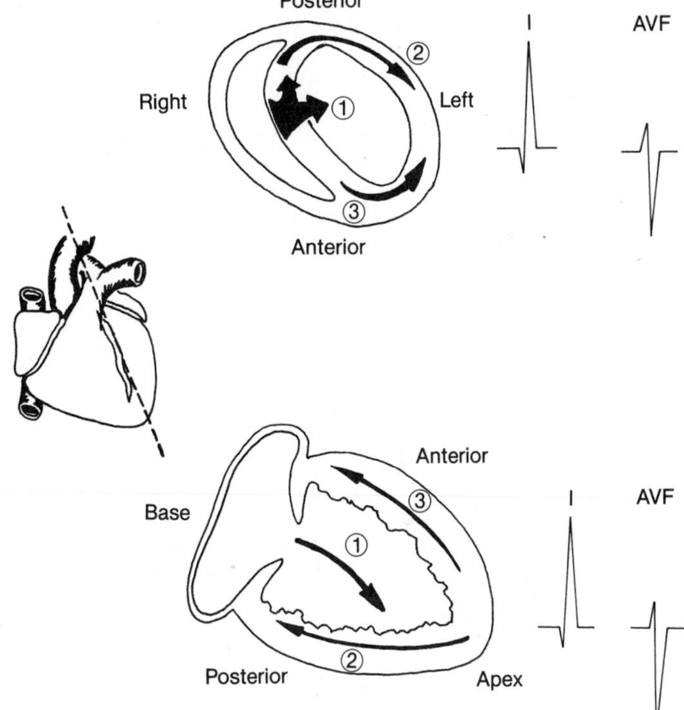

Figure 10–7. This diagram illustrates the abnormalities of depolarization caused by a left anterior hemiblock (see text).

axis deviation is shown in the QRS complexes in leads I and AVF in Figure 10–8.

Since left axis deviation is the major electrocardiographic characteristic of left anterior hemiblock, other conditions that produce left axis deviation cannot be present when one is considering the diagnosis of left anterior hemiblock (see Left Axis Deviation, Table 1, page 25).

In summary, the criteria for the diagnosis of left anterior hemiblock are as follows:

1. Left axis deviation greater than −40°.
2. qR complex in lead I, rS complex in leads II, III and AVF.
3. Normal QRS complex duration.
4. No evidence of other conditions that produce left axis deviation.

Because left anterior hemiblock changes the morphology of the QRS complexes, it can mask or mimic numerous cardiac conditions. In particular, left anterior hemiblock can sometimes be confused with an anterior or lateral myocardial infarction. An anterior myocardial infarction produces Q waves in leads V1 to V4. Similarly, the initial depolarization of the posterior myocardial wall in a left anterior hemiblock may also produce small q waves in these leads. This same reasoning applies in explaining how a left anterior hemiblock may produce Q waves in

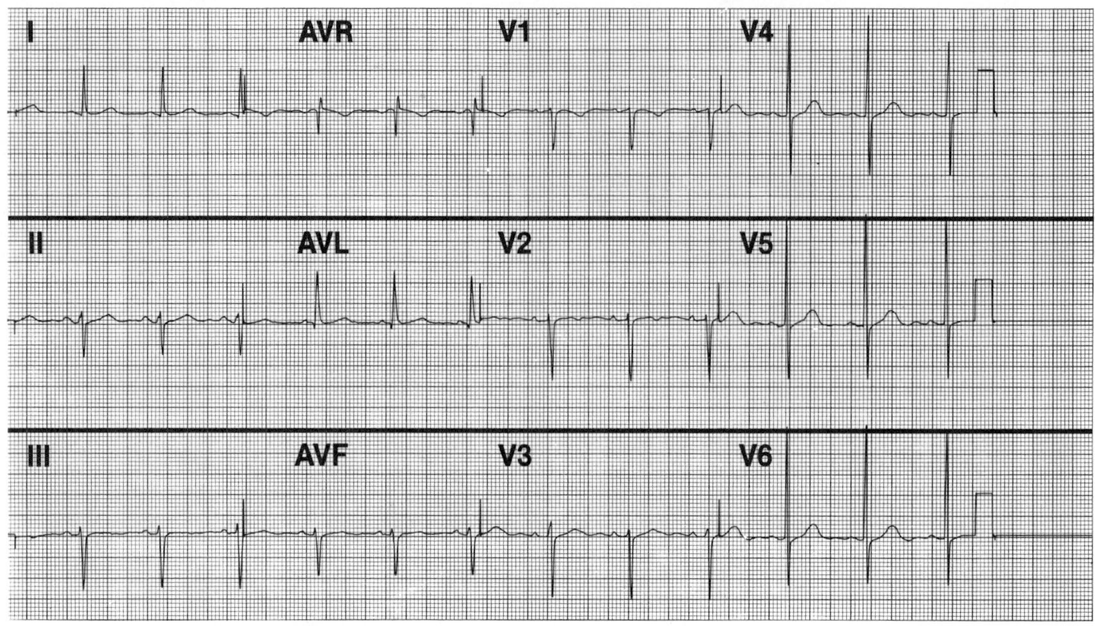

Figure 10–8. **Left anterior hemiblock.** Notice that the mean QRS axis is −50°, and the QRS complex is not widened.

leads II, III and AVF, which may mask the Q waves of an inferior myocardial infarction.

In addition, left anterior hemiblock can mask or mimic left ventricular hypertrophy. Again, the reason for this is found by studying the abnormal route of left ventricular activation caused by left anterior hemiblock. As illustrated in Figure 10–8, the main vector of left ventricular activation in left anterior hemiblock is directed anteriorly and toward the left. This may produce large R voltages in leads I, AVL and the precordial leads that may be mistaken for the large voltages found in left ventricular hypertrophy.

Left Posterior Hemiblock

In *left posterior hemiblock*, the left posterior fascicle is unable to activate its region of the myocardium. This results in left ventricular activation having to proceed solely from the region of the anterior fascicle. Thus, the impulse will be forced to spread from the anterior fascicle in a downward, inferior and rightward direction in order to activate the posterior wall (Fig. 10–9).

The depolarization of the anterior wall and its initial spread along the lateral wall inscribes a small q wave in leads III and AVF. The bulk of the depolarization, however, which is directed downward and to the right, causes the inscription of an S wave in lead I and an R wave in leads III and AVF. Simply by understanding the major direction of the wave of depolarization, one should recognize that the axis should be deviated to the right. Figure 10–10 demonstrates the axis deviation as evidenced by the QRS complexes in leads I and AVF.

Although the most characteristic abnormalities in left posterior hemiblock are seen in the limb leads, all leads of the electrocardiogram demonstrate the effects of the abnormal route of left ventricular depolarization. In particular, the posterior and rightwardly directed main vector of left ventricular depolarization may produce R waves in the right precordial leads. The resulting QRS complexes in these leads may resemble those produced by right ventricular hypertrophy. Likewise, pre-existing right ventricular hypertrophy can mask or mimic left posterior hemiblock; therefore, the diagnosis of left posterior hemiblock cannot be made in the presence of criteria suggestive of right ventricular hypertrophy. In addition, a left posterior hemiblock may mask or mimic an anterior myocardial infarction.

The major characteristics of left posterior hemiblock are as follows:

1. Right axis deviation greater than +120°.
2. rS complex in lead I, qR complex in leads II, III and AVF.
3. Normal QRS complex duration.

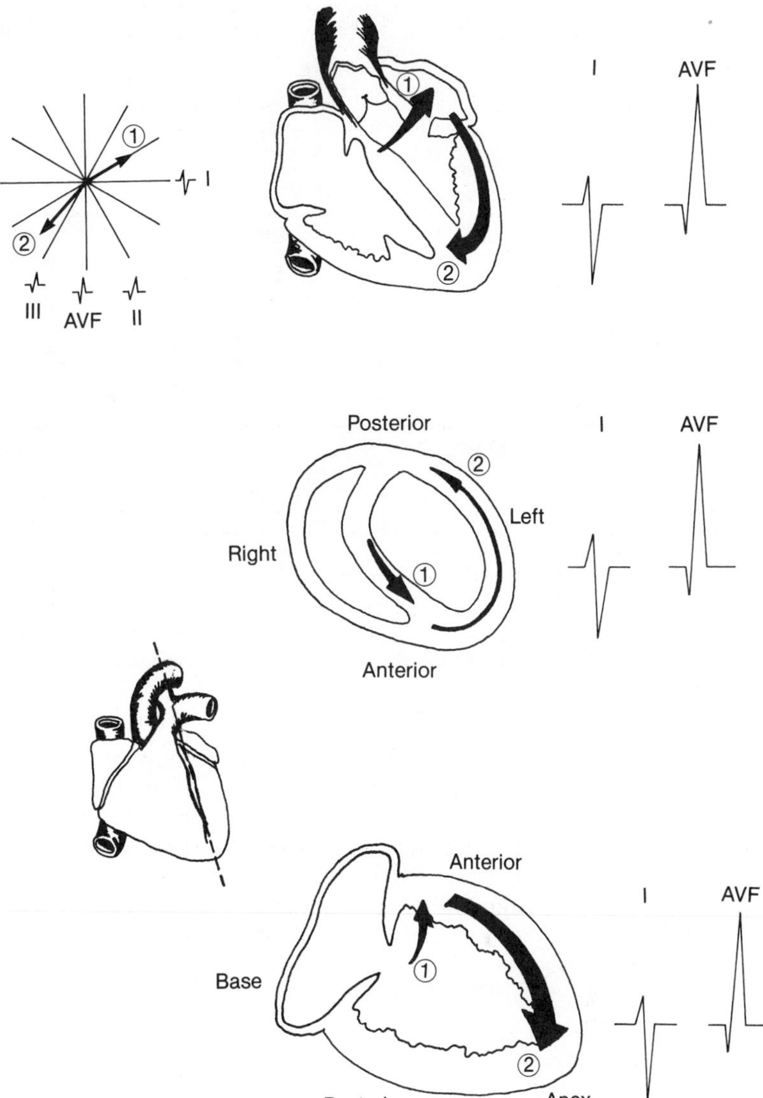

Figure 10–9. This diagram illustrates the abnormalities of depolarization caused by a left posterior hemiblock (see text).

4. No evidence of right ventricular hypertrophy.

Essentially, the characteristic findings of left anterior hemiblock and left posterior hemiblock are mirror images. Left anterior hemiblock demonstrates a left axis deviation by a qR complex in lead I and an rS complex in lead III. In contrast, left posterior hemiblock produces a right axis deviation by an rS in lead I and a qR complex in lead III.

Clinical Significance

Clinically, hemiblocks are not uncommon, especially during an acute myocardial infarction. Left anterior hemiblock is more common than left posterior hemiblock. This is because the posterior fascicle is shorter and thicker than the anterior fascicle, and it receives its blood supply from dual sources.

The causes of hemiblocks include coronary artery disease, hypertension, congenital heart disease and cardiomyopathies. Isolated hemiblocks do not compromise cardiac function. Therapy is directed at treating the underlying etiologic agent.

BIFASCICULAR AND TRIFASCICULAR BLOCKS

Each segment of the conducting system can be considered to be a conducting fascicle.

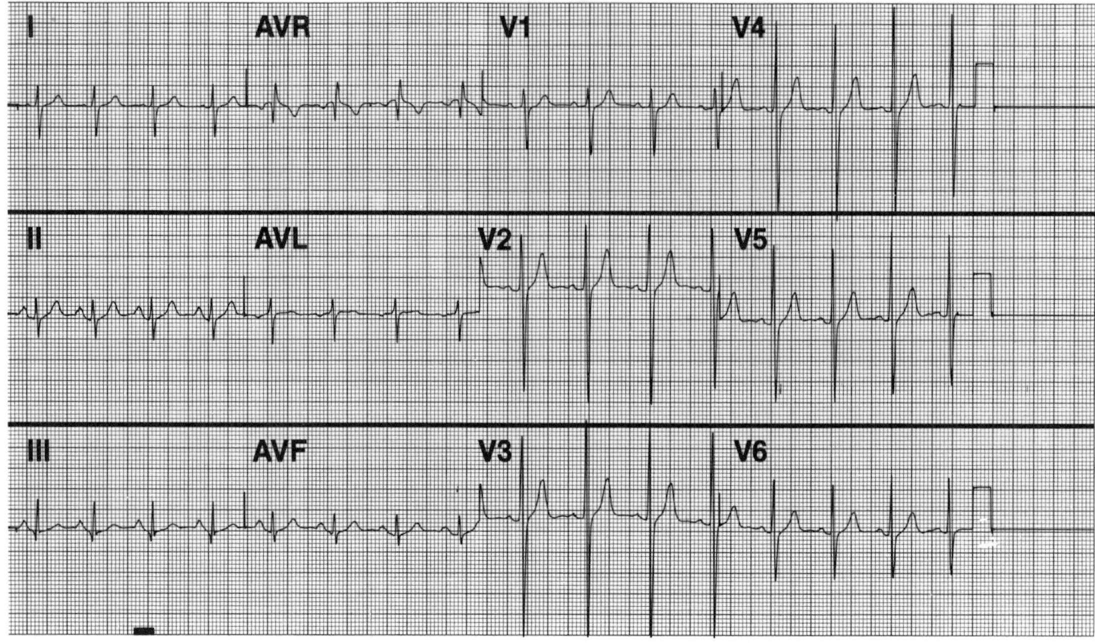

Figure 10–10. **Left posterior hemiblock.** Notice that the mean QRS vector is +130°, and the QRS complex is not widened.

This means that the heart has essentially six conducting fascicles: sinoatrial node, atrioventricular node, bundle of His, right bundle branch, left anterior branch and left posterior branch. *Bifascicular block* refers to slowed conduction in any two segments. The most common bifascicular block is a combination of right bundle branch block and left anterior hemiblock (Fig. 10–11). This type of block frequently occurs in patients suffering from an acute myocardial infarction. The electrocardiogram will demonstrate the characteris-

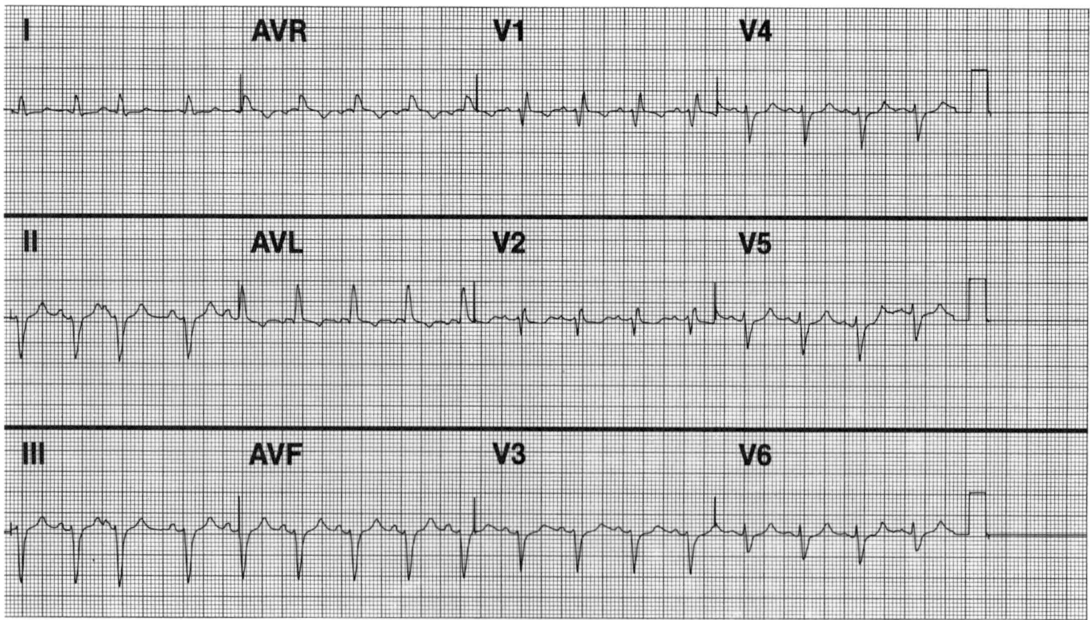

Figure 10–11. **Bifascicular block.** There is an rSR′ complex in leads V1 and V2 together with a slurring of the S waves in leads I and V6. This fulfills the criteria for *right bundle branch block.* In addition, the mean QRS vector has an axis of −70°, resulting in the diagnosis of *left anterior hemiblock.* Therefore, bifascicular block is present.

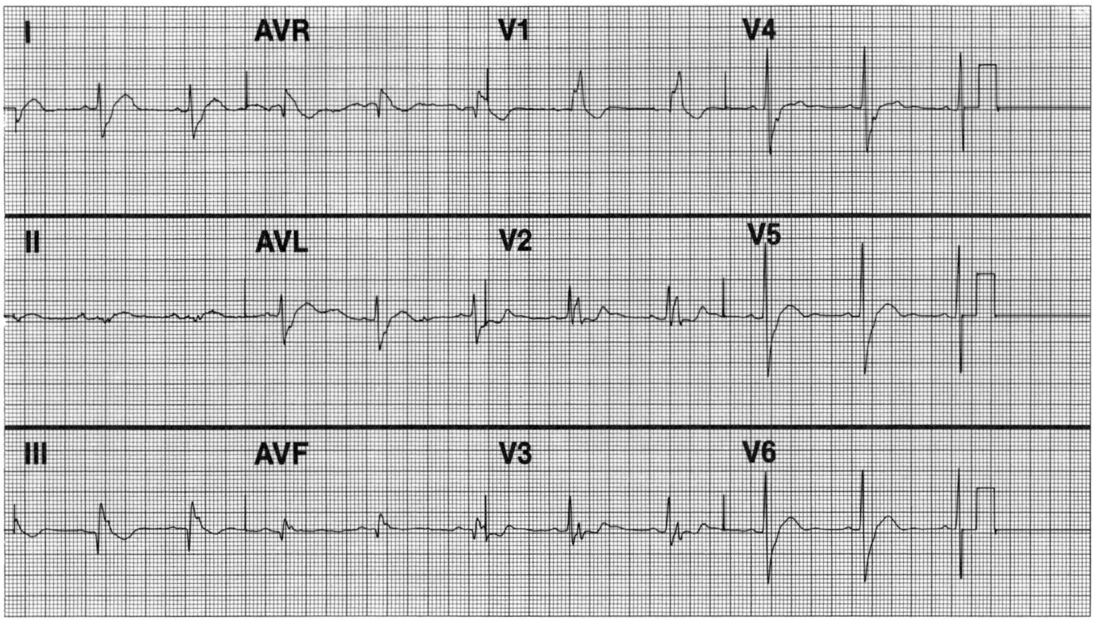

Figure 10–12. **Bifascicular block.** The criteria for *right bundle branch block* and *left posterior hemiblock* are present. These cause the extreme right axis deviation seen in this tracing. In this example, the QRS mean axis is +150°.

tics of the right bundle branch block as well as that of the left anterior hemiblock (i.e., RSR′ complex in lead V1 greater than 0.12 second with a left axis deviation). Bifascicular block involving the right bundle branch and the left posterior fascicle is less common (Fig. 10–12). When present in a patient with an acute myocardial infarction, it indicates that a large area of the myocardium has been infarcted. These patients have a poor prognosis. The electrocardiogram in this type of block will show the characteristics of the right bundle branch block together with a marked right axis deviation.

Technically, blocks that occur in any two conducting fascicles can be considered bifas-

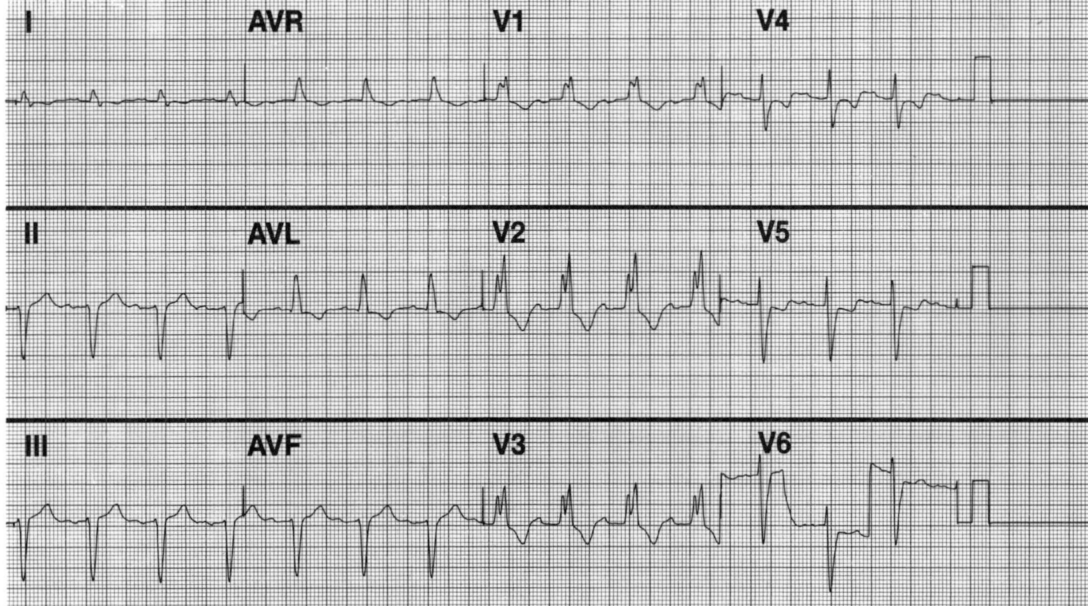

Figure 10–13. **Trifascicular block.** In addition to the abnormalities cited for Figure 10–11, first degree atrioventricular block is also present. The PR interval measures 0.26 second. This results in the diagnosis of trifascicular block.

cicular block; however, these other blocks are most uncommon.

Trifascicular block is block in three of the fascicles. The most common type is right bundle branch block, left anterior hemiblock with first degree atrioventricular block (Fig. 10–13). The electrocardiogram will show a prolonged PR interval, prolonged QRS complex (related to the right bundle branch block), RSR′ complex in lead V1 and a left axis deviation. The occurrence of this triad of blocks is quite common in the elderly population. It is generally associated with myocardial infarction. In individuals who have not suffered a myocardial infarction, aging of the conducting system is thought to be the cause (see Sick Sinus Syndrome, Chapter 9, page 61).

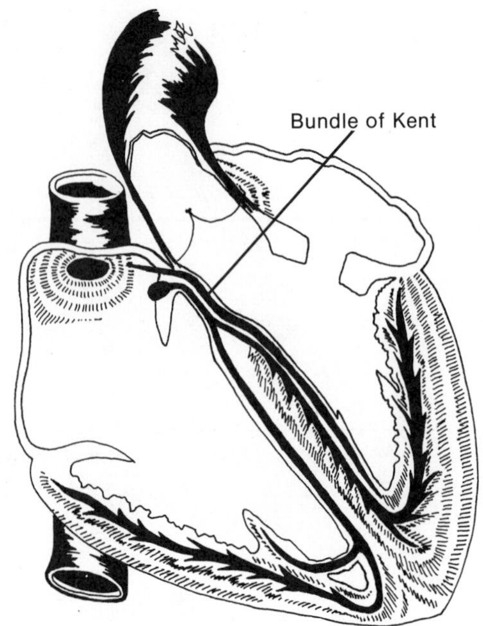

Figure 10–14. This diagram shows the functional anatomy seen in Wolff-Parkinson-White syndrome. Notice that there is an accessory pathway, called the bundle of Kent, which allows impulses to be transmitted to the ventricle without the normal delay in the atrioventricular node.

PRE-EXCITATION SYNDROME

In *pre-excitation syndrome*, the impulse takes an abnormal anatomical pathway to reach the ventricle. The classic example of pre-excitation is the *Wolff-Parkinson-White* syndrome. This syndrome results from an anomalous or accessory pathway known as the *bundle of Kent*, which runs from the atria to the ventricles and bypasses the atrioventricular node (Fig. 10–14). It therefore allows an impulse originating in the atria to avoid the delay encountered in the atrioventricular node. The effect of the transmission of this impulse via the accessory pathway may clearly be seen on the electrocardiogram: Since ventricular depolarization begins earlier than normal, the PR interval will be shortened. However, since the accessory pathway traverses the myocardium, conduction through this pathway is somewhat slower than through the normal conducting system. Consequently, the QRS complex is widened by an early abnormal deflection called a *delta wave* (Fig. 10–15).

Classically, there are two main types of the Wolff-Parkinson-White syndrome based upon the anatomical location of the bypass tract. Type A is defined when the bundle of Kent is left sided near the mitral valve. The delta wave and the remainder of the QRS complex are upright in leads V1 and V6. Type B Wolff-Parkinson-White syndrome occurs when the accessory pathway is right

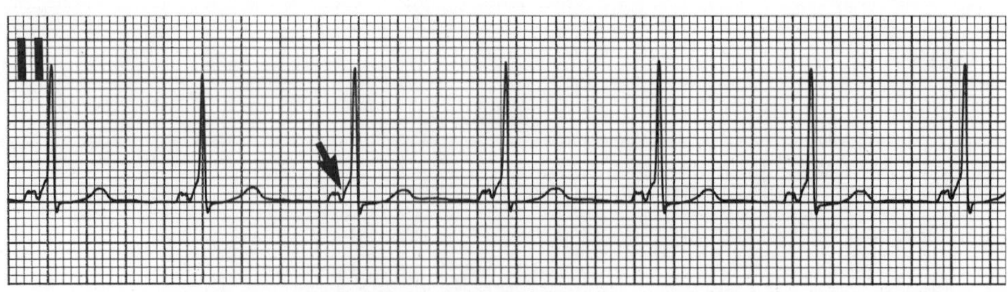

Figure 10–15. **Wolff-Parkinson-White syndrome.** Notice the short PR interval, 0.08 second, as well as the delta wave, indicated by the arrow. The QRS complex is prolonged by the delta wave, which in this example measures 0.11 second.

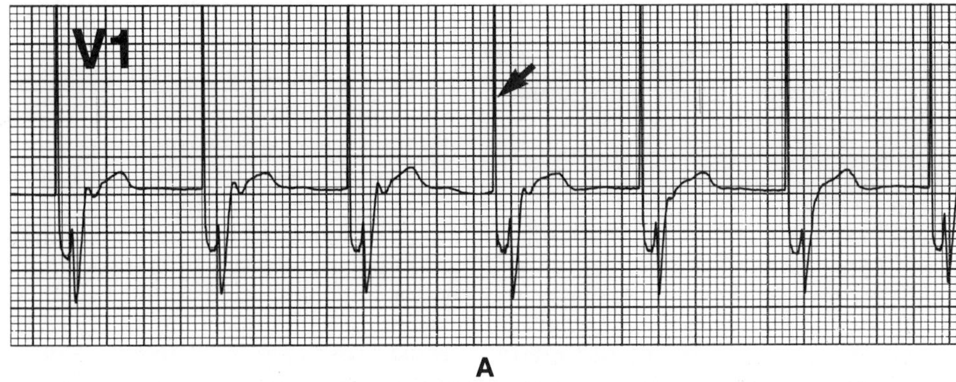

A

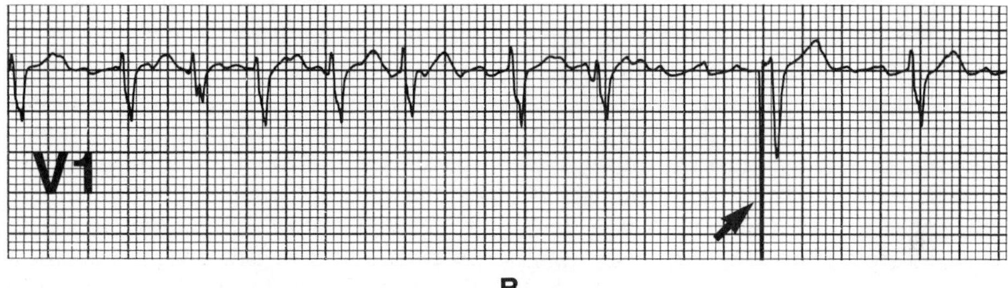

B

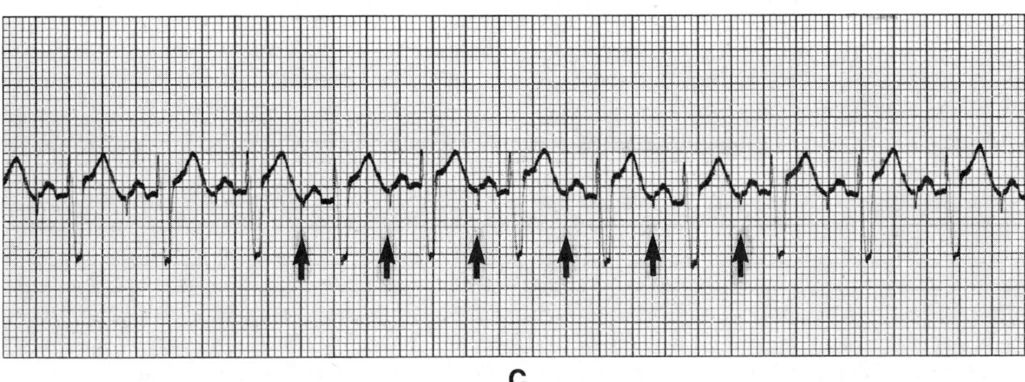

C

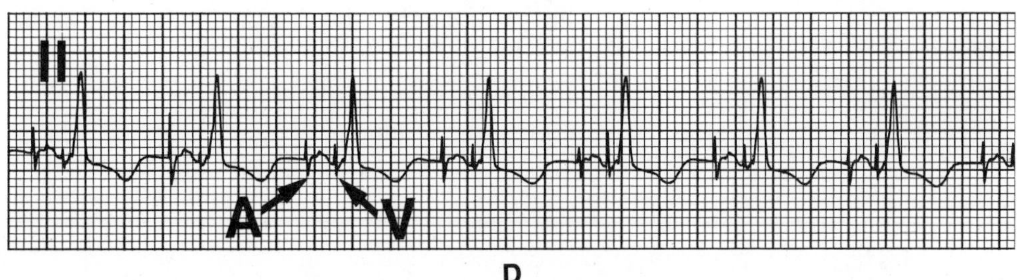

D

Figure 10–16. **Electronic pacemakers.** *A,* A fixed rate ventricular pacemaker. The arrow points to the pacemaker spike, which is set in this patient to occur at 72 times per minute. *B,* A demand ventricular pacemaker. The arrow points to the pacemaker spike. The basic rhythm is atrial fibrillation. *C,* An atrial pacemaker. The arrows again point to the pacemaker spikes. Notice that there is a delay before the QRS complex occurs. This "pacemaker-R" interval is equivalent to the normal PR interval and may be set by the physician. *D,* A dual chamber or sequential pacemaker. There are two spikes for each QRS complex. Arrow "A" points to the atrial component, while arrow "V" points to the ventricular component.

sided. In this case, the QRS complex is inverted in lead V1 but upright in lead V6.

Because of the anomalous pathway, there are a large number of electrocardiographic abnormalities associated with pre-excitation. Type A Wolff-Parkinson-White can produce electrocardiographic abnormalities suggestive of right bundle branch block, right ventricular hypertrophy and inferior myocardial infarction. Type B Wolff-Parkinson-White frequently produces Q waves in the inferior leads II, III and AVF as well as in leads V1 to V3. These can simulate an anterior myocardial infarction or left bundle branch block. These "pseudoinfarction" patterns are quite common with pre-excitation.

Patients with Wolff-Parkinson-White syndrome are extremely vulnerable to episodes of supraventricular tachycardia. This results from re-entry, which is made possible by the retrograde conduction through the accessory pathway back to the atria. In addition, atrial tachycardias that are normally blocked in the slowly conducting atrioventricular node may be transmitted to the ventricle through the accessory tract. This rapid stimulation of the ventricle may produce a very rapid ventricular response, and patients may develop life-threatening ventricular fibrillation. In fact, patients with rapid atrial fibrillation and Wolff-Parkinson-White syndrome are at high risk of sudden death because of rapid stimulation of the ventricles.

There are other syndromes of pre-excitation. The *Lown-Ganong-Levine* syndrome is a type of pre-excitation through an abnormal bundle of James that bypasses the atrioventricular node. This syndrome is characterized by a short PR and a normal QRS complex without a delta wave. The *Mahaim pre-excitation* is characterized by a normal PR interval, a widened QRS complex and a delta wave. A further discussion of pre-excitation is beyond the scope of this book, and the interested reader is referred to the many texts available on pre-excitation.

ELECTRONIC PACEMAKERS

Artificial electrical pacemakers are used in the management of bradycardia and unreliable atrioventricular conduction. Electronic pacemakers are easily recognized by the presence of vertical spikes, which are the electrical impulses released by the pacemaker generator and conducted to the heart. Artificial pacing depends upon the ability of the electronic pacemaker to be able to depolarize an area of myocardium around its electrode.

The scope of pacemakers today is so broad that it is not possible to review all of the electrocardiographic effects of the different types. However, it is important to recognize the more common types of pacemakers. The *fixed rate ventricular pacemaker* continues to discharge at a fixed interval regardless of the appearance of inherent beats (Fig. 10–16*A*). A *demand ventricular pacemaker* is set by the manufacturer to fire after a specified pause. If the demand pacemaker is working properly, it will not discharge unless the asystolic interval exceeds the preset value. Thus, pacemaker spikes are seen only after a long R-R interval (Fig. 10–16*B*).

An *atrial pacemaker* is used when the sinus mechanism is too slow to maintain adequate cardiac output. Atrial pacemakers cannot be used in the presence of atrioventricular block because the block will prevent the impulses generated by the pacemaker from reaching the ventricles. An atrial pacemaker will activate the atria, and a spike can be seen to precede each P wave (Fig. 10–16*C*). The *dual chamber* or *sequential pacemaker* will activate both the atria and ventricles, and a spike will precede each P wave and QRS complex (Fig. 10–16*D*). This type of pacemaker is used in patients who require both the "atrial kick" and ventricular pacing.

11

Chamber Enlargement

Whenever there is a volume or pressure overload in the heart, one or more of the four cardiac chambers will enlarge. Volume overloads tend to increase the diameter of the chamber, and *dilatation* is said to occur. On the other hand, pressure overloads tend to increase the thickness of the chamber wall, and *hypertrophy* results. Actually, even with dilatation there is a need to increase the thickness of the wall, but in order to understand the information in this chapter, this fact is not important.

One usually speaks only of atrial enlargement as a general term meaning both dilatation and hypertrophy have occurred. These terms are more acceptable for the pathological description of ventricular chambers. However, ventricular enlargement implying either hypertrophy or dilatation is also correct.

The electrocardiogram is not generally sensitive enough to be able to differentiate between ventricular dilatation and hypertrophy. All of the criteria for diagnosing enlargement are based on actual hypertrophy of the myocardial wall. However, there are some suggestive signs that help to determine which process may have occurred. These will be discussed later in the chapter.

When a chamber enlarges, it has more surface area. Therefore, the wave of depolarization will not only take longer but the total electrical vectors will be greater. Therefore, atrial or ventricular enlargement is manifested by electrocardiographic evidence of waves of greater duration and magnitude (i.e., the voltage and duration of the P wave in atrial enlargement and the voltage and duration of the QRS complex in ventricular enlargement are increased).

ATRIAL ENLARGEMENT

A diagnosis of atrial enlargement is not always easily made from the electrocardiogram, since a considerable amount of variation in P wave configuration normally exists. Leads II and V1 are most useful in determining atrial enlargement, but leads I, III and AVF are also helpful.

Normally, the right atrium, which is anterior to the left atrium, depolarizes before the left atrium, and the time of left atrial depolarization overlaps with that of the right atrium (Fig. 11–1*A*). This may cause some normal notching of the P wave. This especially occurs in lead II. Lead II usually shows the largest P waves because it is parallel to the axis of the P wave depolarization. The P wave axis can be determined using the same methods outlined previously for the QRS complex axis.

Lead V1 normally shows a diphasic P wave because the left atrium is posterior to the right. The initial positive deflection of the P wave in lead V1 corresponds to right atrial depolarization. The terminal negative deflection in the P wave in lead V1 is a result of left atrial depolarization.

When the left atrium is enlarged, it takes longer to depolarize and shifts the P wave axis more posteriorly. There is also an increase in the time in which the right and left atrial depolarizations overlap. The result is a

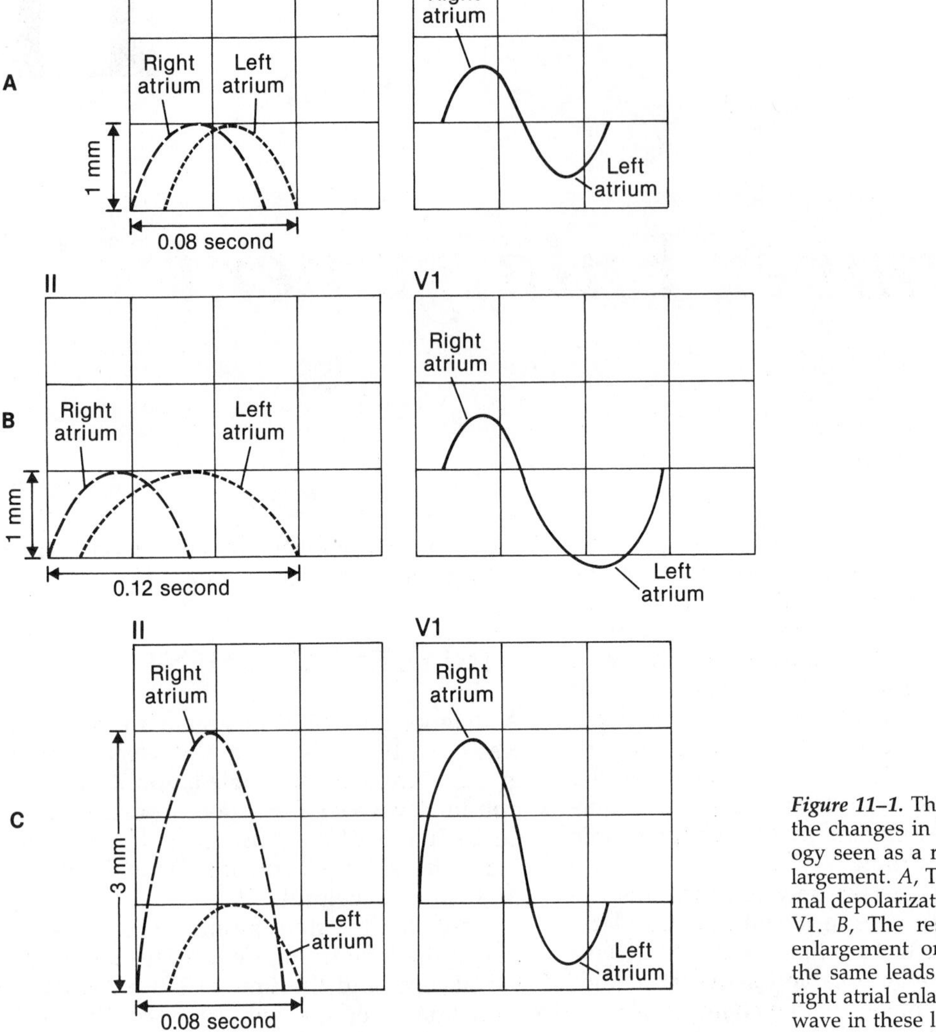

Figure 11–1. This diagram shows the changes in P wave morphology seen as a result of atrial enlargement. *A,* The P wave of normal depolarization in leads II and V1. *B,* The result of left atrial enlargement on the P wave in the same leads. *C,* The result of right atrial enlargement on the P wave in these leads.

widened P wave with enhanced notching, which is best seen in lead II (Fig. 11–1*B*). The left atrial component in lead V1 will also be increased, resulting in a wide, deep terminal component of the P wave. This is caused by the P wave vector moving posteriorly away from lead V1 and recording a large negative wave.

In a similar manner, when the right atrium is enlarged, there will be an increase in the P wave vector directed anteriorly and downward toward lead II. In addition, the time of right atrial depolarization is often increased sufficiently so that it contains the entire time of left atrial depolarization. Thus, the notched P waves in lead II are frequently lost. Instead, tall, slender, peaked P waves are found (Fig. 11–1*C*). In lead V1, the right atrial component will also be increased. This produces a tall, upright initial deflection.

The criteria for left and right atrial enlargement are given as follows:

Left Atrial Enlargement (Fig. 11–2)

1. Wide notched P wave in lead II (also leads I and AVL).
2. P wave duration in lead II ≥ 0.11 second (3 small boxes).

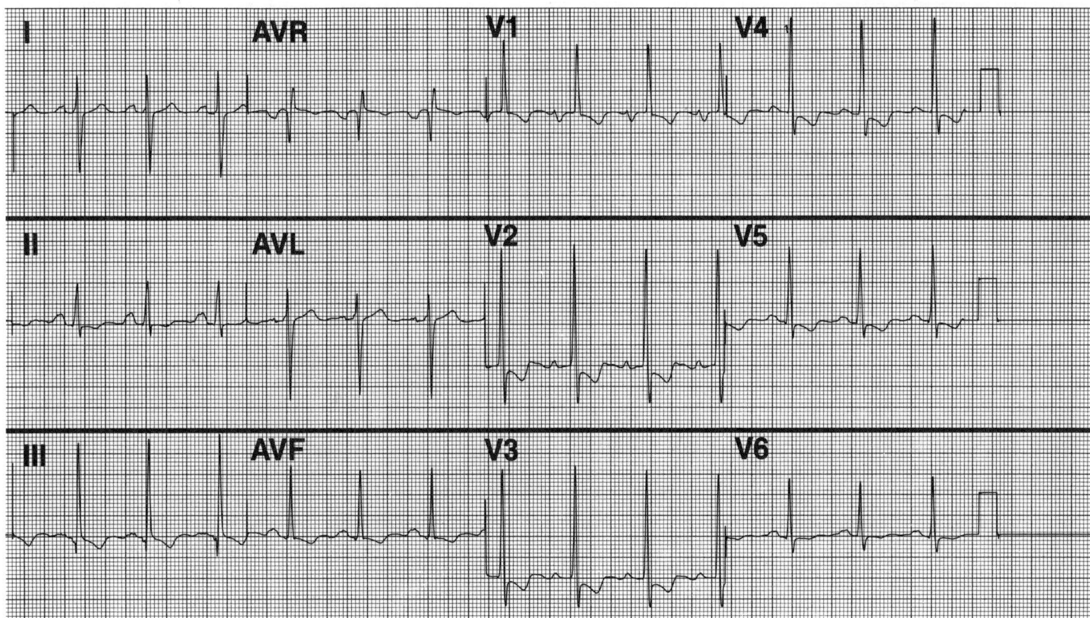

Figure 11–2. **Left atrial enlargement.** Notice the large negative component to the P wave in V1 as well as the broad notched P wave in leads II, III and AVF.

3. Biphasic P wave in lead V1 with a terminal component ≥ 1 small box wide by 1 small box deep.
4. Shift of P wave axis to the left.

Right Atrial Enlargement (Fig. 11–3)

1. Tall, slender, peaked P waves in lead II (also leads III and AVF).
2. P wave height in lead II ≥ 3 mm (3 small boxes).
3. Biphasic P wave in lead V1 with a tall, initial deflection equal to 2 small boxes high.
4. Shift in P wave axis to the right.

In *biatrial enlargement*, the terminal portion of the P wave in lead V1 is equal to or greater

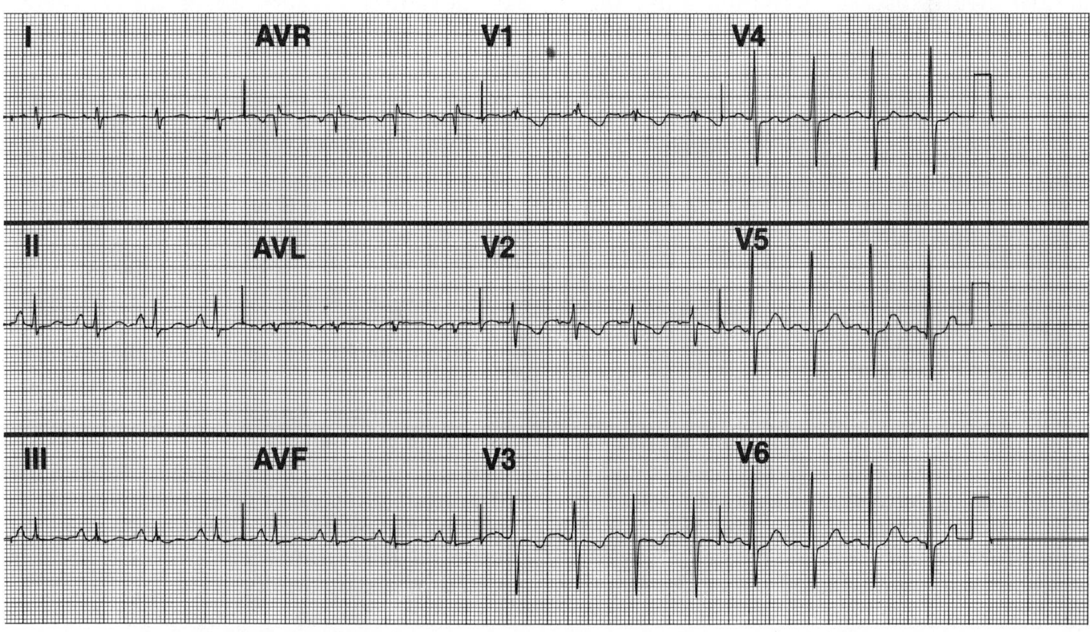

Figure 11–3. **Right atrial enlargement.** Notice the peaked P waves in leads II, III and AVF.

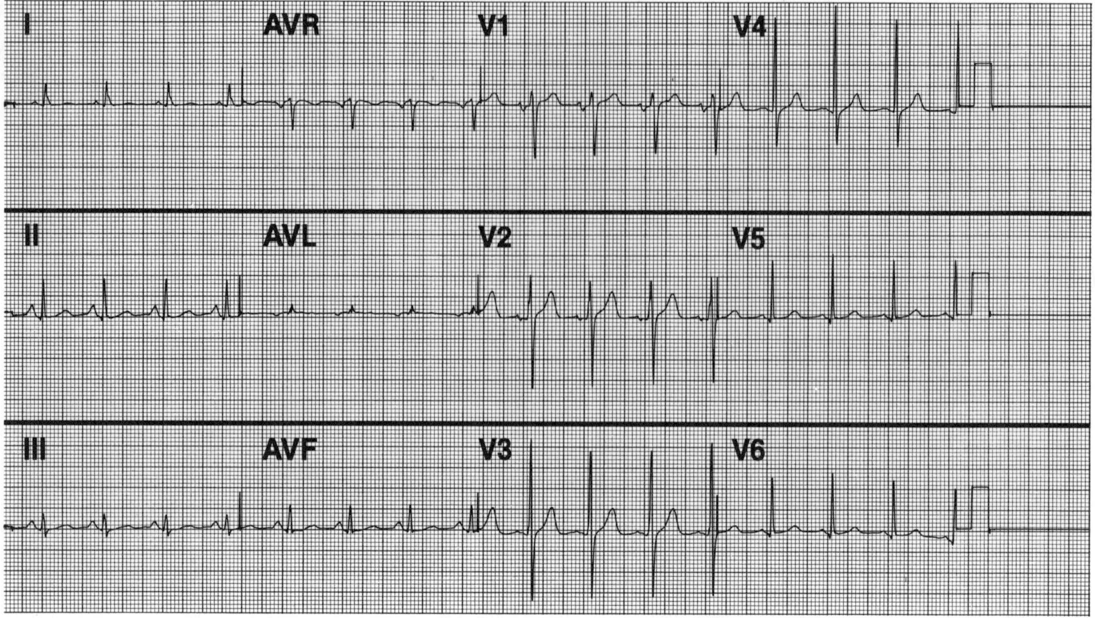

Figure 11–4. **Bi-atrial enlargement.** Notice the large negative component of the P wave in lead V1 and the peaked P wave in lead II.

than 1 small box wide by 1 small box deep (left atrial enlargement), and the P wave in lead II is greater than 2.5 mm (Fig. 11–4). The recognition of biatrial enlargement is generally easy to make, since each atrium affects a different portion of the P wave.

The causes of atrial enlargement include valvular heart disease, hypertension, congenital heart disease and ventricular hypertrophy. One should be aware that a common cause of left atrial enlargement is mitral stenosis, and therefore many physicians refer to left atrial enlargement as "p-mitrale." The peaked P waves in leads II, III and AVF seen as a result of pulmonary disease are referred to as "p-pulmonale."

VENTRICULAR ENLARGEMENT

When the ventricular myocardium sustains a persistent pressure overload, the muscle thickens or hypertrophies. This increases the QRS complex voltage and is often associated with ST segment depression and T wave inversion, sometimes called *ventricular strain.* These changes are termed *secondary repolarization changes.*

Left Ventricular Hypertrophy

The left ventricle is normally about three times as thick as the right ventricle, and this explains the normal axis being directed leftward. In *left ventricular hypertrophy* due to systolic pressure overload, there may be left axis deviation as a result of the increased electrical activity of the increased ventricular mass (Fig. 11–5).

In left ventricular hypertrophy, leads I, AVL and V5 to V6 show the greatest voltages, since they record the wave of depolarization as it moves to the left toward their positive poles. The S wave voltages in leads V1 to V2 will also increase their voltages as the wave of depolarization also moves away from them. In addition, there are repolarization changes caused by the hypertrophic myocardium. These manifest themselves by ST segment depression and T wave inversion seen in the leads demonstrating the voltage changes (Fig. 11–6).

The secondary repolarization changes are important for the diagnosis of left ventricular hypertrophy, since high voltage alone in the precordial leads can occur normally in thin chested or young adults. This is because the chest electrodes are closer to the heart in these patients.

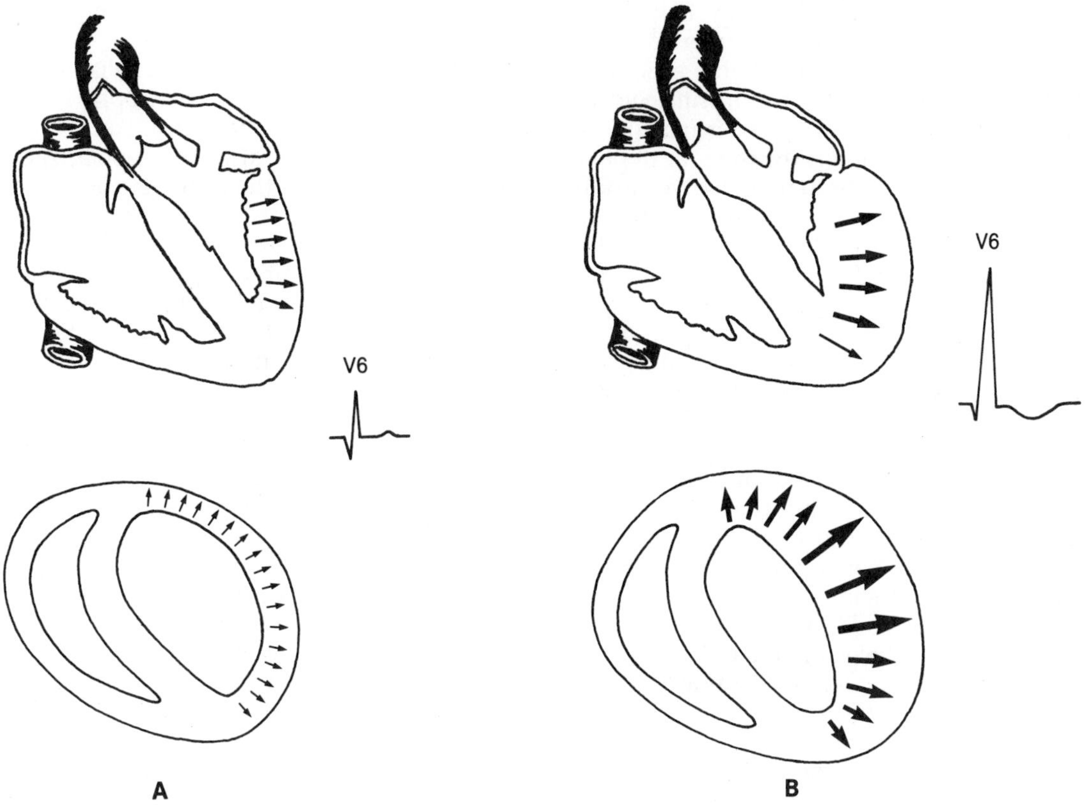

Figure 11–5. A, Cross section of a normal heart and its leftward vectors. *B,* The increase in leftward vectors seen with left ventricular hypertrophy.

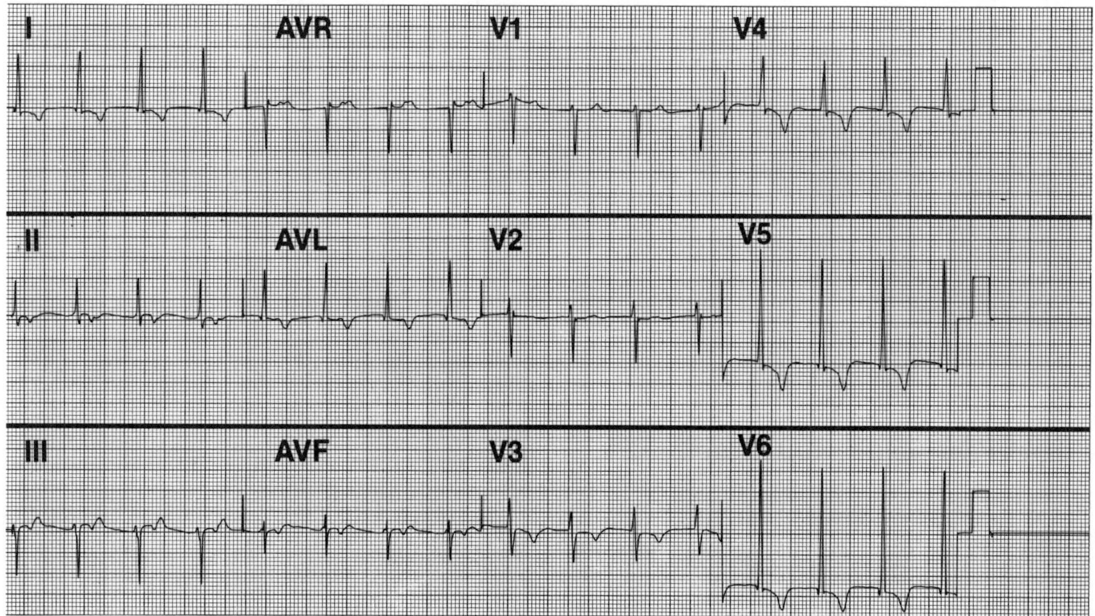

Figure 11–6. **Left ventricular hypertrophy.** The sum of the S wave in lead V1 + the R wave in lead V6 = 40 mm. In addition, there is ST depression and T wave inversion. First degree atrioventricular block is also present in this tracing.

Additional findings that may help in the diagnosis of left ventricular hypertrophy include a more posterior rotational axis deviation and an increase in the intrinsicoid deflection as measured in leads V5 and V6. The intrinsicoid deflection is the time for depolarization to extend through the myocardium and is a measure of ventricular activation time; as the myocardium becomes thicker, the intrinsicoid deflection will increase (see Chapter 4, Review of Complexes).

The electrocardiographic changes of left ventricular hypertrophy are commonly seen in hypertension, aortic stenosis and coarctation of the aorta, since all of these create a pressure overload on the left ventricle.

In left ventricular dilatation due to a diastolic or volume overload, the criteria for left ventricular hypertrophy are also present. However, the secondary repolarization changes do not show a strain pattern. Instead, tall positive T waves in leads V5 to V6 with ST segment elevation may be seen. The causes of diastolic overload include aortic and mitral insufficiency, patent ductus arteriosus and ventricular septal defects.

The criteria for left ventricular hypertrophy or dilatation are outlined as follows (Note: 1 mm = 1 small box):

1. R wave in lead V5 or V6 + S wave in lead V1 > 35 mm.
2. R wave in lead I + S wave in lead III > 25 mm.
3. R wave in lead I > 15 mm.
4. R wave in lead AVL > 11 mm.
5. Intrinsicoid deflection in leads V3 to V6 > 0.05 second.
6. Left axis deviation (occurs in only 50 per cent of cases).
7. Repolarization changes in the left precordial leads.

The most specific sign for left ventricular hypertrophy is an R wave in lead AVL greater than 11 mm.

Right Ventricular Hypertrophy

Since the right ventricle contributes considerably less electrical activity to the electrocardiogram than the left ventricle, it is frequently difficult to diagnose *right ventricular hypertrophy*. In fact, right ventricular hypertrophy may not be detected until the right ventricle hypertrophies enough to become the dominant ventricle.

One of the earliest and most reliable findings in right ventricular hypertrophy is right axis deviation. As the ventricle continues to hypertrophy and the wave of depolarization moves more toward the right ventricle, there is an increase in the R wave height in the right precordial leads (Fig. 11–7). This is associated with a simultaneous decrease in the S wave amplitude in these same leads and an increase in the S waves in the left precordial leads as the mean QRS vector is now directed away from leads V5 and V6. When the R/S ratio is greater than 1, right ventricular hypertrophy may be suspected (Fig. 11–8). In advanced right ventricular hypertrophy, right axis deviation is associated with a tall R wave in lead V1 or a qR complex in lead V1.

Secondary repolarization changes of ST segment depression and T wave inversion may be seen in the right precordial leads when hypertrophy is the result of systolic overload. In cases of diastolic volume overload, resulting in right ventricular dilatation, the ST segment may be elevated. The T waves will be tall and positive, as in the case of diastolic volume overload of the left ventricle.

As the right ventricle becomes more hypertrophied, the time for its depolarization will increase. Thus, the intrinsicoid deflection in leads V1 and V2 will increase, and the QRS complex duration may also increase. This may result in intraventricular conduction defects or a right bundle branch block may actually occur.

The major causes of right ventricular hypertrophy include congenital heart disease, valvular heart disease and chronic lung disease.

The criteria for right ventricular hypertrophy or dilatation are outlined as follows:

1. Right axis deviation of +110° or more.
2. R/S ratio in lead V1 > 1.
3. Deep S waves in leads V5 to V6, I and AVL.
4. rSR′ complex in lead V1 with R′ ≥ 10 mm.
5. qR complex in lead V1.
6. R wave in lead V1 + S wave in lead V6 ≥ 11 mm.
7. Increased intrinsicoid deflection in lead V1 ≥ 0.035 second.
8. Repolarization changes in the right precordial leads.

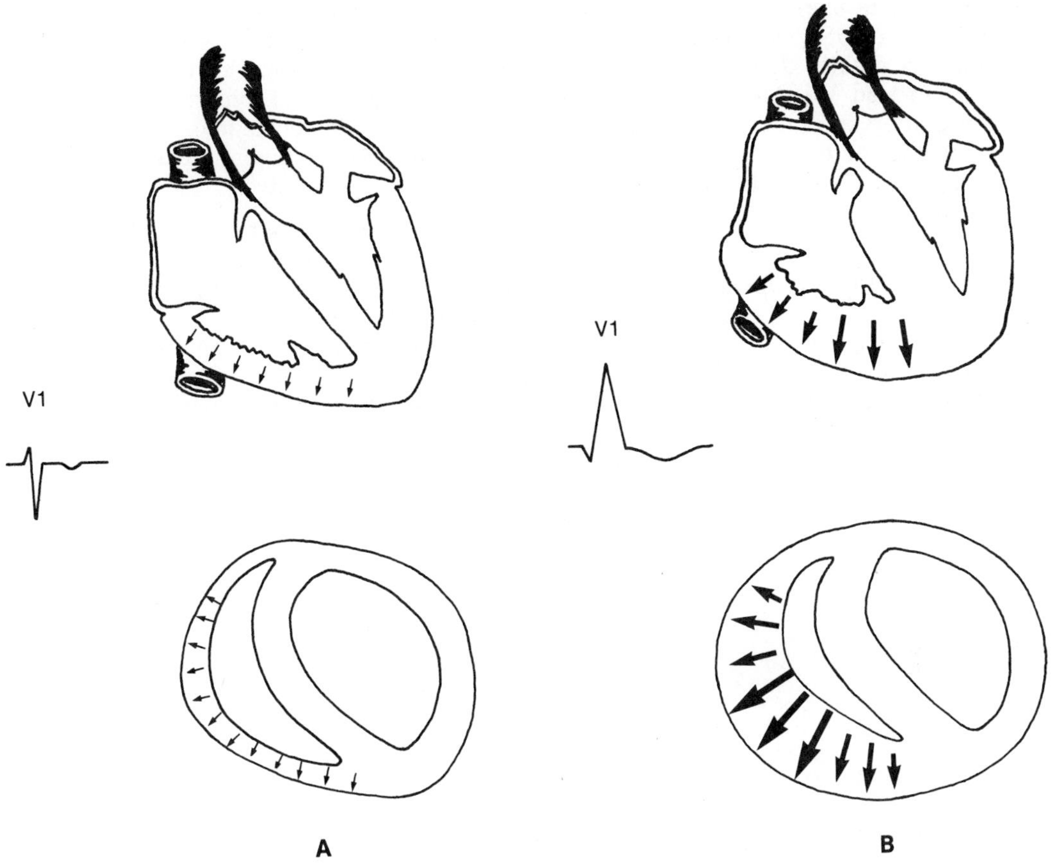

Figure 11–7. *A,* Cross section of a normal heart with only the rightward directed vectors shown. *B,* A heart with right ventricular hypertrophy. Notice the increased forces to the right and the resultant QRS complexes.

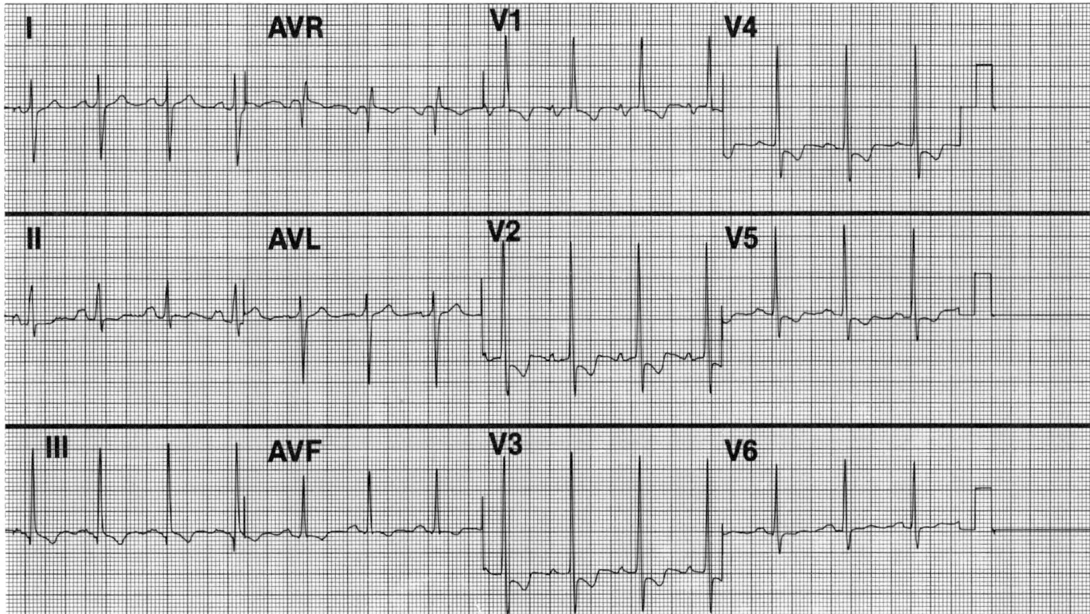

Figure 11–8. **Right ventricular hypertrophy.** The R/S ratio in lead V1 is greater than 1. The R wave in lead V1 + the S wave in lead V6 = 21. In addition, there is right axis deviation, and secondary repolarization changes are present.

The most specific signs of right ventricular hypertrophy are the rSR′ complex in V1, with the R′ complex greater than 10 mm, or the qR complex in lead V1. Abnormal depolarization of the interventricular septum is probably responsible for the initial negativity of the qR complex, although the physiology of this explanation is not clear.

Biventricular Hypertrophy

In *biventricular hypertrophy*, the increased right and left ventricular forces tend to counterbalance each other. Consequently, there may be minimal evidence of hypertrophy on the electrocardiogram. If the hypertrophy is greater for one ventricle, the electrocardiographic signs of that hypertrophy may exist, although to a lesser degree.

The criteria for biventricular hypertrophy are outlined as follows:

1. Diagnostic criteria for isolated left or right ventricular hypertrophy.
2. An equiphasic RS complex throughout the precordial leads.
3. Criteria for left ventricular hypertrophy in the precordial leads and a right axis deviation in the limb leads.

12

Ischemia, Injury and Infarction

Atherosclerosis frequently involves the coronary arteries. Narrowing of these vessels results in a diminished blood supply to the heart muscle. At some point in time, this supply will not be adequate to meet the metabolic demand of the myocardium, and *ischemia* will result. If there is continued ischemia, *injury* to the myocardium will result. Finally, if there is not a return of blood to this area, the tissue will die, and *infarction* is said to have occurred. Patterns of ischemia, injury and infarction on the electrocardiogram represent a continuum of electrical changes that occur as the heart is progressively deprived of an adequate blood supply. Ischemia and injury are reversible conditions; however, infarction is not.

ISCHEMIA

Initially, as the blood supply diminishes, ischemic electrocardiographic changes will occur. These are seen in leads that record the electrical activity over the ischemic area. The findings may be classified as subendocardial, subepicardial or transmural.

Since the subendocardium is farthest away from the coronary arteries, it is at greatest risk; also, subendocardial ischemia is more easily produced than subepicardial ischemia and is often more extensive. The reason for this is simply explained by following the anatomical course of coronary arteries. The coronary arteries first supply the epicardium and then course deep to supply the endocardium. High intraventricular pressure or a thickened myocardium will tend to decrease blood flow to the subendocardial tissue.

The electrocardiographic changes of *ischemia* are transitory ST segment and T wave changes. These are related to a delay in the repolarization process, which is caused by a lack of sufficient energy for repolarization. An electrode that overlies such an ischemic area will record ST segment depression (Fig. 12–1*A*). If the ischemia is only in the subendocardium, there is usually no abnormality of the T wave, as the rest of the myocardial wall balances the effect of the subendocardial ischemia. However, if the ischemia is through the full thickness of the myocardial wall, or *transmural*, T wave inversions will result (Fig. 12–1*B*).

INJURY

In myocardial *injury*, the myocardium is depolarized incompletely. At the end of depolarization, it is more positive than its uninjured neighboring tissue. An electrode overlying the injured myocardium will face this positive charge and will result in ST segment elevation (Fig. 12–2). An electrode overlying the uninjured myocardium opposite will face a negative charge and will therefore record ST segment depression.

Two classifications for myocardial injury exist: subendocardial injury and subepicardial injury. *Subendocardial injury* produces ST segment depression that is greater than 1

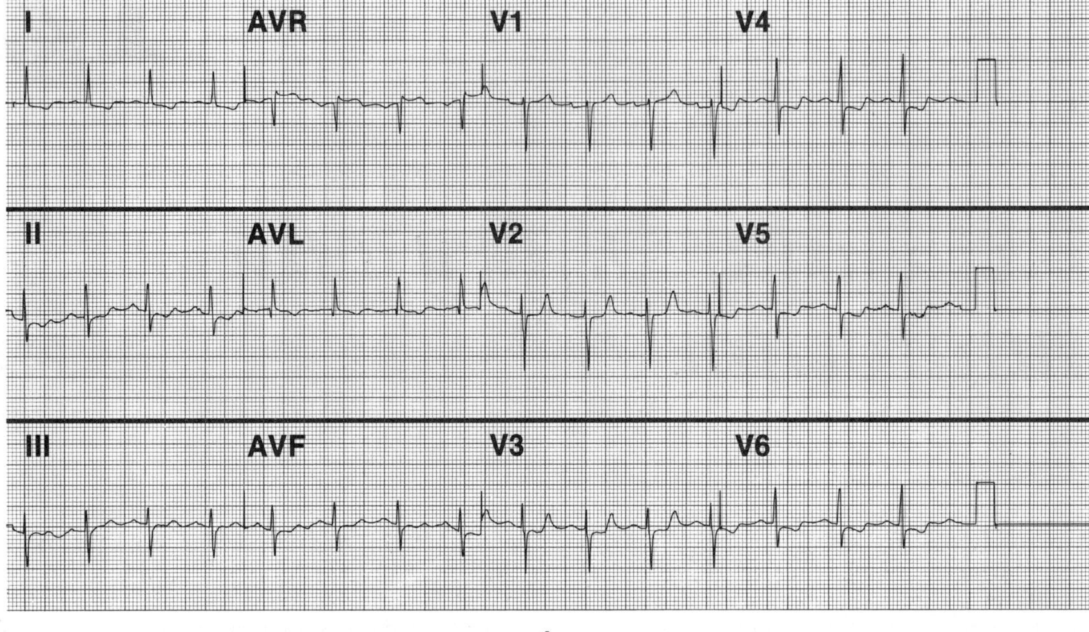

A

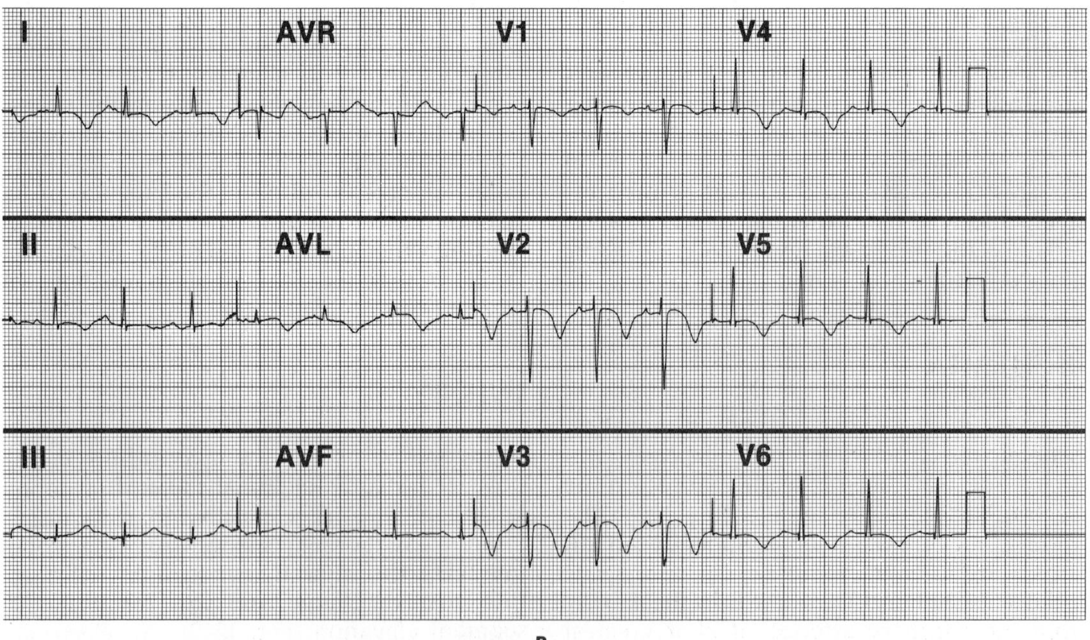

B

Figure 12–1. **Ischemia.** *A,* 2-mm ST segment depression and T wave inversion in leads II, III, AVF and V4 to V6 indicative of inferolateral ischemia. *B,* Symmetric T wave inversions mostly in leads V1 to V6 indicative of anterolateral ischemia. The symmetric inversion of T waves is usually the result of ischemia.

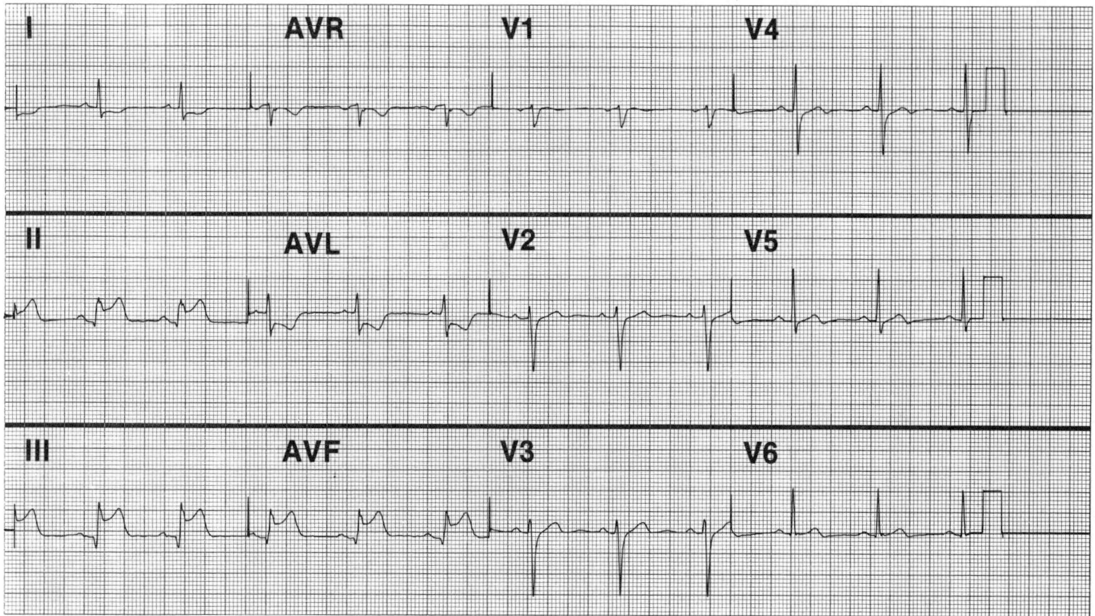

Figure 12–2. **Inferior injury pattern.** Notice the 4-mm ST elevation in leads II, III and AVF. In fact, this patient has suffered an acute inferior myocardial infarction. The Q waves have already developed. In addition, notice the reciprocal ST segment depression in leads I and AVL.

mm. It commonly occurs during episodes of chest pain. Patients with compromised coronary artery circulation and angina pectoris will show ST segment depression during an exercise test. In most cases, ST segment depression is transient, and a return to baseline occurs when the pain subsides. If the ST segment depression persists, one should suspect subendocardial infarction.

Subepicardial injury is less common than subendocardial injury. It produces ST segment elevation, and is found in patients with atypical or Prinzmetal's angina. More importantly, subepicardial injury often precedes myocardial infarction. In these cases the subepicardial injury usually subsides in a few days. If ST segment elevation persists for more than a few months after the infarction, one should suspect a ventricular aneurysm. Diffuse ST segment elevation is seen in acute pericarditis (Fig. 12–3), but in this condition reciprocal ST segment depression in opposing leads is not generally seen. The electrocardiographic findings in ischemia and injury are summarized in Figure 12–4.

INFARCTION

Infarction results in death of tissue. In a myocardial infarction, the area of necrosis is electrically silent. The vector forces tend to point away from this area, as the potential of the opposite wall is not counterbalanced by any forces in the infarcted zone. Thus, an electrode facing an area of infarcted myocardium will record an abnormal negative deflection during depolarization. This is because the electrode appears to be looking through the infarction to the endocardial surface of the opposite wall. Since depolarization proceeds from endocardium to epicardium, this electrode now records the vector going away in the opposite wall; thus, the generation of the Q wave. Abnormal Q waves stem from the loss of electrical activity in the damaged muscle, which normally balances the electrical action of the tissue diametrically opposite. It is the depolarization of the unopposed healthy tissue that produces the Q waves in the leads over the infarction. In addition, the electrode that overlies the healthy myocardium records larger than normal R waves. This is caused by the lack of vector forces in the area of the infarcted myocardium, which would normally reduce this R wave voltage (Fig. 12–5). This is an example of the concept of reciprocal changes.

The concept of *reciprocal changes* in the electrocardiogram is very important in determining the significance of many findings. Once one is aware that such changes can

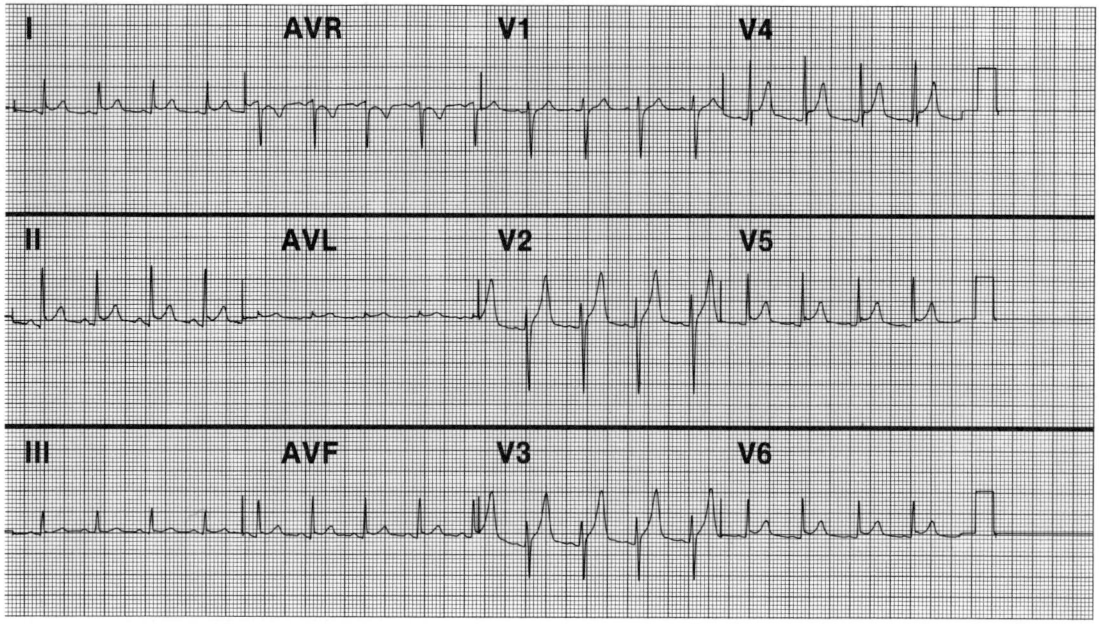

Figure 12–3. **Acute pericarditis.** Notice the diffuse ST segment elevation present in all leads except lead AVR, which shows reciprocal ST segment depression.

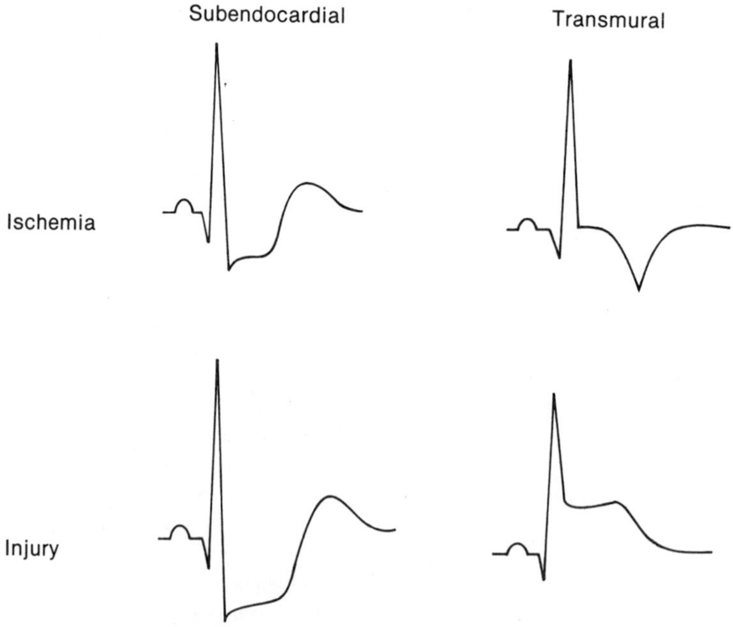

Figure 12–4. **Summary of electrocardiographic findings in ischemia and injury.** Note that both subendocardial ischemia and injury produce ST segment depression of greater than 1 mm. Transmural ischemia is characterized by symmetrically inverted T waves. Transmural injury demonstrates ST segment elevation of greater than 1 mm.

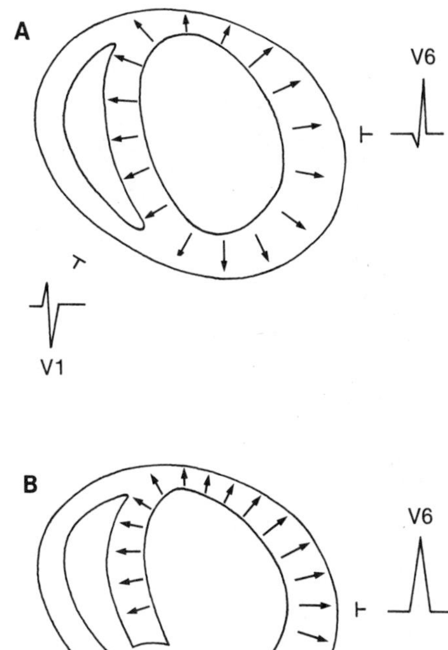

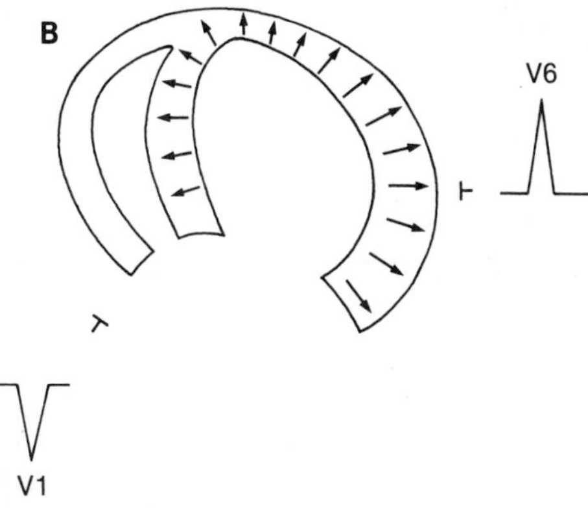

Figure 12–5. **The concept of the Q wave.** *A,* A cross section of the heart with the normal QRS patterns in leads V1 and V6. *B,* The result of a myocardial infarction. In this example, the rS complex in lead V1 has been replaced by a QS complex, and the septal Q wave in lead V6 is no longer present. Notice that the electrode records the vectors as if there were no myocardium present in the area of the infarction (see text).

occur, there will be much less confusion by the variety of changes seen in a tracing. Essentially, this concept is very simple. ST segment elevation in one lead will be recorded by an opposite lead as ST segment depression, since each lead is looking at the vector from different viewpoints (Fig. 12–2). Another important use of this concept is the electrical activity recorded from the posterior myocardium. Since no lead records it directly, we can see the changes in the anterior precordial leads as reciprocal changes. A posterior wall infarction produces tall R waves in leads V1 to V3. When an electrocardiographic abnormality is suspected, the presence of reciprocal changes will help determine that the changes are real.

The serial changes associated with an acute myocardial infarction are shown in Figure 12–6. The first indication of an acute myocardial infarction is injury. This is manifested by ST segment elevation in the area overlying the injury, with reciprocal changes in the opposite leads. Peaking of the T waves occurs within minutes to hours after the infarction. Abnormal Q waves usually appear within several hours to days after the onset of the infarction. Within 1 to 2 days, the T waves return to normal, and within 2 weeks the ST segment elevation resolves. The abnormal Q wave, a sign of transmural infarction, persists indefinitely.

The electrocardiographic findings in a myocardial infarction include abnormal Q waves that are greater than 0.04 second (1 small box). The tissues surrounding the infarction usually show ischemic changes (i.e., ST segment changes), and leads that face the tissue opposite the infarction will show reciprocal changes. In scanning the tracing for signs of infarction, the reader should be aware that at least two leads must show the proper findings. Lead III alone will often show Q waves, but these are frequently related to respiration and electrical positioning of the heart and not to infarction. Also, remember that as one goes from leads V1 to V6, a q wave, indicative of septal activation, will develop. This septal Q wave is normal and should not be mistaken for a Q wave of infarction.

Transmural myocardial infarctions can occur in any area of the myocardium. An occlusion of the left anterior descending artery

Text continued on page 100

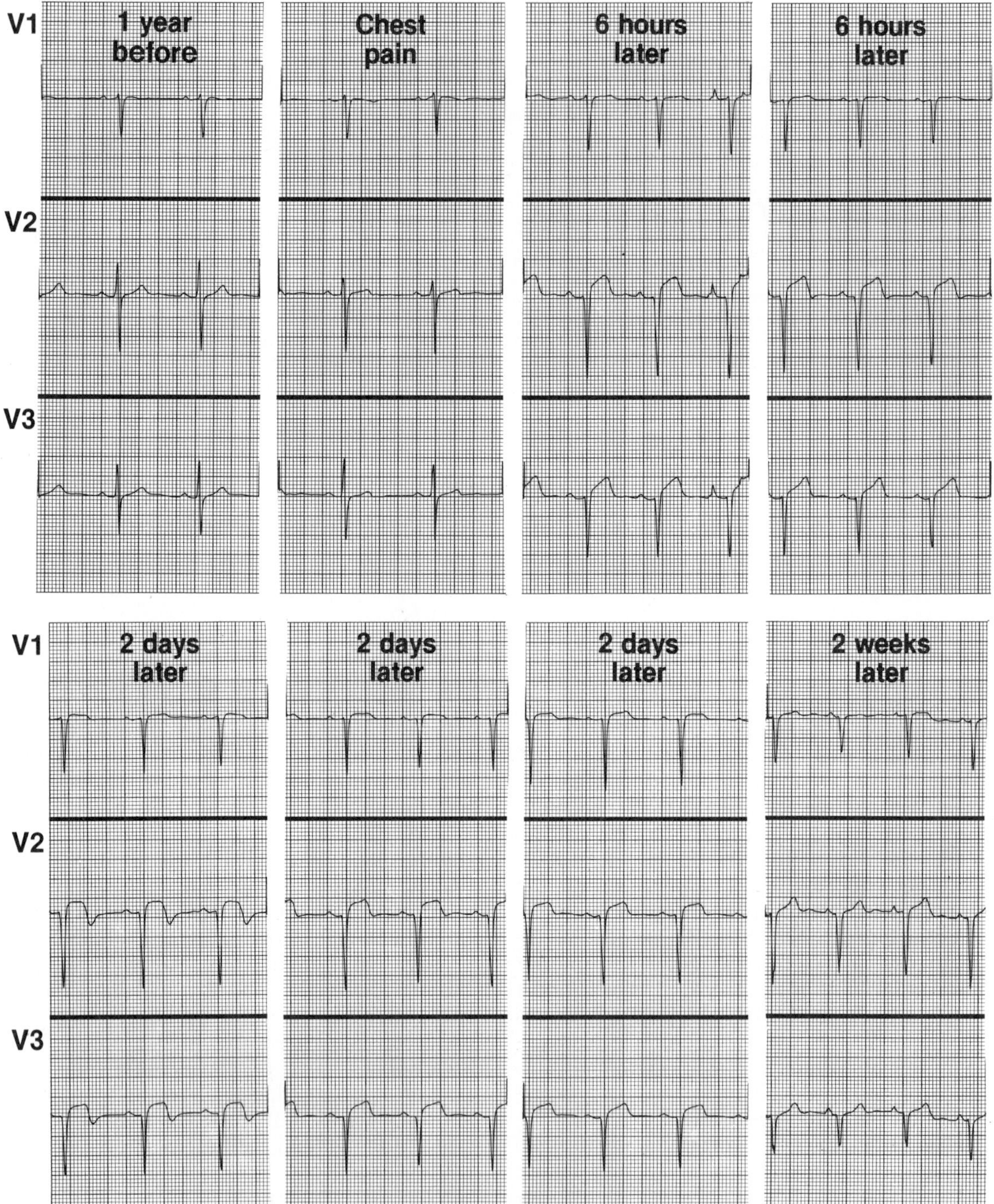

Figure 12–6. **Serial changes associated with an acute anteroseptal myocardial infarction.** Notice the loss of the R wave voltages associated with the development of the QS wave in its place. The ST segment elevation is followed by T wave inversion. The last segment shows the return of the ST segment to its normal position and the T wave to its normal upright position. The QS complex remains as the marker of the infarction.

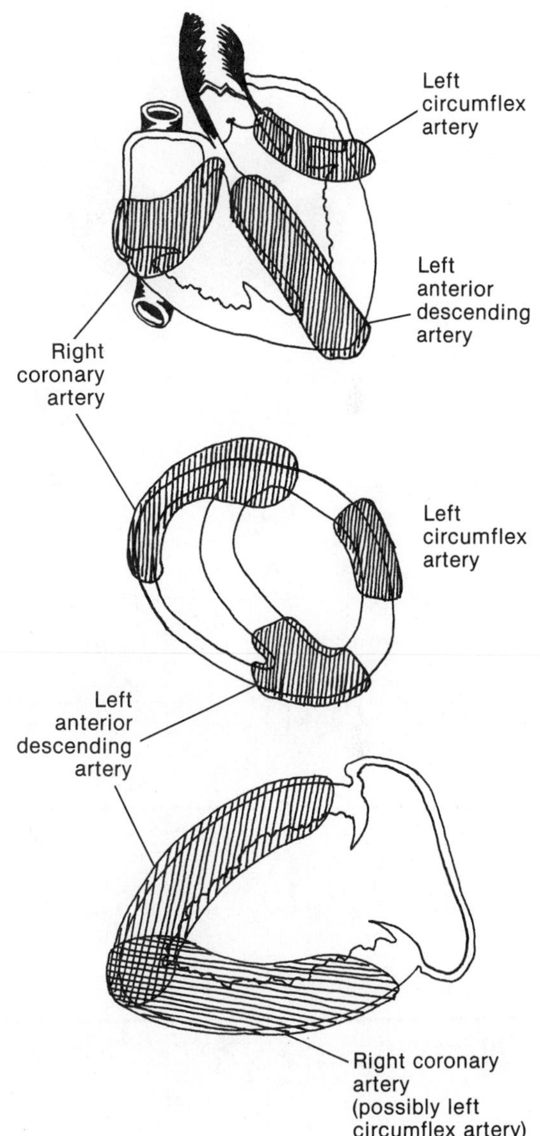

Figure 12–7. This diagram illustrates the locations of various myocardial infarctions based upon occlusions of the coronary artery supplying the area (see text).

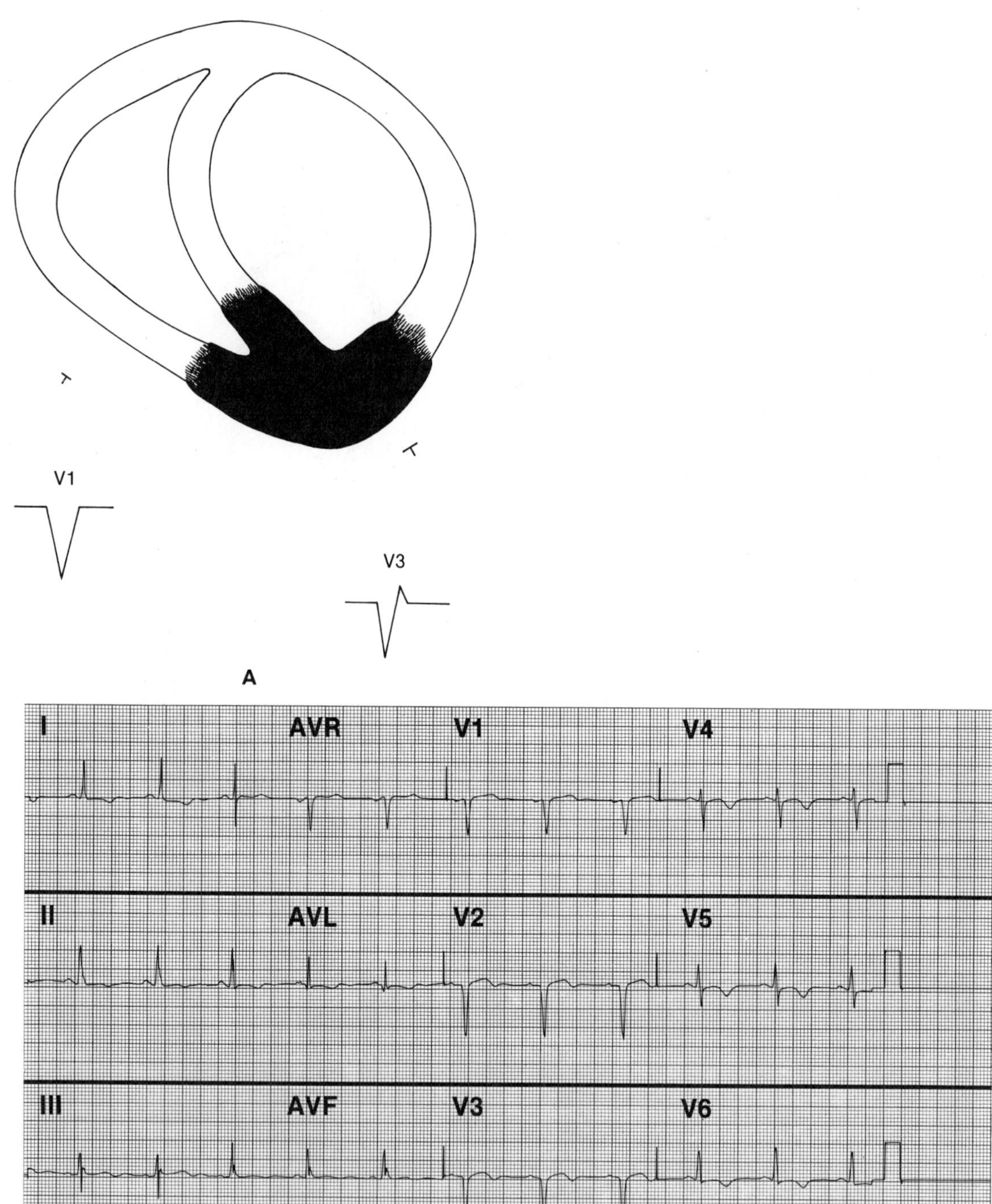

Figure 12–8. **Anteroseptal myocardial infarction.** *A,* Diagram of the location of the myocardial infarction and the resulting QRS patterns. *B,* Actual tracing. Notice the Q waves in leads V1 to V3.

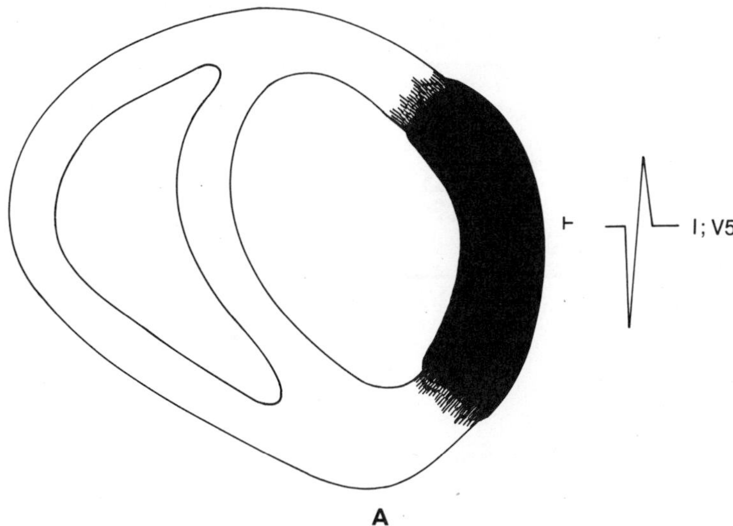

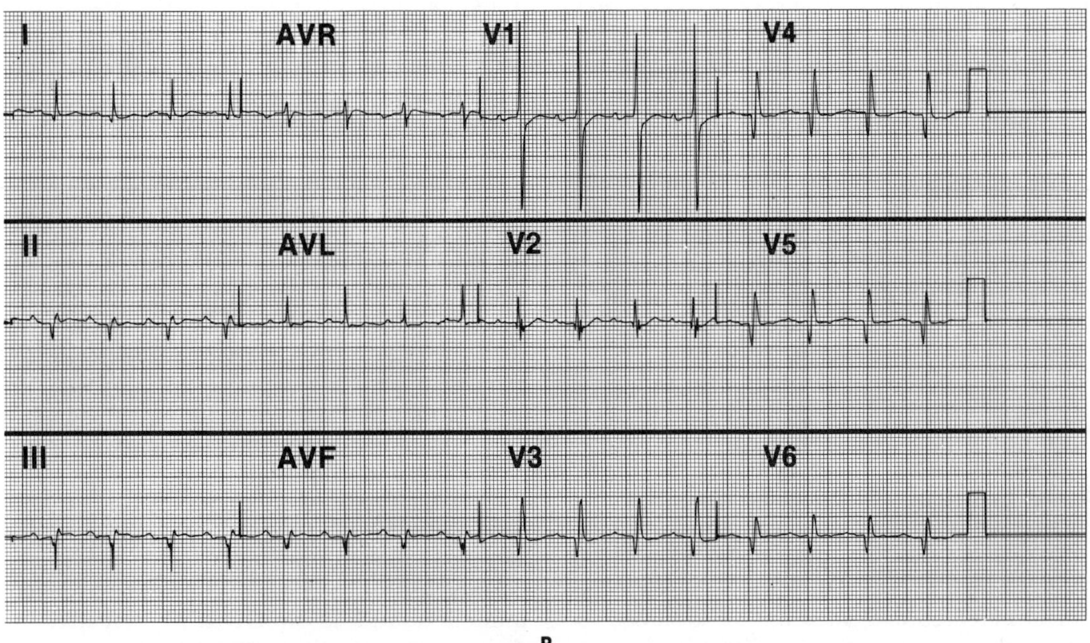

Figure 12–9. **Anterolateral and high lateral myocardial infarction.** *A,* The location of a lateral myocardial infarction and the resulting QRS patterns. *B,* An anterolateral myocardial infarction. Notice the deep Q waves in leads V4 to V6. This patient also has Q waves in leads II, III and AVF indicative of an inferior myocardial infarction (see Fig. 12–10). C, A high lateral myocardial infarction. Notice the deep Q waves in leads I and AVL.

Illustration continued on following page

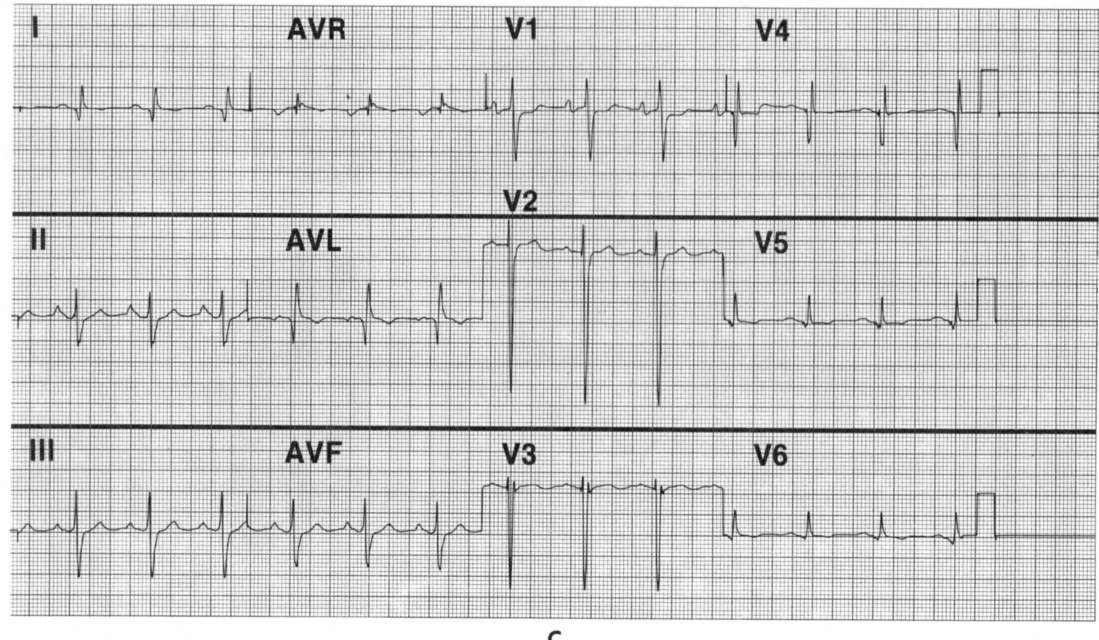

C

Figure 12–9. Continued.

may result in an anterior or anteroseptal infarction. A blockage of the left circumflex artery produces a high lateral or anterolateral infarction, while occlusion of the right coronary artery causes an inferior or posterior infarction (Fig. 12–7).

The criteria for localization of the infarcted area are as follows:

Anteroseptal	Leads V1 to V3 (Fig. 12–8)
Anterolateral Leads	V4 to V6 (Fig. 12–9)
High lateral	Leads I, AVL (Fig. 12–9)
Inferior (diaphragmatic)	Leads II, III, AVF (Fig. 12–10)
Posterior	Tall R waves in leads V1 to V2 (Fig. 12–11)
Subendocardial	ST segment and T wave changes only; no Q waves (Fig. 12–12)

The infarcted area may not be localized to one of these areas, and so various leads may show Q waves. The more extensive the infarction, the more leads will generally show Q waves. For instance, an extensive anterior infarction may show Q waves in leads V1 to V6 as well as in leads I and AVL.

The age of a transmural myocardial infarction is often difficult to assess. Therefore, one often uses the term "age undetermined" to describe a myocardial infarction. However, if there are pathological Q waves present and they are associated with ST segment and T wave changes, one can suggest that the infarction is "possibly acute."

The term *subendocardial infarction* refers to infarction involving only the inner half of the myocardial wall. Approximately 25 per cent of all myocardial infarctions are subendocardial. Since only one half of the wall is necrotic, the remaining portion is depolarized normally, and therefore no Q waves result. As can be expected, if only one half of the wall is electrically active, the R wave recorded from an electrode overlying this area may be smaller than normal. In addition, ST segment depression and T wave inversion in the leads facing the infarction will result.

The diagnosis of infarction using electrocardiographic evidence is only 85 per cent accurate. In addition, the electrocardiogram is only useful in diagnosing left ventricular infarction and is much more sensitive in detecting transmural infarction than subendocardial infarction. Since no electrode faces the true posterior wall of the myocardium, it is also difficult to diagnose a true posterior wall infarction; we can only use the precordial leads and look for reciprocal changes.

Left bundle branch block can also make the diagnosis of a myocardial infarction difficult, since both conditions interfere with the initial segment of the QRS vector. If a

Text continued on page 104

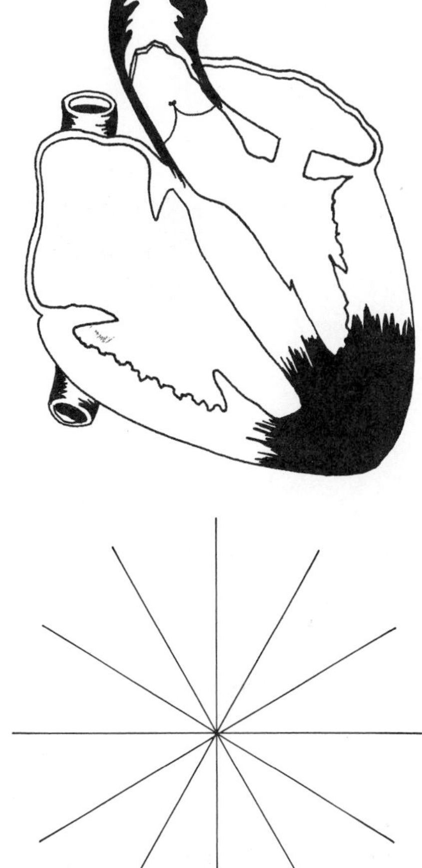

Figure 12–10. **Inferior myocardial infarction.** *A,* The location of the myocardial infarction and resulting QRS pattern. *B,* Actual tracing. Notice the Q waves in leads II, III and AVF as well as the ST segment elevation and T wave inversions in the same leads. In addition, there is a 2-mm ST elevation in leads V4 to V6 also associated with T wave inversions. This patient has developed an acute inferolateral myocardial infarction—a type of infarction that is the result of occlusion of either the right coronary artery or the left circumflex artery.

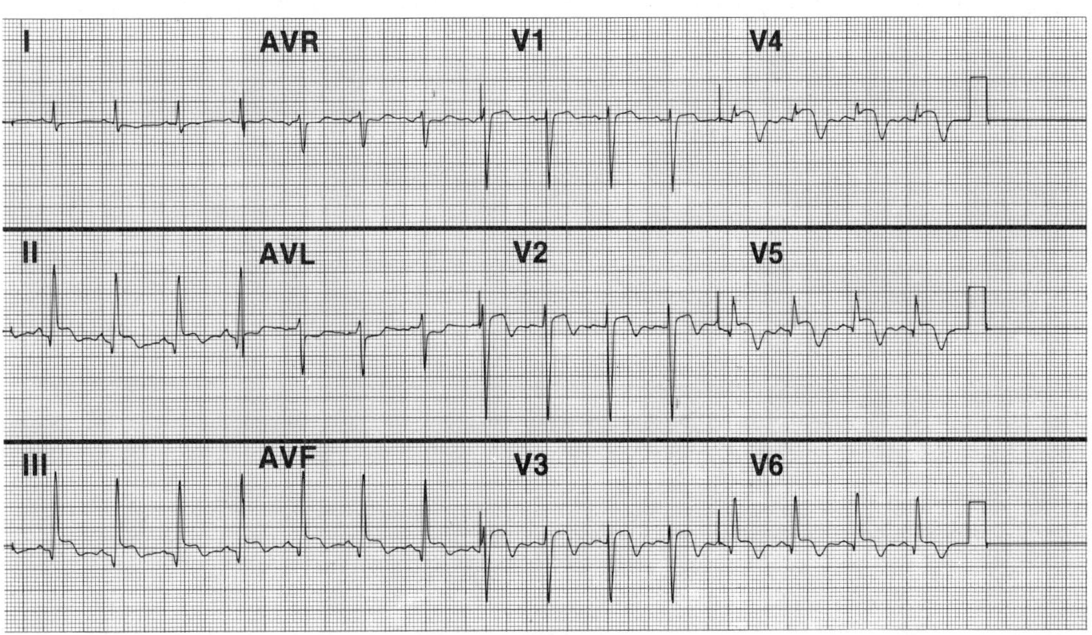

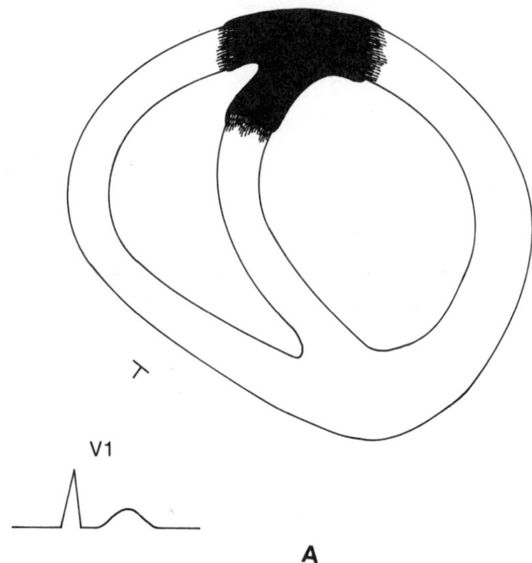

A

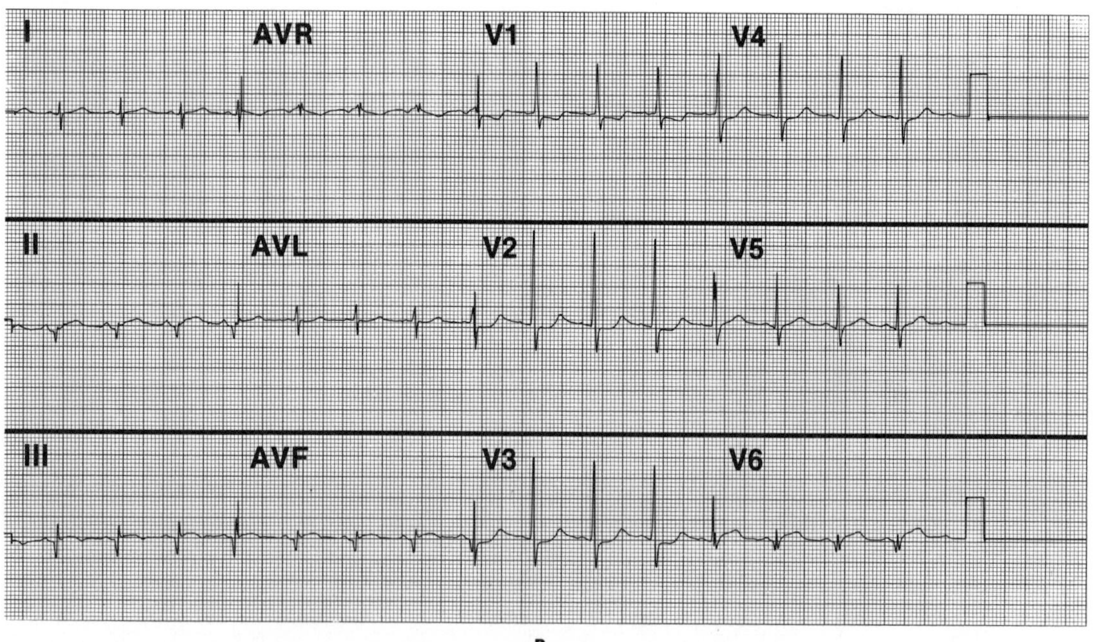

B

Figure 12–11. **Inferior myocardial infarction with posterior extension.** *A,* The location of the myocardial infarction and the resulting QRS patterns. *B,* An actual tracing. Notice the 12-mm R wave in lead V1 associated with ST segment depression and T wave inversion.

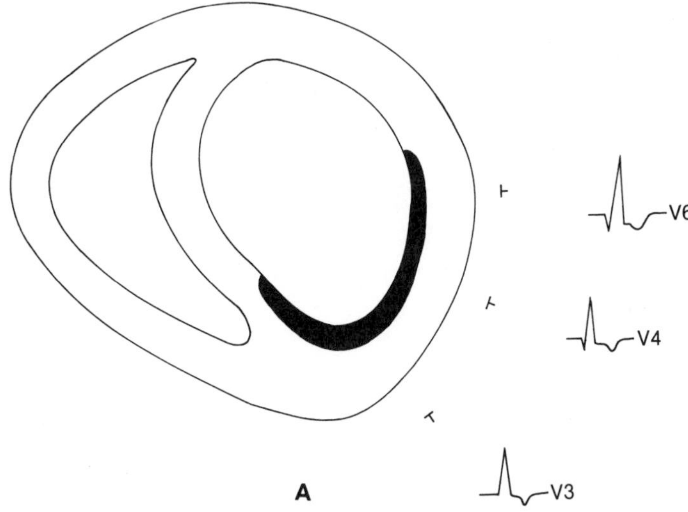

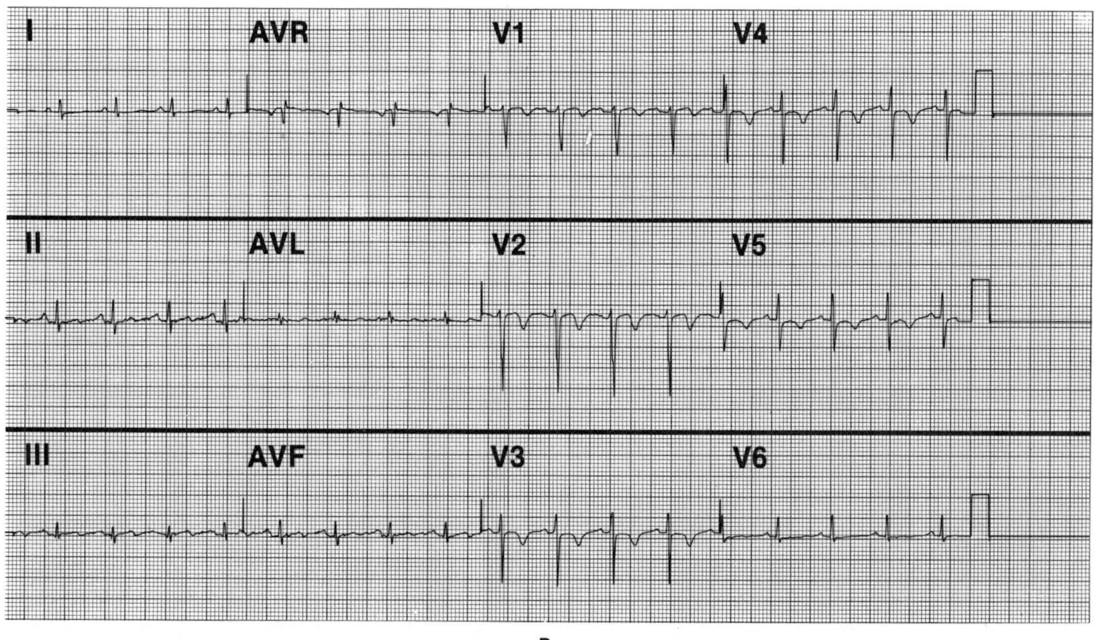

Figure 12–12. **Subendocardial myocardial infarction.** *A,* The location of the myocardial infarction and the resulting QRS patterns. *B,* An actual tracing. Notice the symmetric T wave inversions in leads V1 to V6.

serial tracing shows the same left bundle branch block pattern, a more accurate diagnosis can be made if the Q waves are present in only one of the tracings. Old infarctions and hypertrophy are other instances in which serial tracings are a valuable aid in the diagnosis of infarction.

With these limitations on the electrocardiographic diagnosis of myocardial infarction, it is of paramount importance to correlate the patient's clinical status with the electrocardiogram. If a patient shows clinical signs of infarction, one should look for subtle changes in the electrocardiogram, which may indicate an infarction. Since subendocardial infarctions often precede transmural infarctions, one should pay significant attention to any ST segment or T wave changes. ST elevation can represent subepicardial damage, and ST depression can mean subendocardial damage. Some physicians believe that ST segment elevation alone suggests infarction, but this is not diagnostic.

13

Pulmonary Pathology

Lung disease usually produces abnormalities in the electrocardiogram by changing the intrathoracic volume, resistance to outflow to the lungs or impairment of oxygen supply.

In chronic obstructive lung disease, the hyperinflation of the lungs tends to push the diaphragm inferiorly. As a result, the heart is rotated clockwise and assumes a more vertical position. The electrocardiogram, therefore, shows a rightward shift of the P wave and QRS complex axes. The P wave becomes smaller in lead I and larger in leads II, III and AVF. In addition, the hyperinflation of the lungs tends to reduce the voltage in all leads, since the lung is a poor conductor of the electrical impulse (Fig. 13–1). Chronic lung disease also causes hypoxia, which induces arrhythmias, and can also result in pulmonary hypertension. The most useful criteria in detecting these abnormalities include tall, peaked P waves in leads II, III and AVF; large R waves in leads V1 to V3; ST

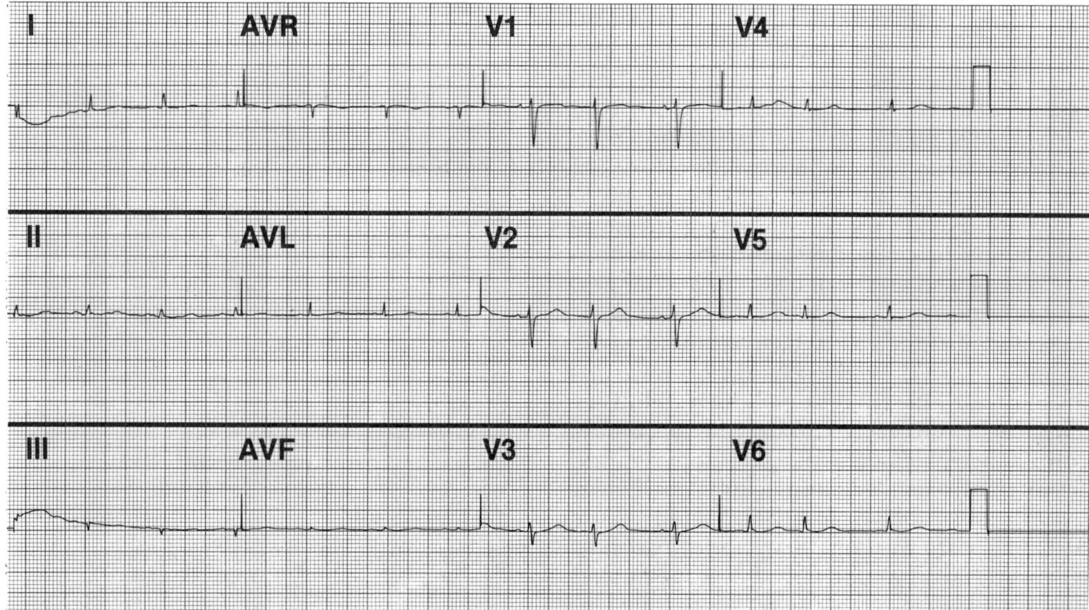

Figure 13–1. **Low voltage.** Notice that all of the R wave voltages are less than 10 mm. This satisfies the criteria for low voltage. This finding is seen in pulmonary disease, pericardial effusion or cardiomyopathy. It may occasionally be seen as a normal variant.

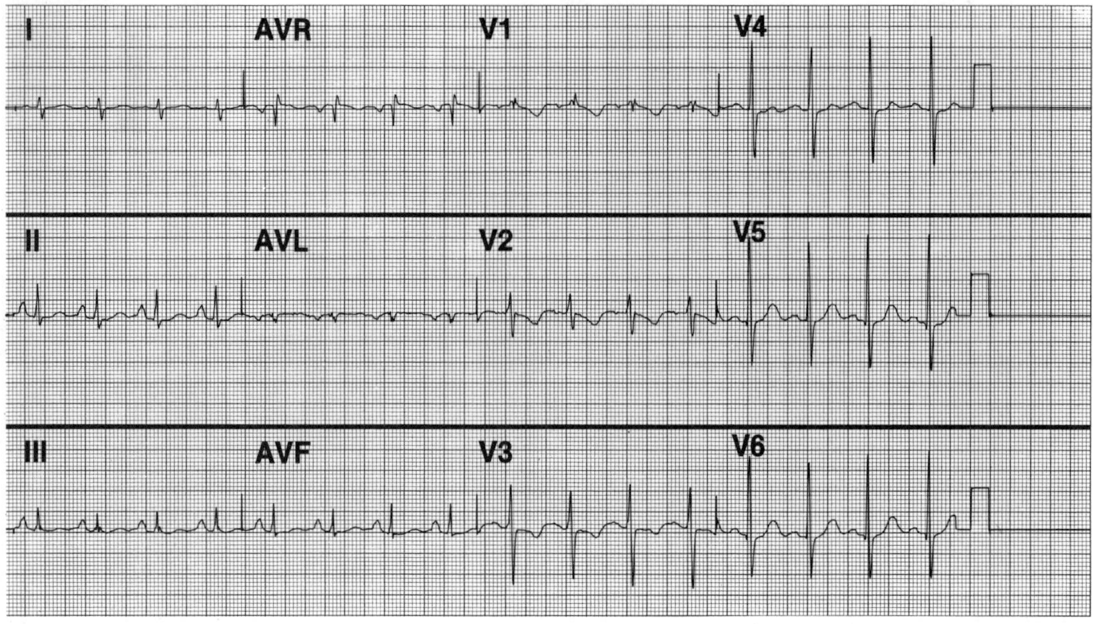

Figure 13–2. **Pulmonary disease.** A right axis together with prominent S waves in leads V4 to V6 and repolarization changes in leads V1 to V3 suggests right ventricular hypertrophy. An incomplete right bundle branch block is also present. The P waves are peaked in leads II, III and AVF, indicative of right atrial enlargement. This group of findings is suggestive that this patient has pulmonary disease.

segment changes; inverted T waves; intraventricular conduction defect; low voltage; right axis deviation and right ventricular hypertrophy (Fig. 13–2). The right atrial abnormalities are generally secondary to the noncompliant, hypertrophic right ventricle and are referred to as "P pumonale."

Patients with pulmonary hypertension, chronic cor pulmonale and pulmonary embolization may also present with these findings. However, only one third of patients with acute pulmonary embolization have electrocardiographic abnormalities. All of these changes result from right heart strain. They are usually transient, lasting no more than hours to a few days, and include nonspecific as well as specific electrical changes. The nonspecific changes are the most common and include sinus tachycardia and ST segment and T wave changes; however, these are of little help in making a definitive diagnosis. The less common but more specific changes include acute-peaking P waves, acute right axis deviation, right ventricular hypertrophy, atrial fibrillation and acute S1-Q3-T3 pattern (large S wave in lead I, Q wave in lead III and inverted T wave in lead III). In addition, there may be a transient right bundle branch block.

There may also be electrocardiographic signs of anoxia to the left ventricle as a result of pulmonary disease. These changes are manifested by primary T wave inversions indicative of ischemia.

A summary of the electrocardiographic findings associated with pulmonary disease is shown in Table 2.

Table 2. SUMMARY OF ELECTROCARDIOGRAPHIC FINDINGS IN PULMONARY DISEASE*

Cor pulmonale	Tall peaked P waves in leads II, III and AVF
	T wave inversions
	ST segment changes
	Right axis deviation
	Right ventricular hypertrophy
	Low voltages
	Intraventricular conduction defect
Pulmonary embolus	
Nonspecific	ST segment and T wave changes, acute
	Sinus tachycardia
Specific	Peaked P waves, acute
	Atrial fibrillation
	S1-Q3-T3, acute
	Right bundle branch block, acute

*Leads II, III, V1 to V3.

14

Effects of Drugs

DIGITALIS

Digitalis has direct and indirect actions on the cardiovascular system that make it useful in the treatment of congestive heart failure and supraventricular tachycardias. The pharmacological actions that make it useful as an antiarrhythmic agent include lengthening of atrioventricular nodal conduction time (increases the PR interval) and an increase in its refractory period, both attributable to increased vagal tone. This increased vagal tone also causes a decrease in the refractory period of the atrial muscle. The direct effect of digitalis is to decrease the refractory period of the ventricular myocardium.

Based on these pharmacological actions, we can predict some of the toxic effects of digitalis. Supraventricular arrhythmias, premature ventricular contractions and paroxysmal atrioventricular tachycardias are the most common. Paroxysmal atrioventricular tachycardia is a result of the direct effect of high doses of digitalis, which tend to excite the atrioventricular node and hence increase its automaticity. This is unlike the effect of digitalis at therapeutic doses, which tends to suppress atrioventricular conduction. The hallmark of digitalis toxicity is evidence of increased automaticity and blocks.

Extracardiac manifestations of digitalis toxicity commonly include anorexia, nausea, visual disturbances, fatigue and headaches. Depending upon the digitalis preparation, these symptoms may precede the cardiac arrhythmias. It is very important to note serum potassium levels in patients given digitalis therapy, since hypokalemia can predispose to digitalis toxicity. A summary of the findings in digitalis toxicity is shown in Table 3.

Table 3. SUMMARY OF FINDINGS IN DIGITALIS TOXICITY

Electrocardiographic	
ST segment and T wave	ST segment sagging T wave flattening QT shortening
Arrhythmias	Frequent premature ventricular contractions Ventricular tachycardia Paroxysmal atrioventricular tachycardia Sinus bradycardia
Blocks	Sinoatrial block Atrioventricular block
Extracardiac	Anorexia, nausea Visual disturbance—halos Fatigue, headache

ST segment and T wave changes also occur with digitalis therapy and are not necessarily an indication of toxicity but rather of therapeutic effect. These changes include a sagging of the ST segment and a flattening of the T waves.

Table 4. SUMMARY OF THERAPEUTIC AND TOXIC EFFECTS OF QUINIDINE

THERAPEUTIC DOSE	TOXIC DOSE
PR increased	Sinoatrial block
QRS complex increased	Atrioventricular block
QT increased	Intraventricular block
ST segment depression	Ectopic beats
T inversion	Ventricular tachycardia

QUINIDINE

Quinidine is useful in the treatment of ectopic arrhythmias. It has both vagolytic and direct actions that decrease myocardial excitability. Toxic effects may be a result of decreased intraventricular conduction or of increased ventricular automaticity. Low serum potassium antagonizes the therapeutic effects of quinidine, whereas digitalis toxicity and hyperkalemia may contribute to quinidine toxicity. Quinidine is absolutely contraindicated in a patient with atrioventricular block and an atrioventricular nodal pacemaker, since quinidine will suppress the pacemaker's action. The electrocardiographic changes due to quinidine are summarized in Table 4.

PROPRANOLOL

Propranolol is a beta-blocking agent that has direct quinidine-like effects on the heart. It depresses the automaticity of the sinoatrial node, prolongs atrioventricular conduction and prolongs the refractory period of the atrioventricular node. Therapeutic doses will decrease the sinus rate without any other significant effect on the electrocardiogram.

ANTIPSYCHOTROPIC AGENTS

Phenothiazines and other antipsychotropic drugs have electrophysiological effects similar to those of quinidine. The most common electrocardiographic changes include widening and flattening or inversion of the T wave with QT prolongation. In overdoses of these drugs, cardiac arrhythmias, including ventricular tachycardia, are common.

15

Electrolytes

The electrocardiogram is a useful clinical tool for the recognition of electrolyte abnormalities. Once the diagnosis has been made, the electrocardiogram may provide a rapid guide to the status of the imbalance during therapy.

POTASSIUM

Intracellular potassium concentration is 30 times greater than its extracellular concentration. It is this gradient that establishes the resting membrane potential of myocardial cells (see Chapter 2, The Action Potential). Changes in potassium concentration affect the resting potential and result in cardiac arrhythmias. The effects of potassium on cardiac function are best determined using the electrocardiogram, as serum potassium may not reflect the K^+ gradient accurately.

Hyperkalemia commonly results from renal insufficiency and inappropriate intravenous fluid administration. High serum K^+ increases the extracellular K^+ concentration and produces a decrease in resting membrane potential (i.e., makes it less negative). This change in membrane potential results in decreased atrial and intraventricular conduction as well as a decrease in the effective refractory period. Normal serum potassium is 3.5 to 5.0 mEq per liter. At plasma levels of 5.8 to 6.2 mEq per liter, atrioventricular conduction is accelerated. However, at levels above 6.5 mEq per liter, atrioventricular conduction is depressed.

The earliest change of hyperkalemia on the electrocardiogram is peaking of the T waves, best seen in the precordial leads (Fig. 15–1*A*). As the serum K^+ level continues to rise, the P waves flatten, and the PR interval is prolonged. This is followed by a widening of the QRS complex (Fig. 15–1*B*) and the development of a sine wave configuration of all complexes (Fig. 15–1*C*). Ultimately, if left uncorrected, ventricular fibrillation and cardiac standstill occur (Fig. 15–1*D*). The electrocardiographic changes associated with hyperkalemia are summarized in Figure 15–2.

Hypokalemia is frequently caused by diuretic therapy and intestinal loss by vomiting, diarrhea and fistulae. Hypokalemia increases the resting membrane potential, making it more negative, which increases myocardial excitability. This can lead to ectopic beats and tachyarrhythmias. In addition, hypokalemia predisposes to digitalis intoxication. In fact, during digitalis therapy arrhythmias may occur at serum K^+ levels that would otherwise be considered normal. This discrepancy between serum K^+ and cardiac dysfunction makes serum determinations less helpful than the electrocardiographic findings of hypokalemia.

The electrocardiographic changes characteristic of hypokalemia include the following: prominent U waves, ST segment changes and ectopic tachyarrhythmias (Fig. 15–3). If a U wave is superimposed on a T wave, the electrocardiogram may appear to have a prolonged QT interval, and confusion with hypocalcemia may occur. The electrocardiographic evidence of hypokalemia is summarized in Figure 15–4.

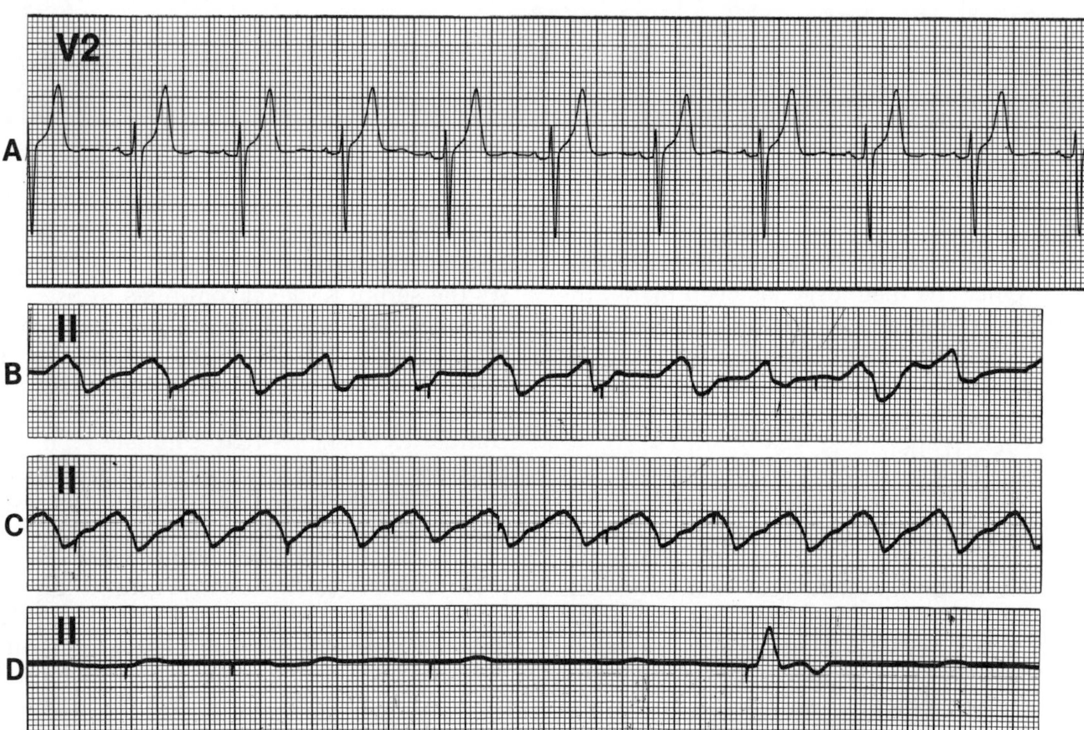

Figure 15–1. **Hyperkalemia.** *A,* The peaking of the T waves in a patient with a serum K^+ level of 6.1 mEq/l. *B, C* and *D,* Another patient who previously had an implanted pacemaker, renal failure and refractory hyperkalemia. *B* shows a marked widening of the QRS complex when the serum K^+ was 7.3 mEq/l. *C* shows a sine wave pattern as the serum K^+ rose to 8.9 mEq/l. *D* shows a terminal rhythm with only the pacemaker spikes seen and a rare captured wide QRS complex. The serum K^+ at this time was 9.4 mEq/l.

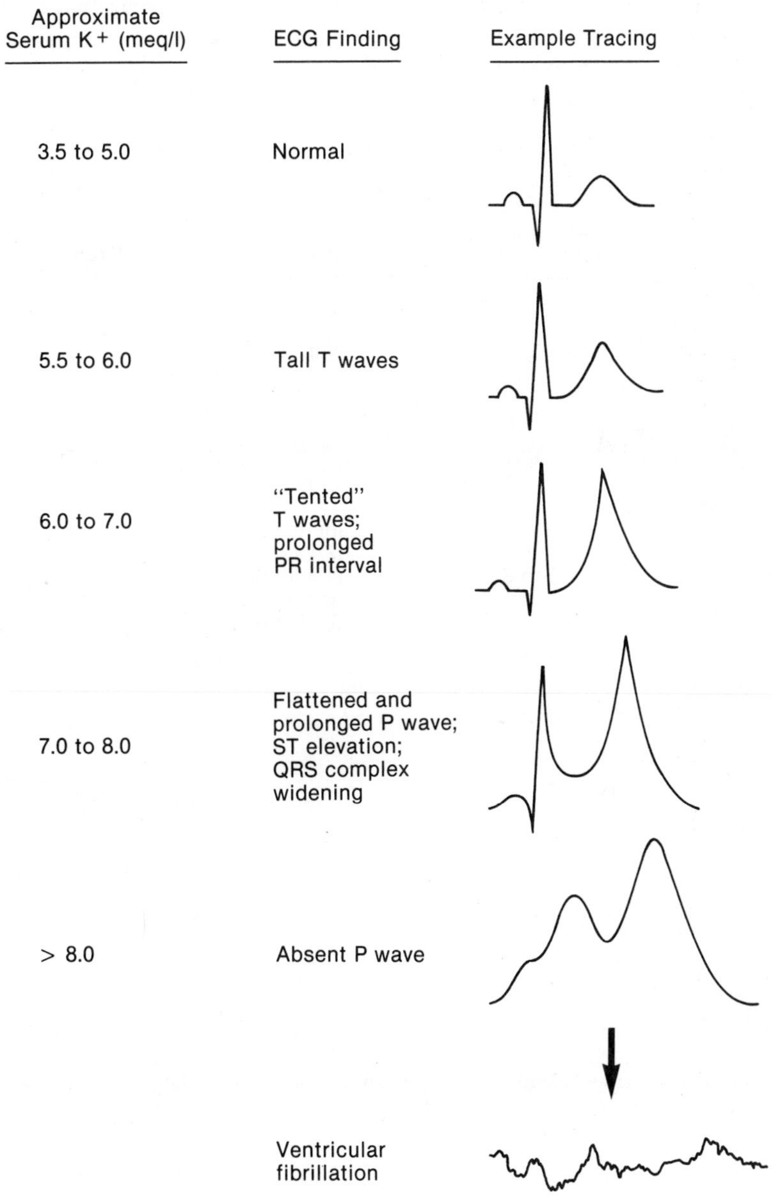

Approximate Serum K+ (meq/l)	ECG Finding	Example Tracing
3.5 to 5.0	Normal	
5.5 to 6.0	Tall T waves	
6.0 to 7.0	"Tented" T waves; prolonged PR interval	
7.0 to 8.0	Flattened and prolonged P wave; ST elevation; QRS complex widening	
> 8.0	Absent P wave	
	Ventricular fibrillation	

Figure 15–2. **Hyperkalemia.** This figure illustrates the electrocardiographic findings associated with hyperkalemia.

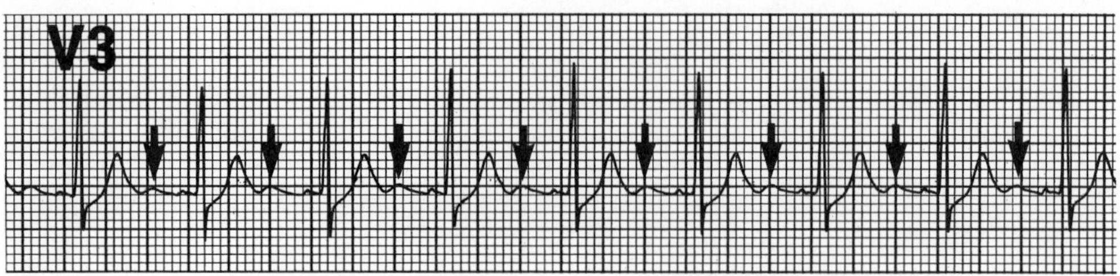

Figure 15–3. **Hypokalemia.** The arrows point to the U waves in this electrocardiogram taken on a patient with mild hypokalemia. The serum K^+ was 2.2 mEq/l.

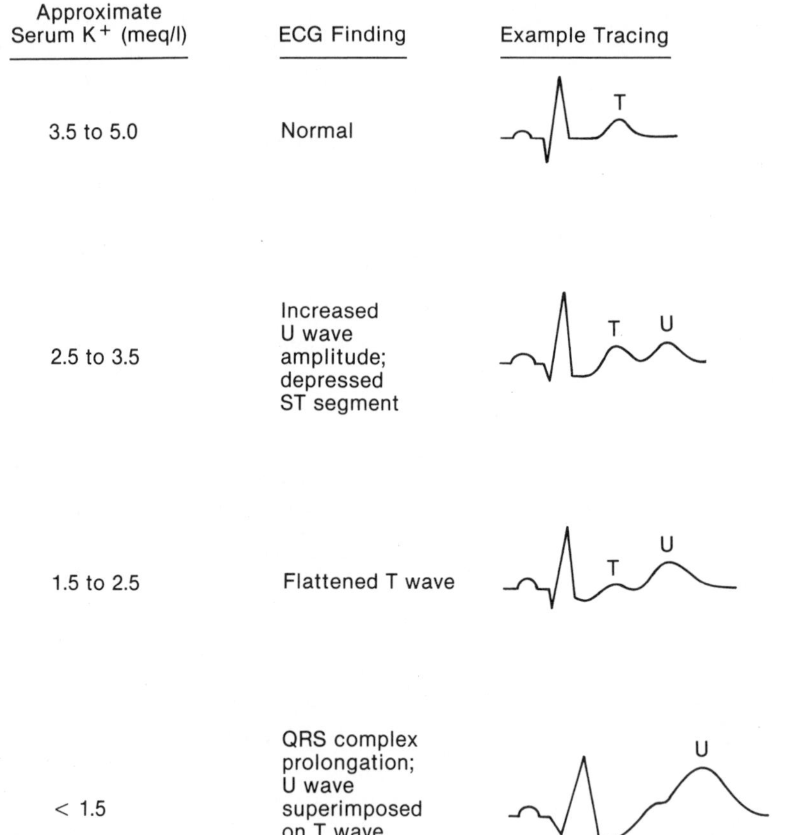

Approximate Serum K^+ (meq/l)	ECG Finding	Example Tracing
3.5 to 5.0	Normal	T
2.5 to 3.5	Increased U wave amplitude; depressed ST segment	T U
1.5 to 2.5	Flattened T wave	T U
< 1.5	QRS complex prolongation; U wave superimposed on T wave	U

Figure 15–4. **Hypokalemia.** This figure shows the electrocardiographic findings associated with hypokalemia.

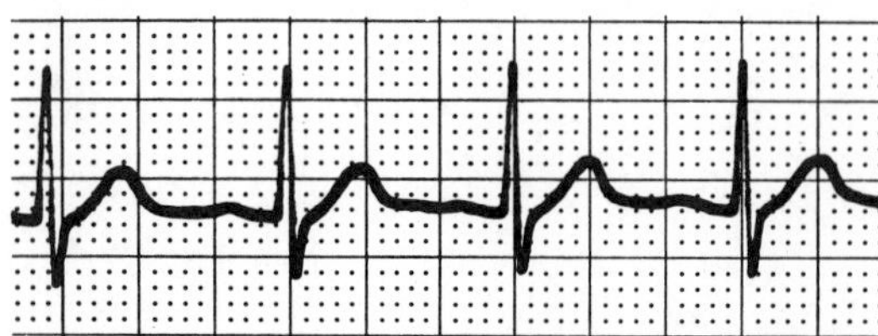

Figure 15–5. **Hypercalcemia.** Notice the shortened QT interval, which is shortened as a result of the shortened ST segment. This is characteristic of hypercalcemia.The serum Ca^{++} was 14.2 mEq/l.

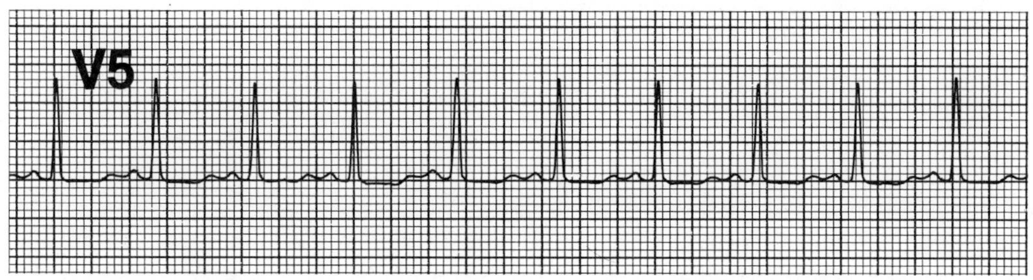

Figure 15–6. **Hypocalcemia.** Notice the prolonged QTc interval. The QT interval measures 0.40 seconds, and when corrected for the rate of 112 beats per minute, the QTc measures 0.53 second. The QT interval is increased as a result of prolongation of the ST segment. This is characteristic of hypocalcemia. The serum Ca^{++} was 6.8 mEq/l.

CALCIUM

Hypercalcemia can be caused by hyperparathyroidism, tumors, especially breast and lung, and also excessive vitamin D. Myocardial contractility is determined in part by calcium concentration. Hypercalcemia increases contractility and reduces the threshold potential (making it less negative) (see Chapter 2, The Action Potential). The electrocardiogram will show a shortening of the QT interval (Fig. 15–5). In addition, the QRS complex may widen because of conduction disturbances. Premature ventricular contractions may also occur.

Hypocalcemia often results from intestinal malabsorption, pancreatitis, renal insufficiency and hypoparathyroidism. Hypocalcemia will increase the threshold potential (making it more negative). The electrocardiographic changes most characteristic are the opposite of those seen in hypercalcemia; i.e., the QTc interval is prolonged (Fig. 15–6). Severe hypercalcemia may produce inverted T waves and may thus simulate myocardial ischemia and hypokalemia. Arrhythmias are not as common in this condition; however, the prolonged QTc interval may induce the R on T phenomenon, which may result in ventricular tachycardia (see Ventricular Tachycardia, page 52 and Chapter 4, Review of Complexes).

MAGNESIUM

Abnormal magnesium concentrations can affect cardiac function. Although the exact mechanism is unknown, magnesium acts on the Na^{+}-K^{+} pump and can interfere with the concentrations of these ions. *Hypomagnesemia* can produce arrhythmias and can predispose to digitalis toxicity. The electrocardiogram in hypomagnesemia may resemble that of hypokalemia.

Hypermagnesemia will slow the upstroke velocity of phase 0 (see Chapter 2, The Action Potential) and will decrease atrioventricular conduction.

Both hypermagnesemia and hypomagnesemia may produce QTc prolongation. This may predispose to the R-on-T phenomenon, which can result in ventricular tachycardia (see Ventricular Tachycardia, page 52 and Chapter 4, Review of Complexes).

16

Systematic Approach to Interpretation

An outline for the clinical interpretation of electrocardiograms is provided in Appendix B. Each topic has been discussed in the preceding chapters and is summarized for easy future reference.

Rate should be determined for both atria and ventricles. Differences in atrial and ventricular rates reflect conduction disturbances, especially atrioventricular block or dissociation.

Rhythm determinations are made by assessing the regularity of the P wave and the QRS complex and the relationship between them. The PR interval, QRS complex duration and QT intervals must always be measured to assess conduction and rhythm.

Although each arrhythmia is different, there is a common guideline that one should use in approaching an arrhythmia:

1. Is the QRS complex rhythm regular or irregular?
2. If the QRS complex rhythm is irregular, is there any regularity or repetition to this irregularity?
3. What is the P wave-QRS complex relationship? Is there a P wave prior to each QRS complex?
4. Are the P waves that precede the QRS complexes related to them or are they independent?
5. If the P waves are related to the QRS complex, is the PR interval fixed? Is there a progressive increase in the PR intervals with a decrease in the R-R intervals?
6. If the QRS complexes are without a P wave, are the QRS complexes ectopic or are the P waves hidden?
7. If the QRS complexes are ectopic, where is the focus? A narrow QRS complex is of supraventricular origin. A widened QRS complex may be ventricular or supraventricular with aberrancy in etiology.
8. If the P waves are absent, is the atrial rhythm fibrillation or flutter?
9. Are there any premature events?
10. Are there any pauses or late events?
11. Are there any unexpected events?

When one analyzes the pauses and late events, it is important to recognize that several mechanisms may be responsible. The pause may be a result of the following:

1. A dropped beat from second degree sinoatrial block.
2. A dropped beat resulting from second degree atrioventricular block.
3. A blocked atrial premature contraction.
4. A blocked or nonconducted atrioventricular nodal extrasystole.
5. Marked sinus arrhythmia.

Axis is also always assessed. Variations from normal axis are often part of the criteria for a definitive diagnosis (e.g., right ventricular hypertrophy, pulmonary disease, left anterior hemiblock), or they may be a clue to evolving disease. Most clinicians approximate the axis to within 15 degrees.

Enlargement of the atria is assessed by looking at the configuration of the P waves in leads II and V1. Determination of ventricular hypertrophy requires an assessment of voltage, but axis deviations and ST segment and T wave changes also contribute to a definitive diagnosis.

Infarction can be determined by the presence of Q waves. However, one should remember that since no electrode records the posterior myocardium directly, one should look for reciprocal changes in the anterior precordial leads (e.g., tall R waves in lead V1).

Ischemia and *injury* are assessed by the structure and polarity of the ST segment and T waves. A rule of thumb is that the T wave has the same polarity as the QRS complex and is normally upright in leads I, II and V3 to V6. The QT interval, ST segment and T wave assessment can also reveal *pulmonary, electrolyte* and *drug effects*.

II

Practice Tracings

Interpretation of Electrocardiograms

The following list should be used as a guide for the analysis of every electrocardiogram. You should begin by looking at the whole tracing, then analyze each complex in each lead and describe the findings. Use a ruler or caliper to measure all the intervals and complexes. Finally, try to synthesize a diagnosis based upon the smaller details. It is important to be precise and to follow the guide for each electrocardiogram regardless of how simple the tracing may appear. A detailed discussion of each abnormality will be found in Part I of this book. Appendix B summarizes the major characteristics of some common and important rhythm disturbances.

Each electrocardiogram is presented for your analysis, and an objective review is provided for your study. Please note that an electrocardiogram is no substitute for the clinical assessment of the patient. Many of the analyses, particularly those of infarction, will state nonspecific changes. If a patient presented with these same electrocardiographic abnormalities and symptoms suggestive of a myocardial infarction, one would be inclined to consider these changes significant.

OUTLINE FOR CLINICAL INTERPRETATION

1. Rate:
   a. Atrial
   b. Ventricular
2. Rhythm: Always measure PR interval, QRS complex duration and QT interval.
   a. Supraventricular rhythms
   b. Ventricular rhythms
3. Conduction abnormalities:
4. QRS mean axis:
5. Chamber enlargement:
   a. Atrial: Look at P wave configuration.
   b. Ventricular: Check voltage criteria and look at ST segment and T wave for evidence of hypertrophy.
6. Infarction: Look for Q waves. For posterior infarction, look for tall R waves in leads V1 to V2.
7. ST segment and T wave abnormalities: Look for ST segment and T wave changes.
8. Other findings:
   a. QT interval
   b. Pulmonary pathology
   c. Drug effects
   d. Electrolytes

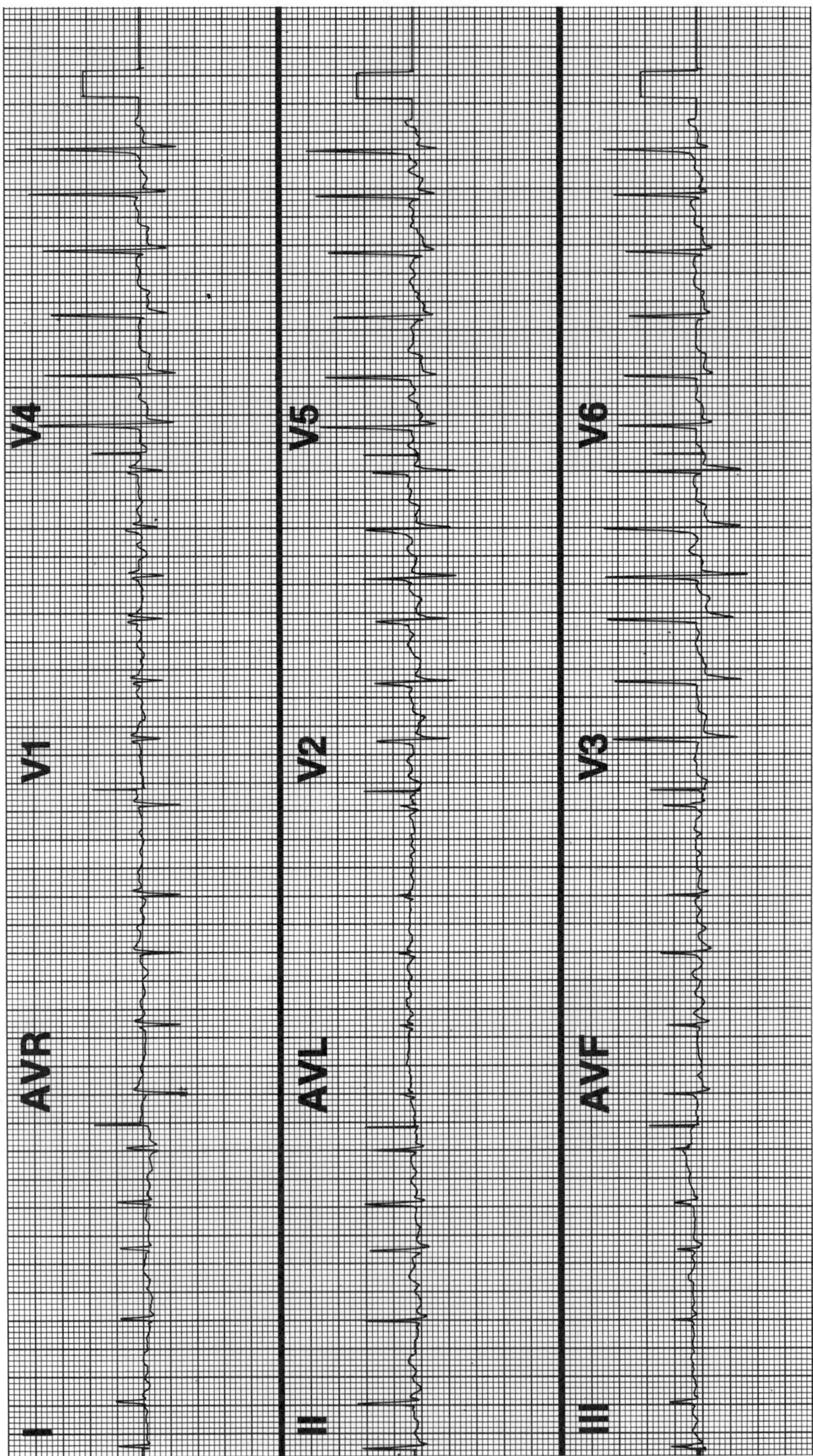
I
AVR
V1
V4
II
AVL
V2
V5
III
AVF
V3
V6

Electrocardiogram #1

Atrial Rate	—	**Beats/Minute**
Ventricular Rate	140	**Beats/Minute**
PR Interval	—	**Second**
QRS Duration	0.09	**Second**
QT-QTc	0.26–0.40	**Second**
QRS Complex Axis	50	**Degrees**

Rate: The average ventricular rate is 140 beats per minute.

Rhythm: The rhythm is grossly irregular, and fine fibrillatory waves may be seen throughout. No P waves are seen. The rhythm is atrial fibrillation with a rapid ventricular response.

Conduction Abnormalities: There is a rSr′ complex in lead V1 suggestive of a right bundle branch block. However, the QRS complex is only 0.09 second. Therefore, one can only suggest that the RSR′ complex is a manifestation of a right ventricular conduction delay.

QRS Complex Axis: The mean QRS is 50°. Notice that the QRS complex is upright in both leads I and AVF, making the mean QRS complex axis between 0 and 90°. When one evaluates lead AVL, one sees that the QRS complex is almost equiphasic in this lead; therefore, the mean QRS complex axis is perpendicular to lead AVL, which would place it parallel to lead II. However, since lead AVL is slightly positive, the mean QRS complex axis is slightly less, therefore, +50°.

Chamber Enlargement: No criteria present in this electrocardiogram.

Infarction: No criteria present in this electrocardiogram.

ST Segment and T Wave Abnormalities: There are diffuse ST segment and T wave abnormalities.

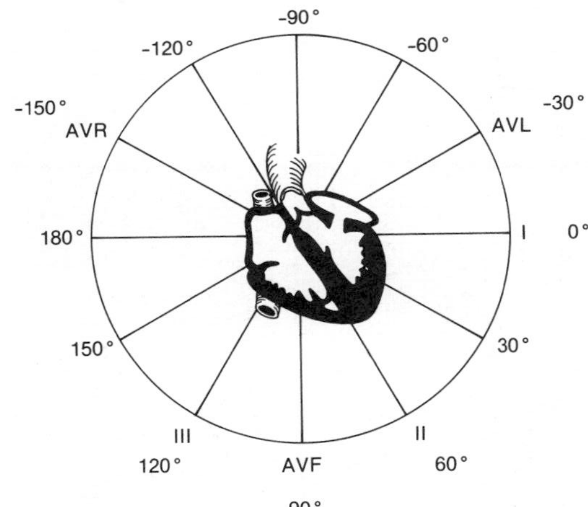

Summary

Atrial fibrillation

RSR′ complex in lead V1 suggestive of a right ventricular conduction delay

Nonspecific ST segment and T wave abnormalities

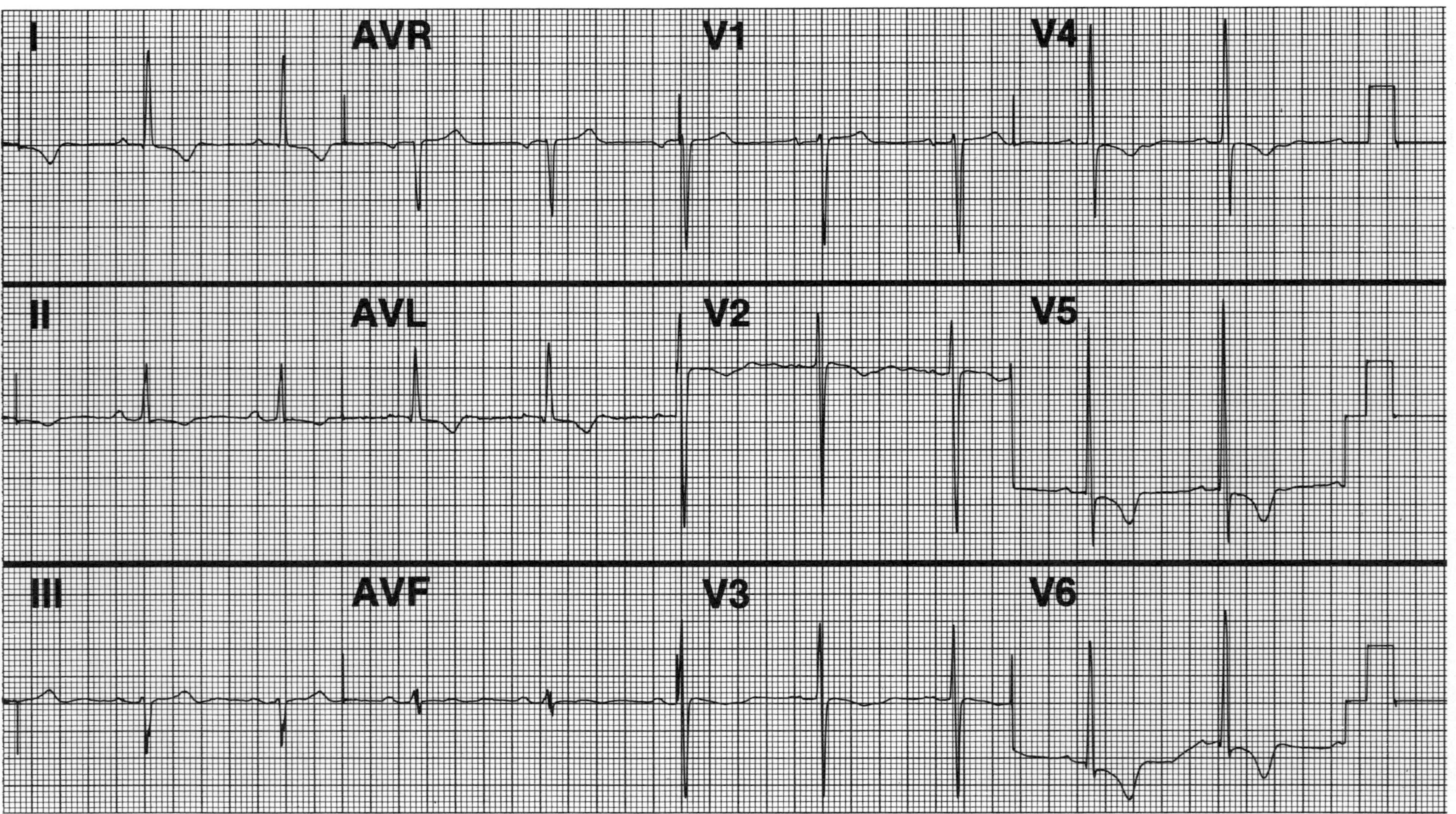
I
AVR
V1
V4
II
AVL
V2
V5
III
AVF
V3
V6

Electrocardiogram #2

Atrial Rate	**63**	**Beats/Minute**
Ventricular Rate	**63**	**Beats/Minute**
PR Interval	**0.16**	**Second**
QRS Duration	**0.09**	**Second**
QT-QTc	**0.42–0.41**	**Second**
QRS Complex Axis	**0**	**Degrees**

Rate: The atrial and ventricular rates are 63 beats per minute.

Rhythm: The PR interval is 0.16 second and constant. The rhythm is normal sinus rhythm.

Conduction Abnormalities: No criteria present in this electrocardiogram.

QRS Complex Axis: The mean QRS complex axis is 0°. The QRS complex in lead AVF is equiphasic. Therefore, the mean QRS vector is perpendicular to lead AVF. Since it is positive in lead I, the mean QRS complex axis is 0°.

Chamber Enlargement: The voltage in lead AVL is 18 mm. An R wave voltage of 13 mm in lead AVL is the most significant and specific criterion for left ventricular hypertrophy based on post-mortem studies.

Infarction: No criteria present in this electrocardiogram.

ST Segment and T Wave Abnormalities: The ST segment and T wave changes are secondary changes to left ventricular hypertrophy, and together with the presence of voltage criteria, the diagnosis of left ventricular hypertrophy should be made.

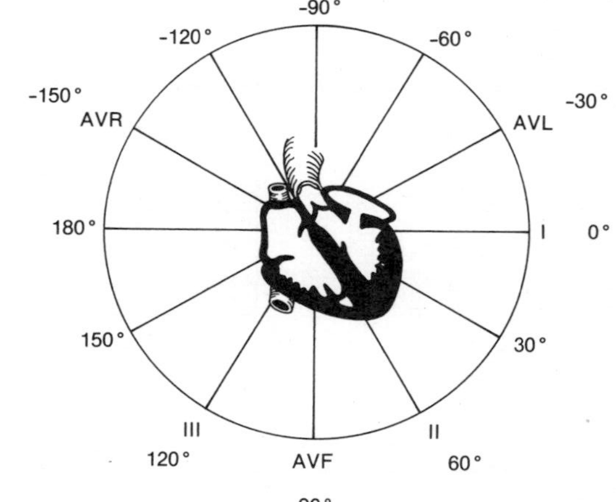

Summary

Normal sinus rhythm

Left ventricular hypertrophy

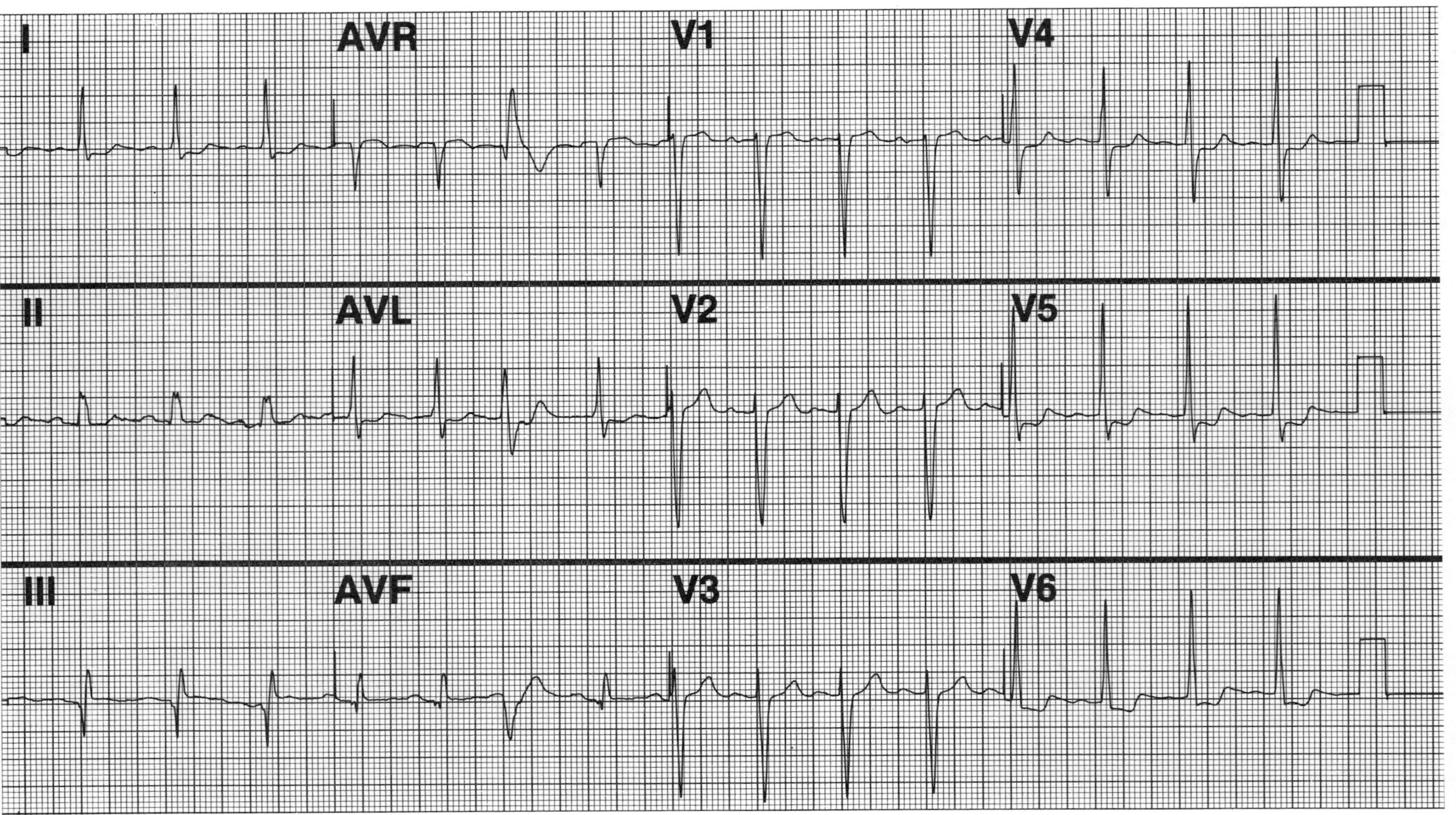
I
AVR
V1
V4
II
AVL
V2
V5
III
AVF
V3
V6

Electrocardiogram #3

Atrial Rate	96	**Beats/Minute**
Ventricular Rate	96	**Beats/Minute**
PR Interval	0.20	**Second**
QRS Duration	0.10	**Second**
QT-QTc	0.35–0.44	**Second**
QRS Complex Axis	10	**Degrees**

Rate: The atrial and ventricular rates are 96 beats per minute.

Rhythm: The rhythm is regular with a PR interval of 0.20 second. There is an occasional premature ventricular contraction as noted in leads AVR, AVL and AVF. The third QRS complex is widened and bizarre in comparison to the QRS complex that precedes and follows it; therefore, the QRS complex is a premature ventricular contraction.

Conduction Abnormalities: The QRS complex duration is 0.11 seconds. The QRS complex in leads I and V6 shows an initial delay. There is an absence of the normal septal Q wave in leads I and V6. Therefore, the diagnosis of incomplete left bundle branch block should be made.

QRS Complex Axis: The mean QRS complex axis is 10°.

Chamber Enlargement: The S wave voltage in lead V1 and the R wave voltage in lead V5 exceed 35 mm. Therefore, the diagnosis of left ventricular hypertrophy should be suspect.

Infarction: No criteria present in this electrocardiogram.

ST Segment and T Wave Abnormalities: The ST segment and T wave abnormalities are secondary repolarization changes, and, together with the voltage criteria, the diagnosis of left ventricular hypertrophy should be made.

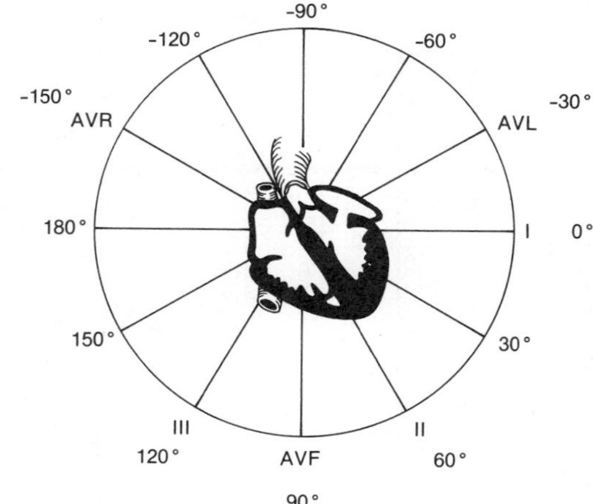

Summary

Normal sinus rhythm with occasional premature ventricular contractions

Incomplete left bundle branch block

Left ventricular hypertrophy with secondary repolarization changes

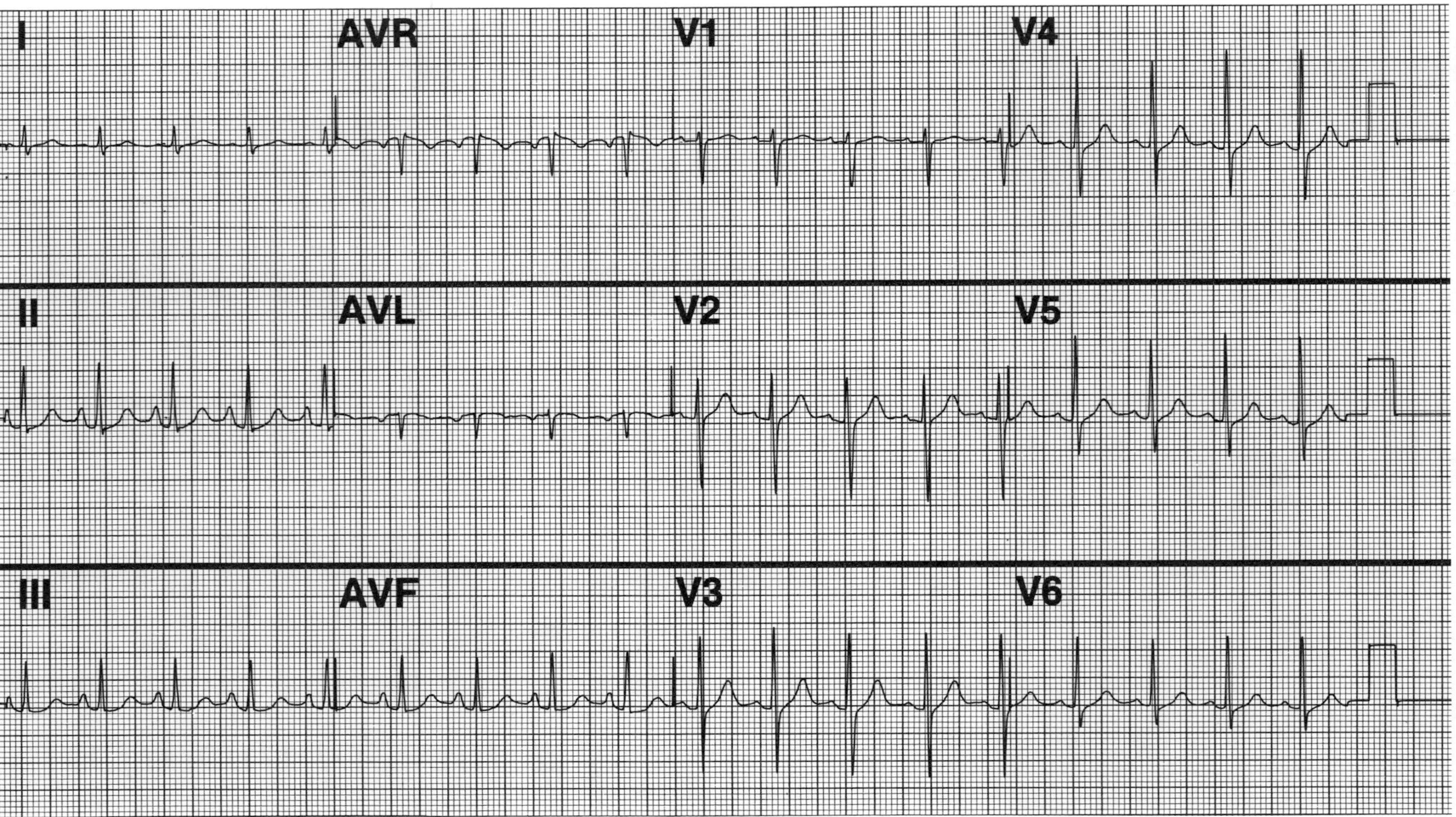
I
AVR
V1
V4
II
AVL
V2
V5
III
AVF
V3
V6

Electrocardiogram #4

Atrial Rate	**115**	**Beats/Minute**
Ventricular Rate	**115**	**Beats/Minute**
PR Interval	**0.15**	**Second**
QRS Duration	**0.07**	**Second**
QT-QTc	**0.32–0.43**	**Second**
QRS Complex Axis	**80**	**Degrees**

Rate: The atrial and ventricular rates are 115 beats per minute.

Rhythm: The PR interval is 0.15 second and constant. The rhythm is normal sinus tachycardia.

Conduction Abnormalities: No criteria present in this electrocardiogram.

QRS Complex Axis: The mean QRS complex axis is 80°.

Chamber Enlargement: Although this appears to be a normal electrocardiogram, there is a strong suggestion of right atrial enlargement. Notice the P wave configuration in leads II, III and AVF. The P wave in lead II measures 3 mm and tends to be peaked. The diagnosis of right atrial enlargement should be made.

Infarction: No criteria present in this electrocardiogram.

ST Segment and T Wave Abnormalities: No criteria present in this electrocardiogram.

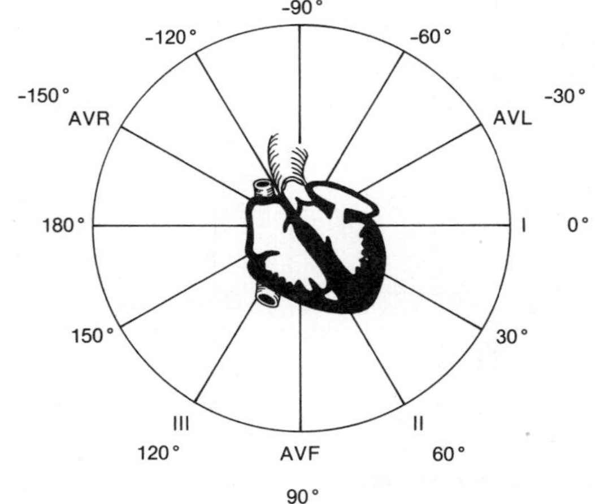

Summary

Sinus tachycardia

Right atrial enlargement

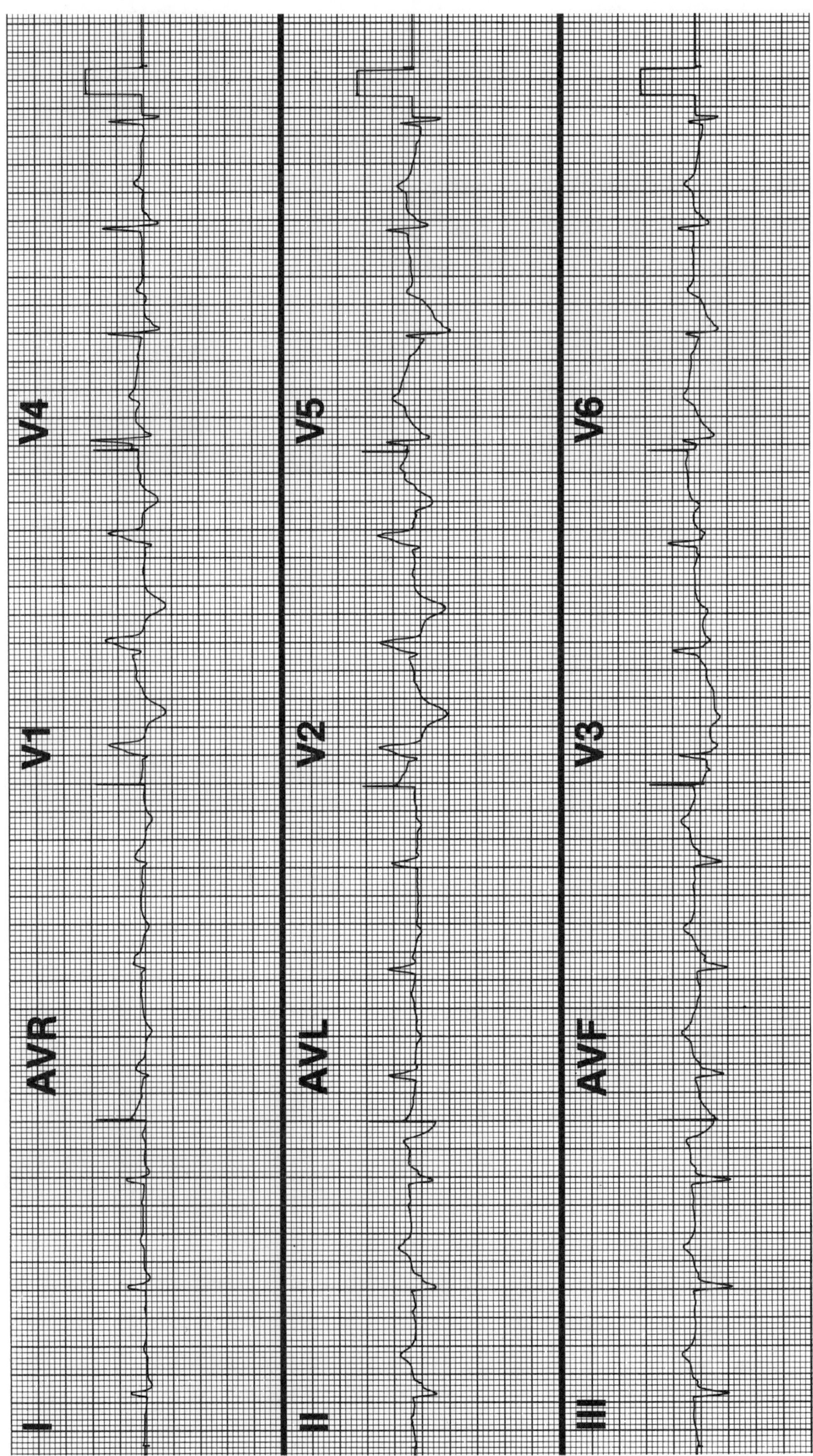
I
AVR
V1
V4
II
AVL
V2
V5
III
AVF
V3
V6

Electrocardiogram #5

Atrial Rate	**81**	**Beats/Minute**
Ventricular Rate	**81**	**Beats/Minute**
PR Interval	**0.19**	**Second**
QRS Duration	**0.16**	**Second**
QT-QTc	**0.40–0.46**	**Second**
QRS Complex Axis	**−70**	**Degrees**

Rate: The atrial and ventricular rates are 81 beats per minute.

Rhythm: The PR interval is 0.19 second and constant. The rhythm is normal sinus rhythm.

Conduction Abnormalities: One should immediately notice that the QRS complex duration is prolonged. Each QRS complex comprises four small boxes; therefore, the QRS complex duration is 0.16 second. One should also notice that the QRS complex has a slurred S wave in leads I, V5 and V6. Although an RSR′ complex is not seen in lead V1, it is clear that there is a notching in the R wave in leads V1 and V2. The diagnosis of a right bundle branch block should still be made.

QRS Complex Axis: The deflection is positive in lead I and negative in lead AVF, which places the mean QRS complex axis between 0 and −90°. Since the complex is almost equiphasic in lead AVR, it is therefore perpendicular to this lead; consequently, the mean QRS complex axis is approximately −60°. However, since the QRS complex is slightly positive in lead AVR, the mean QRS complex axis is still more negative, making it approximately −70°.

Chamber Enlargement: No criteria present in this electrocardiogram.

Infarction: There is a singificant Q wave measuring 0.04 second in duration and greater than 25 per cent of the QRS complex in leads V1 and V2. Therefore, the diagnosis of an anteroseptal wall infarction, age undetermined, should be made. In addition, the absence of R waves in leads II, III and AVL should make one suspicious that an inferior wall myocardial infarction is present as well.

ST Segment and T Wave Abnormalities: There are ST segment and T wave abnormalities seen in the anterior right precordial leads that are secondary to the conduction abnormality.

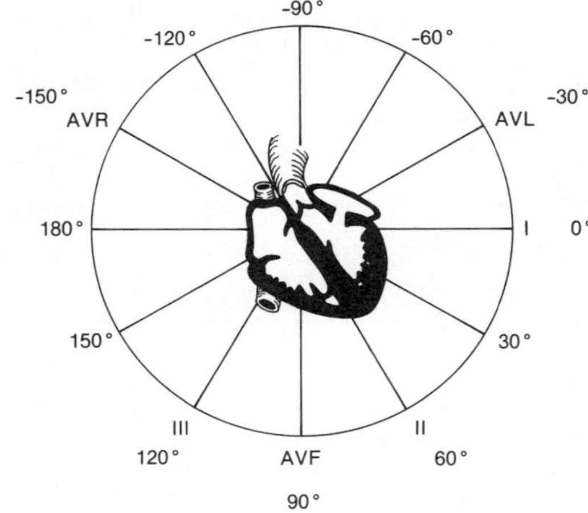

Summary

Normal sinus rhythm

Right bundle branch block

Anteroseptal myocardial infarction

Cannot rule out an inferior myocardial infarction

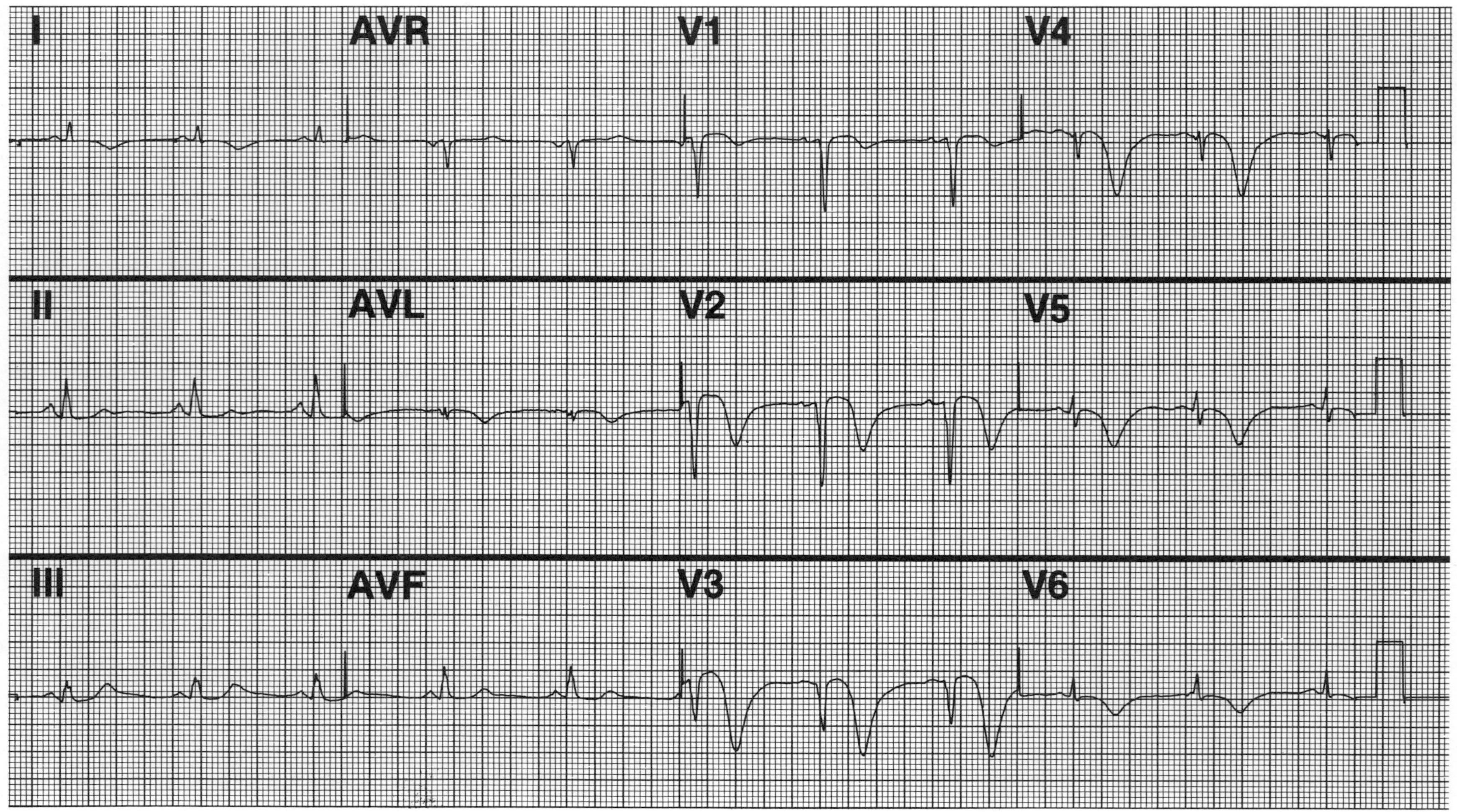
I
AVR
V1
V4
II
AVL
V2
V5
III
AVF
V3
V6

Electrocardiogram #6

Atrial Rate	67	**Beats/Minute**
Ventricular Rate	67	**Beats/Minute**
PR Interval	0.14	**Second**
QRS Duration	0.09	**Second**
QT-QTc	0.52–0.54	**Second**
QRS Complex Axis	60	**Degrees**

Rate: The atrial and ventricular rates are 67 beats per minute.

Rhythm: The PR interval is 0.14 second and constant. The rhythm is normal sinus rhythm.

Conduction Abnormalities: No criteria present in this electrocardiogram.

QRS Complex Axis: The mean QRS axis is perpendicular to the most equiphasic QRS complex, which is lead AVL in this tracing. This means that the mean QRS complex axis is either +60° or −120°. However, lead AVF is positive. Therefore, the QRS axis must be +60°.

Chamber Enlargement: No criteria present in this electrocardiogram.

Infarction: The QS complex in leads V1 to V3 and the Q wave in lead V4 are diagnostic of an anteroseptal myocardial infarction.

ST Segment and T Wave Abnormalities: The marked T wave inversions are ischemic changes secondary to the myocardial infarction. Notice the symmetry of the T waves, which are diagnostic of ischemia.

Other Findings: The QTc is prolonged secondary to the infarction.

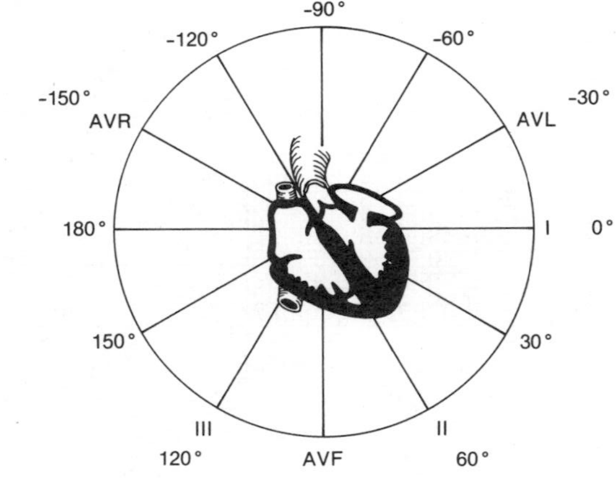

Summary

Normal sinus rhythm

Anteroseptal myocardial infarction, possibly acute

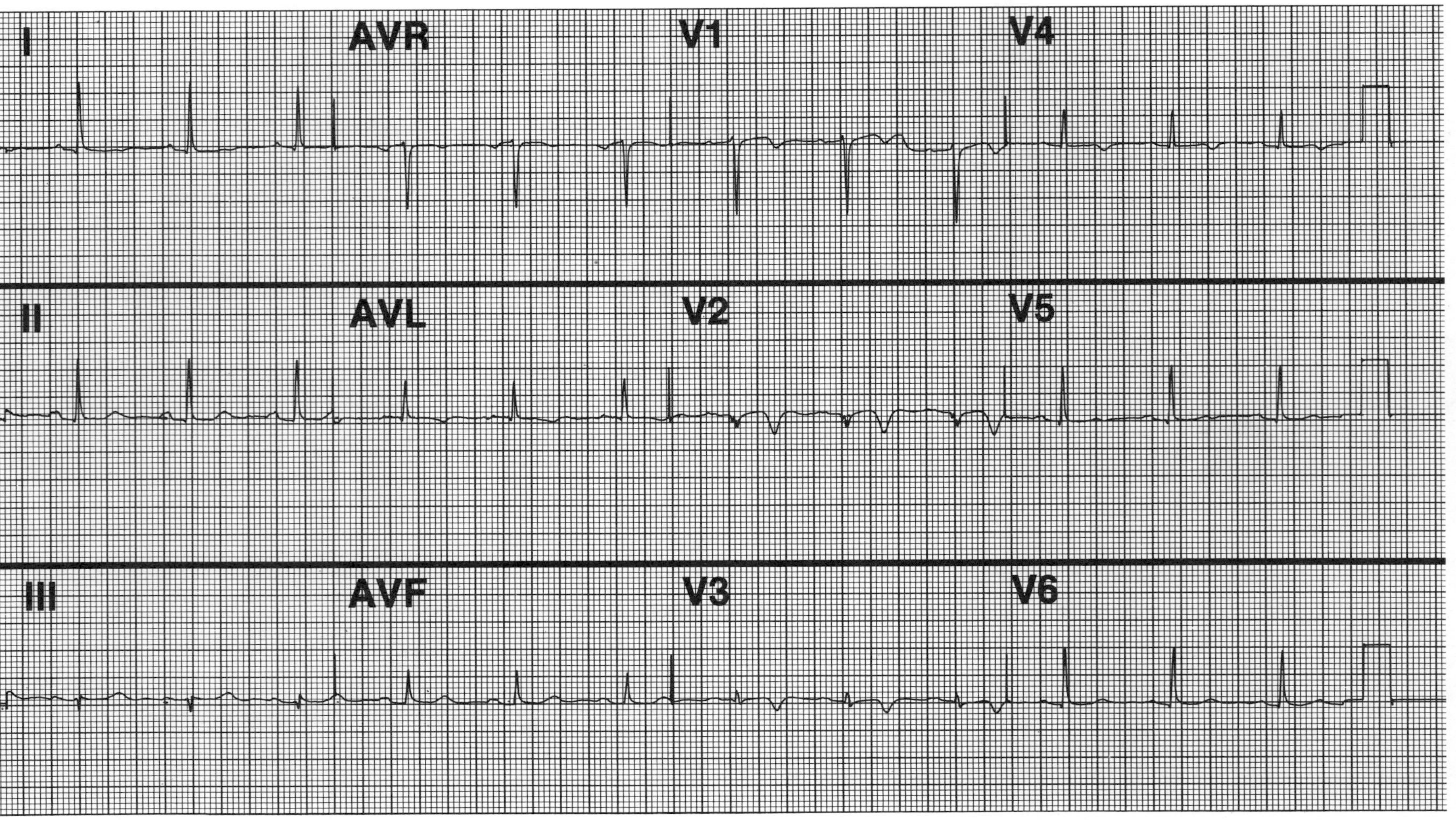
I
AVR
V1
V4
II
AVL
V2
V5
III
AVF
V3
V6

Electrocardiogram #7

Atrial Rate	77	**Beats/Minute**
Ventricular Rate	77	**Beats/Minute**
PR Interval	0.17	**Second**
QRS Duration	0.08	**Second**
QT-QTc	0.40–0.45	**Second**
QRS Complex Axis	20	**Degrees**

Rate: The atrial and ventricular rates are 77 beats per minute.

Rhythm: The PR interval is 0.17 second and constant. The rhythm is normal sinus rhythm.

Conduction Abnormalities: No criteria present in this electrocardiogram.

QRS Complex Axis: The mean QRS axis is approximately perpendicular to lead III, which makes the axis 30°. However, since it is slightly positive in lead III, the mean QRS complex axis is slightly less, therefore, 20°.

Chamber Enlargement: No criteria present in this electrocardiogram.

Infarction: The striking feature of this electrocardiogram is the absence of normal ventricular forces in leads V1 to V3. If one examines the selected electrocardiogram still further, one notices a micro R wave of 1 mm in lead V1 and a Q wave of a 0.04 second duration in lead V2 indicative of an anteroseptal infarction.

ST Segment and T Wave Abnormalities: There are ST segment elevations and symmetric T wave inversions in leads V1 to V3. These changes are indicative of ischemia, related to the infarction or to a new event.

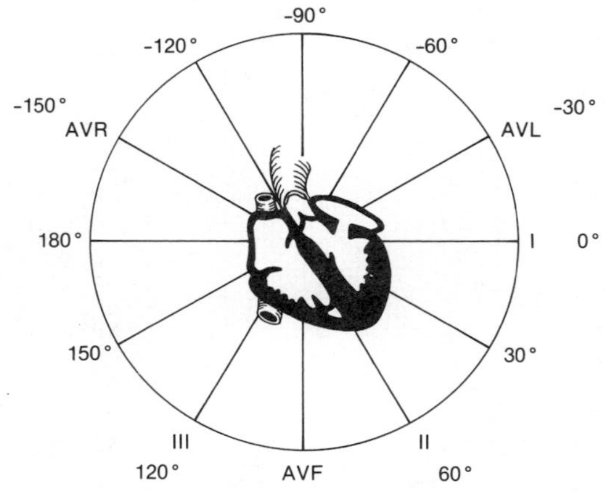

Summary

Normal sinus rhythm

Anteroseptal myocardial infarction, age undetermined

Anterior ischemia

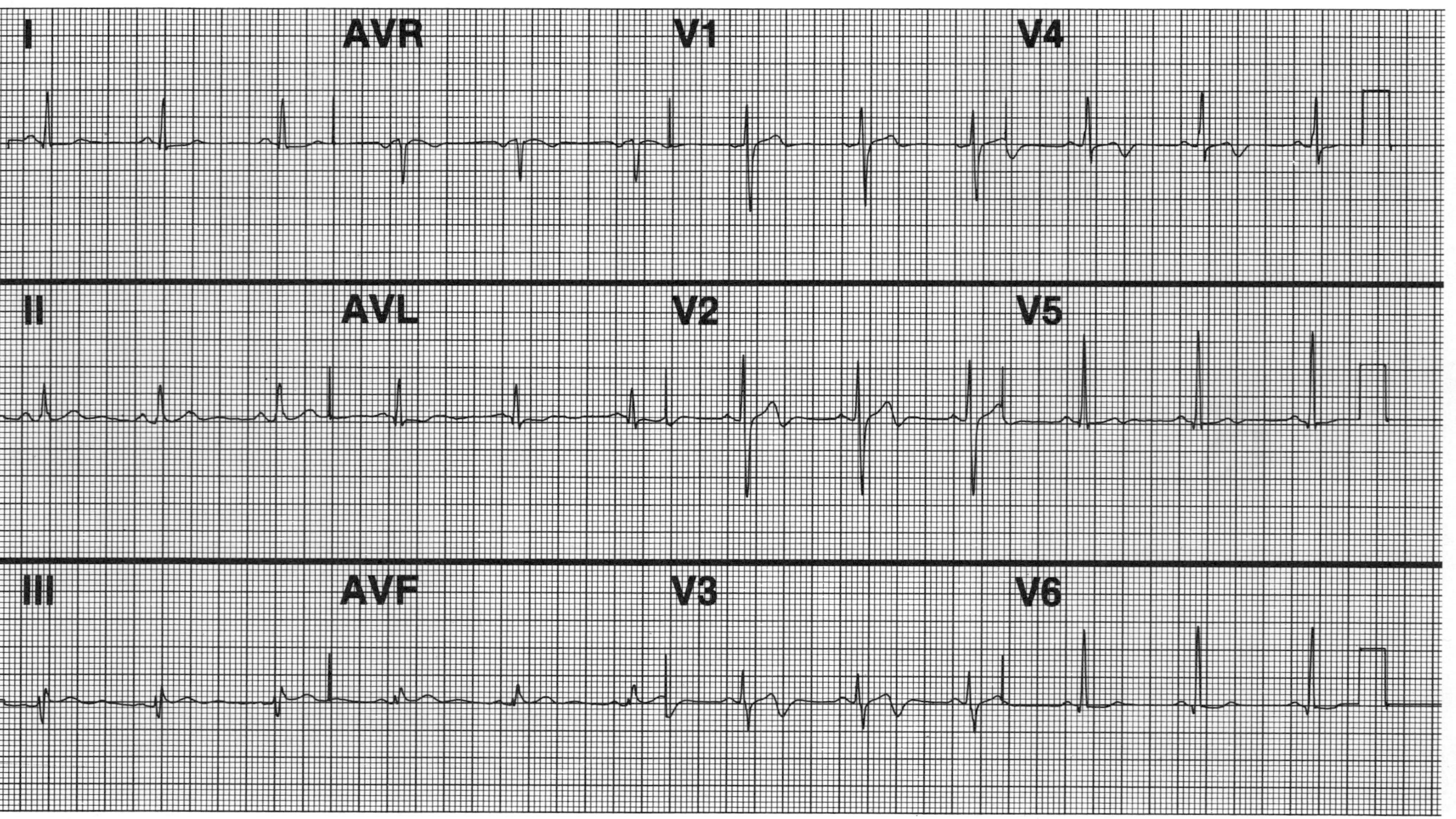
I
AVR
V1
V4
II
AVL
V2
V5
III
AVF
V3
V6

Electrocardiogram #8

Atrial Rate	**75**	**Beats/Minute**
Ventricular Rate	**75**	**Beats/Minute**
PR Interval	**0.14**	**Second**
QRS Duration	**0.09**	**Second**
QT-QTc	**0.40–0.45**	**Second**
QRS Complex Axis	**30**	**Degrees**

Rate: The atrial and ventricular rates are 75 beats per minute.

Rhythm: The PR interval is 0.14 second and constant. The rhythm is normal sinus rhythm.

Conduction Abnormalities: No criteria present in this electrocardiogram.

QRS Complex Axis: The mean QRS complex axis is perpedicular to lead III, therefore, 30°.

Chamber Enlargement: No criteria present in this electrocardiogram.

Infarction: No criteria present in this electrocardiogram.

ST Segment and T Wave Abnormalities: One should note immediately that there is ST segment elevation in leads V1 to V3 together with biphasic T waves in leads V2 and V3 and T wave inversions in lead V4. In addition, the T waves in leads V5 and V6 tend to be quite flattened. The T wave morphology should follow that of the preceding R wave. Consequently, as the R waves increase in amplitude from leads V1 through V6, so should the T waves. In this tracing, however, the T wave is flatter in lead V6 than it is in lead V1, which is abnormal and indicative of ischemia. This electrocardiogram therefore illustrates anterior ischemia.

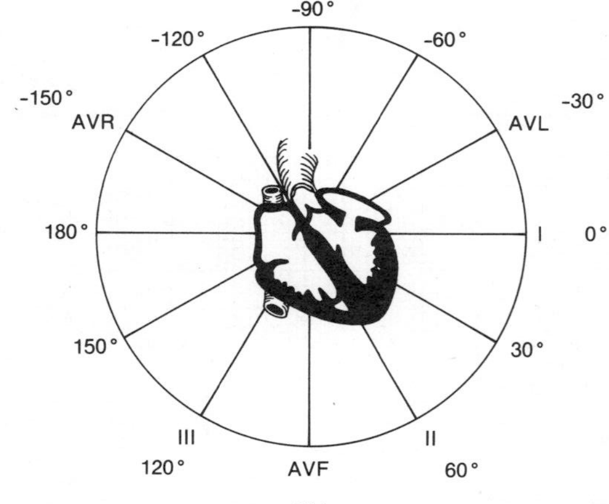

Summary

Normal sinus rhythm

Anterior ischemia

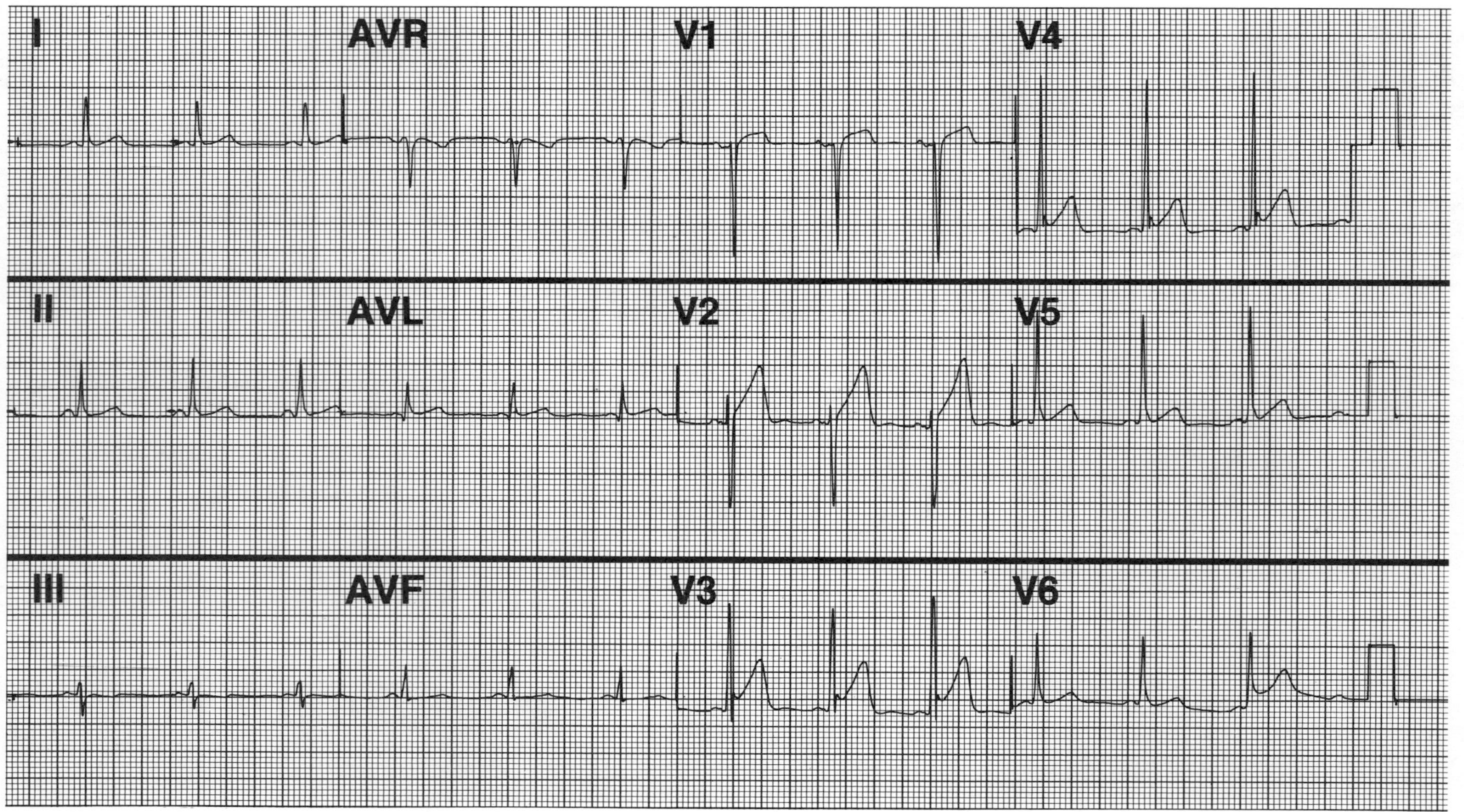
I
AVR
V1
V4
II
AVL
V2
V5
III
AVF
V3
V6

Electrocardiogram #9

Atrial Rate	**79**	**Beats/Minute**
Ventricular Rate	**79**	**Beats/Minute**
PR Interval	**0.13**	**Second**
QRS Duration	**0.08**	**Second**
QT-QTc	**0.36–0.40**	**Second**
QRS Complex Axis	**30**	**Degrees**

Rate: The atrial and ventricular rates are 79 beats per minute.

Rhythm: The PR interval is 0.13 second and constant. The rhythm is normal sinus rhythm.

Conduction Abnormalities: No criteria present in this electrocardiogram.

QRS Complex Axis: The mean QRS complex axis is approximately perpendicular to lead III, or 30°.

Chamber Enlargement: Although the voltages are high, neither the voltage criteria for hypertrophy nor the repolarization changes are present.

Infarction: No criteria present in this electrocardiogram.

ST Segment and T Wave Abnormalities: The interesting feature of this electrocardiogram is the J point elevation seen in leads V1 to V4. You can notice in lead V2 that the J point and the take off of the ST segment occur approximately 2 mm above the isoelectric portion of the electrocardiogram. This is also clearly seen in lead V3, in which the take off occurs approximately 4 mm above the isoelectric segment. This type of electrocardiogram may be a normal variant and is termed early repolarizaton. However, it could be consistent with the diagnosis of pericarditis. One must carefully correlate the clinical findings with the electrocardiograms. This electrocardiogram, however, is frequently found in young black or hispanic men.

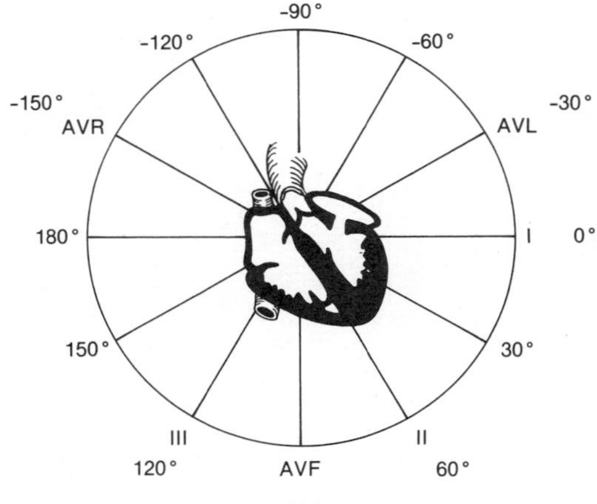

Summary

Normal sinus rhythm

Early repolarization

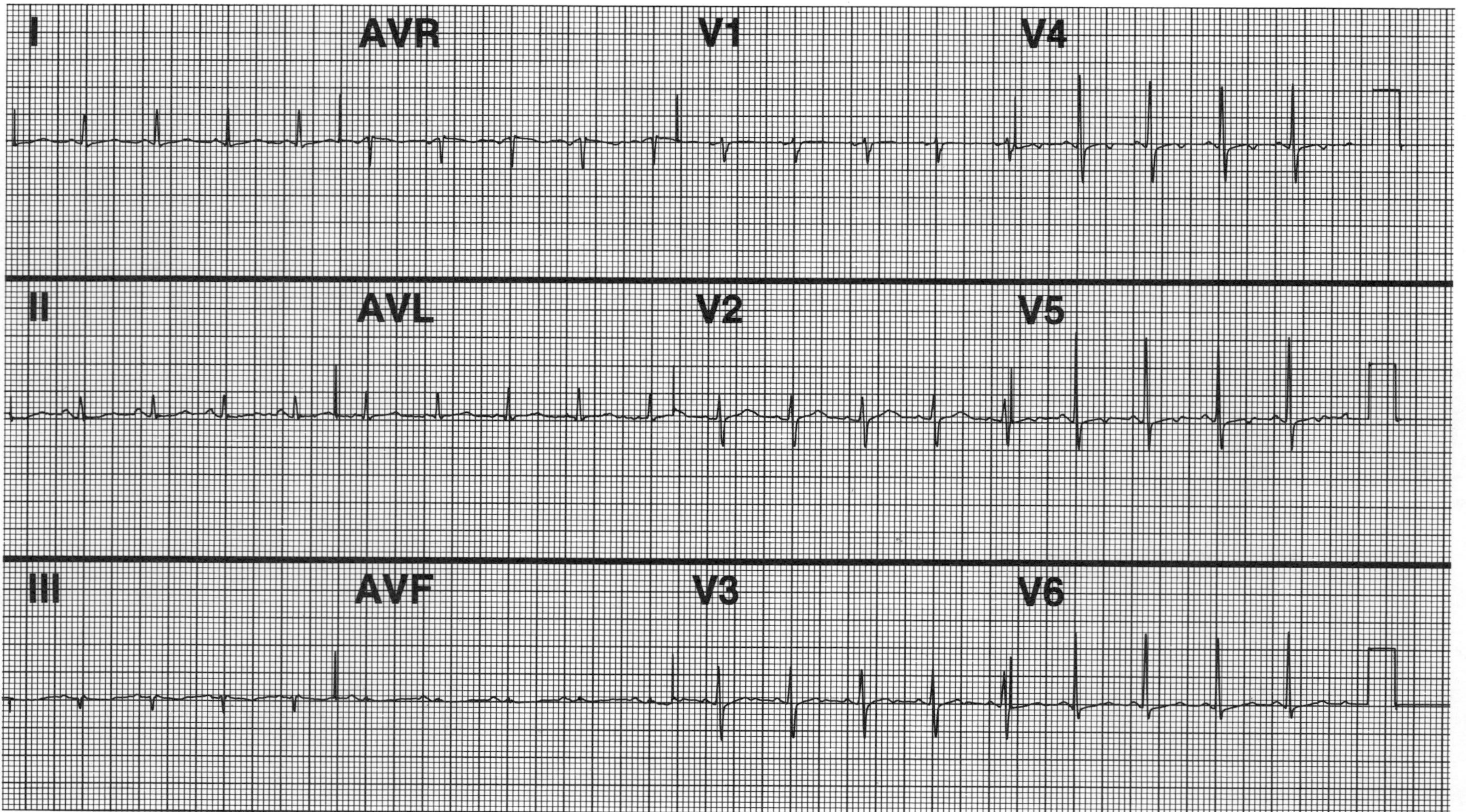
I
AVR
V1
V4
II
AVL
V2
V5
III
AVF
V3
V6

Electrocardiogram #10

Atrial Rate	**120**	**Beats/Minute**
Ventricular Rate	**120**	**Beats/Minute**
PR Interval	**0.11**	**Second**
QRS Duration	**0.07**	**Second**
QT-QTc	**0.32–0.43**	**Second**
QRS Complex Axis	**0**	**Degrees**

Rate: The atrial and ventricular rates are 120 beats per minute.

Rhythm: The PR interval is 0.11 second and constant. The rhythm is sinus tachycardia with a short PR interval.

Conduction Abnormalities: No criteria present in this electrocardiogram.

QRS Complex Axis: The complex in lead AVF is approximately equiphasic; therefore, the mean QRS complex axis is 0°. This type of axis is referred to as a horizontal axis. The heart tends to be horizontal, and this type of axis may be seen in obese individuals in whom the diaphragm tends to be elevated.

Chamber Enlargement: No criteria present in this electrocardiogram.

Infarction: No criteria present in this electrocardiogram.

ST Segment and T Wave Abnormalities: No criteria present in this electrocardiogram.

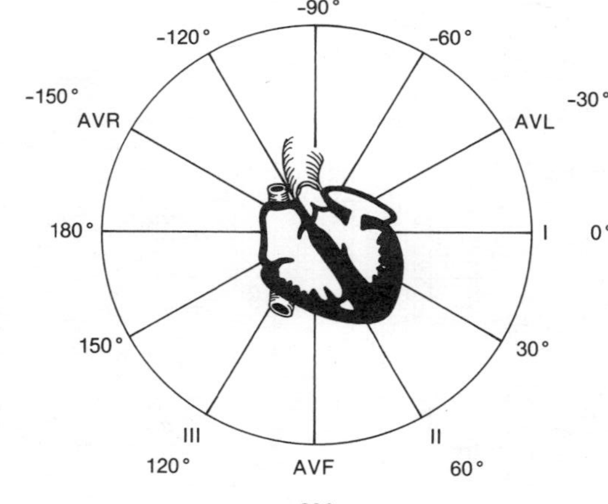

Summary

Sinus tachycardia with a short PR interval

Otherwise normal electrocardiogram

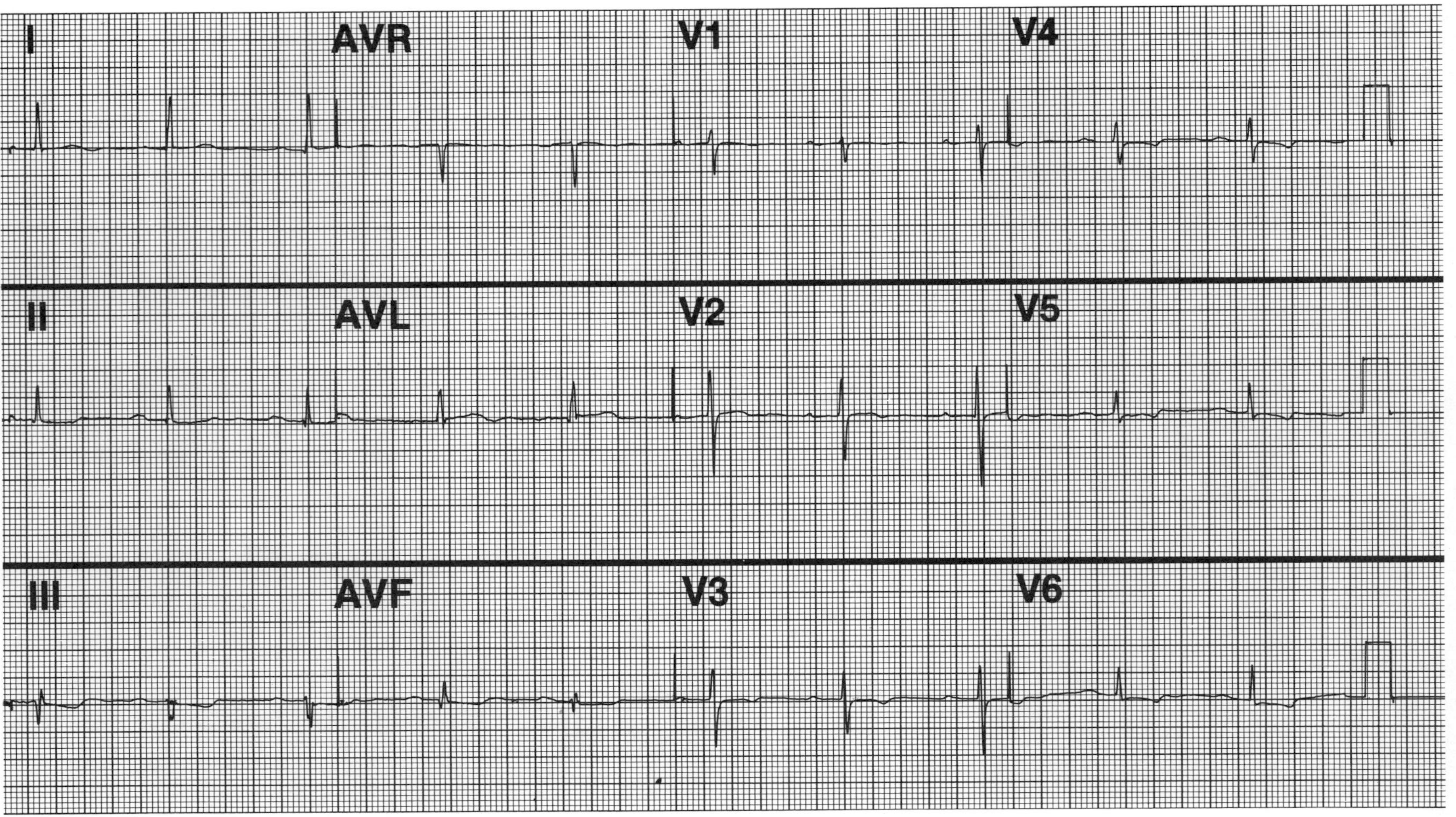
I
AVR
V1
V4
II
AVL
V2
V5
III
AVF
V3
V6

Electrocardiogram #11

Atrial Rate	**64**	**Beats/Minute**
Ventricular Rate	**64**	**Beats/Minute**
PR Interval	**0.25**	**Second**
QRS Duration	**0.09**	**Second**
QT-QTc	**0.40–0.40**	**Second**
QRS Complex Axis	**10**	**Degrees**

Rate: The atrial and ventricular rates are 64 beats per minute.

Rhythm: The PR interval is 0.25 second and constant. The diagnosis of normal sinus rhythm (borderline sinus bradycardia).

Conduction Abnormalities: Since the PR interval is prolonged and constant, the diagnosis of first degree atrioventricular block should be made.

QRS Complex Axis: The mean QRS complex axis is 10°.

Chamber Enlargement: No criteria present in this electrocardiogram.

Infarction: No criteria present in this electrocardiogram.

ST Segment and T Wave Abnormalities: There are nonspecific ST segment changes. One should note there is a flattening of the T waves together with T wave inversions across the mid and left precordium. These changes are suggestive of lateral wall ischemia.

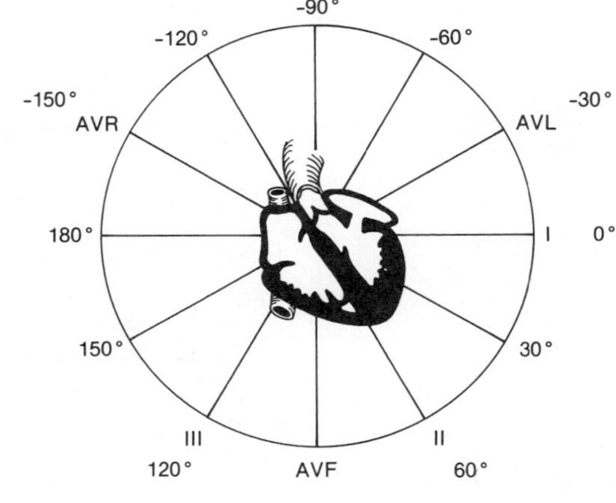

Summary

Sinus bradycardia with first degree atrioventricular block

Lateral wall ischemia

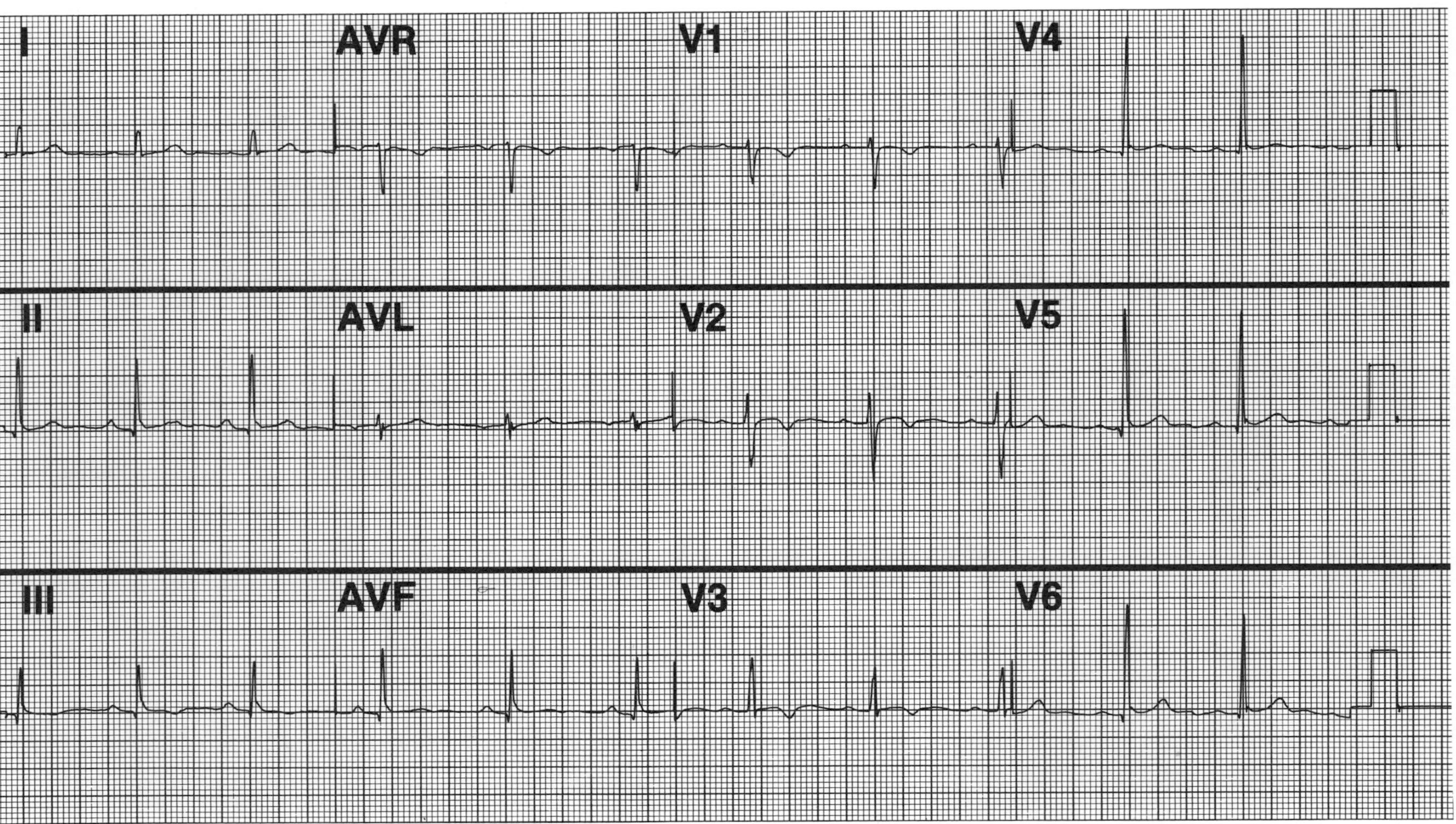
I
AVR
V1
V4
II
AVL
V2
V5
III
AVF
V3
V6

Electrocardiogram #12

Atrial Rate	68	**Beats/Minute**
Ventricular Rate	68	**Beats/Minute**
PR Interval	0.20	**Second**
QRS Duration	0.09	**Second**
QT-QTc	0.38–0.40	**Second**
QRS Complex Axis	70	**Degrees**

Rate: The atrial and ventricular rates are 68 beats per minute.

Rhythm: The PR interval is 0.20 second and constant. The rhythm is normal sinus rhythm.

Conduction Abnormalities: No criteria present in this electrocardiogram.

QRS Complex Axis: The mean QRS complex axis is 70°.

Chamber Enlargement: No criteria present in this electrocardiogram.

Infarction: No criteria present in this electrocardiogram.

ST Segment and T Wave Abnormalities: Although the T waves are normal in the lateral left precordium, they are abnormal in leads V1 to V3. This abnormality of T wave inversions is commonly called a persistent juvenile T wave abnormality. The term juvenile T wave pattern is used to define any T wave negativity in the right precordium even if only in leads V1 and V2. Occasionally, it may be seen persisting through leads V3 and V4. It is termed a juvenile T wave pattern because in children the T wave is normally negative in the right precordium. Generally, however, by the time adolescence has been reached, the T wave is rarely negative beyond lead V1. Various maneuvers can normalize the juvenile T wave pattern (make the T wave upright). Frequently, deep breathing will normalize the juvenile pattern into the adult pattern. It is most important to recognize juvenile T pattern and differentiate it from other ischemic and nonischemic T wave abnormalities.

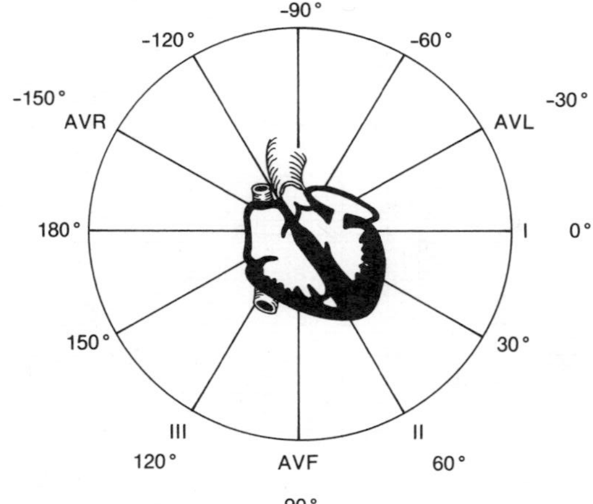

Summary

Normal sinus rhythm

Persistent juvenile T wave pattern

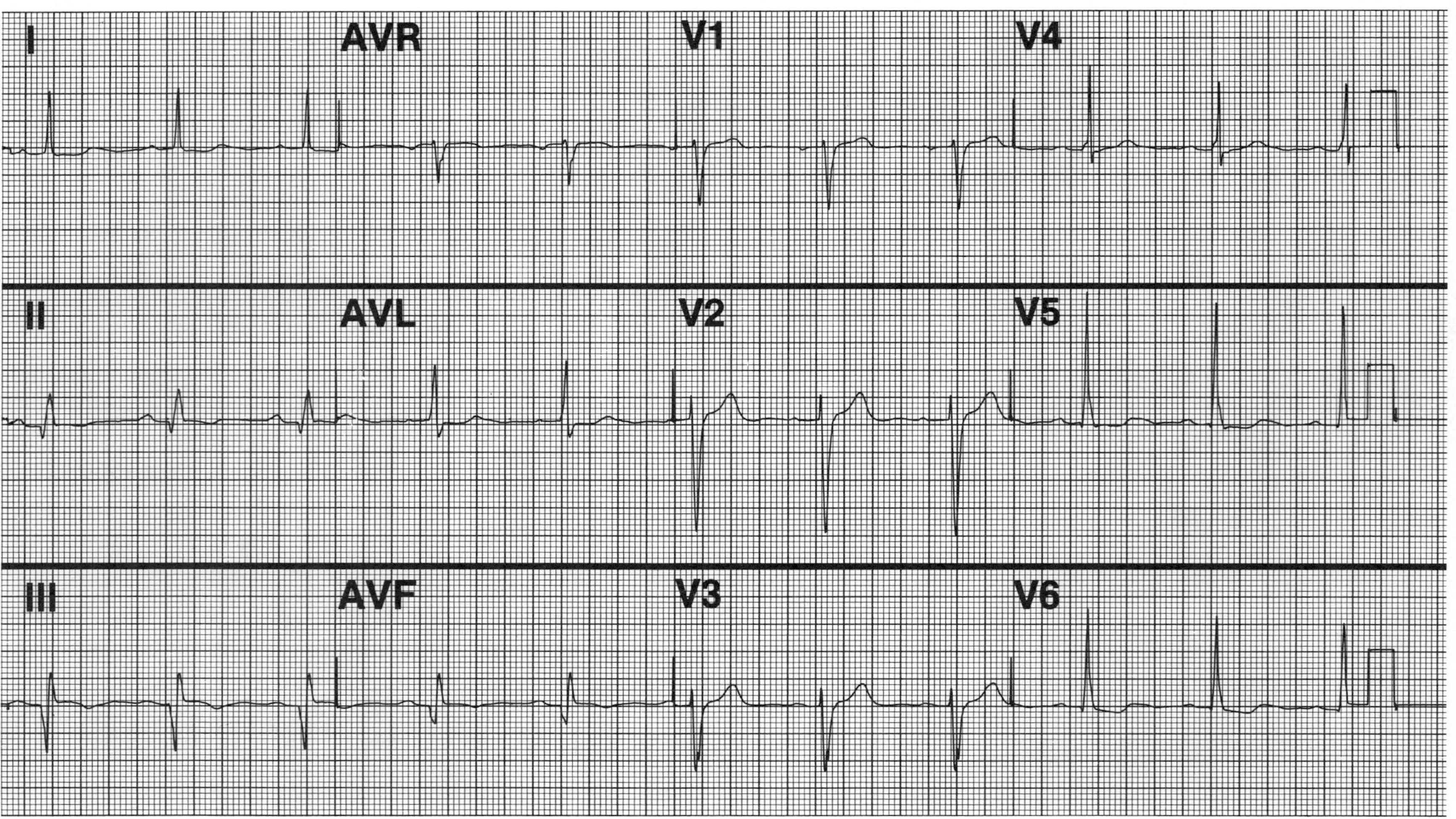
I
AVR
V1
V4
II
AVL
V2
V5
III
AVF
V3
V6

Electrocardiogram #13

Atrial Rate	**67**	**Beats/Minute**
Ventricular Rate	**67**	**Beats/Minute**
PR Interval	**0.22**	**Second**
QRS Duration	**0.13**	**Second**
QT-QTc	**0.40–0.42**	**Second**
QRS Complex Axis	**5**	**Degrees**

Rate: The atrial and ventricular rates are 67 beats per minute.

Rhythm: The PR interval is 0.22 second and constant. The diagnosis is normal sinus rhythm.

Conduction Abnormalities: Since the PR interval is prolonged and constant, the diagnosis of first degree atrioventricular block should be made. The QRS complex duration is prolonged at 0.13 second. However, there are no other criteria for either a left or right bundle branch block; therefore, a nonspecific intraventricular conduction delay exists.

QRS Complex Axis: The QRS complex axis is slightly positive in lead AVF; therefore, the mean QRS complex is 5°.

Chamber Enlargement: Although this electrocardiogram displays high voltages, it does not meet the criteria for left ventricular hypertrophy.

Infarction: The salient feature of this electrocardiogram is the wide and deep Q wave seen in leads II, III and AVF. These leads also show a 1-mm ST segment elevation and T wave inversions indicative of an inferior infarction, age undetermined.

ST Segment and T Wave Abnormalities: No criteria present in this electrocardiogram.

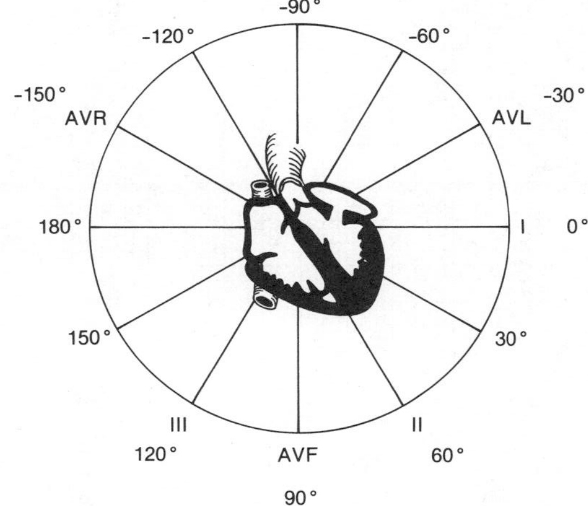

Summary

Normal sinus rhythm with first degree atrioventricular block

Nonspecific intraventricular block

Inferior myocardial infarction, age undetermined

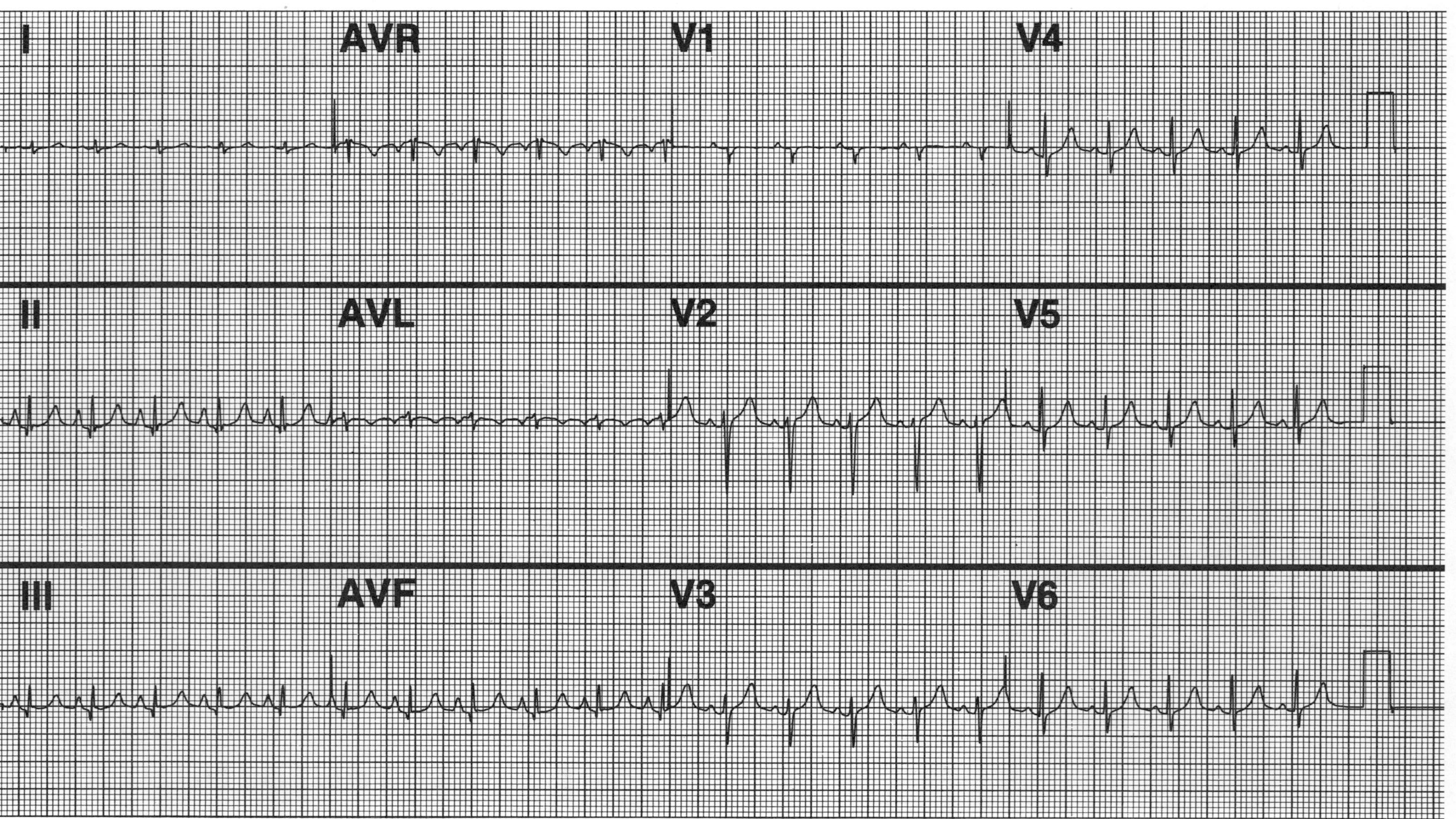
I
AVR
V1
V4
II
AVL
V2
V5
III
AVF
V3
V6

Electrocardiogram #14

Atrial Rate	**163**	**Beats/Minute**
Ventricular Rate	**163**	**Beats/Minute**
PR Interval	**0.11**	**Second**
QRS Duration	**0.07**	**Second**
QT-QTc	**0.30–0.42**	**Second**
QRS Complex Axis	**90**	**Degrees**

Rate: The atrial and ventricular rates are 163 beats per minute and are regular.

Rhythm: The PR interval is 0.11 second and constant. The rhythm is sinus tachycardia.

Conduction Abnormalities: No criteria present in this electrocardiogram.

QRS Complex Axis: The mean QRS complex axis is approximately perpendicular to lead I; therefore, the QRS is 90°. This type of axis, which is termed a vertical axis, is seen in tall, thin individuals in which the diaphragm tends to be displaced downward and the heart's axis tends to be more vertical.

Chamber Enlargement: One should note the very prominent P waves in the inferior leads II, III and AVF. The P waves in lead II are 4 mm in height. These peaked P waves are strongly suggestive of p pulmonale or right atrial enlargement.

Infarction: No criteria present in this electrocardiogram.

ST Segment and T Wave Abnormalities: No criteria present in this electrocardiogram.

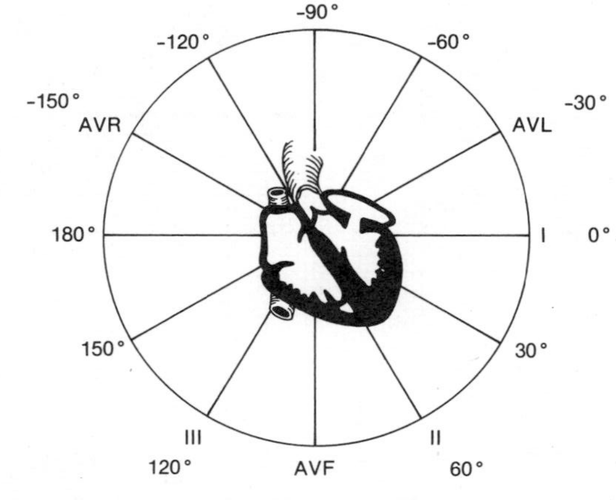

Summary

Sinus tachycardia

Right atrial enlargement

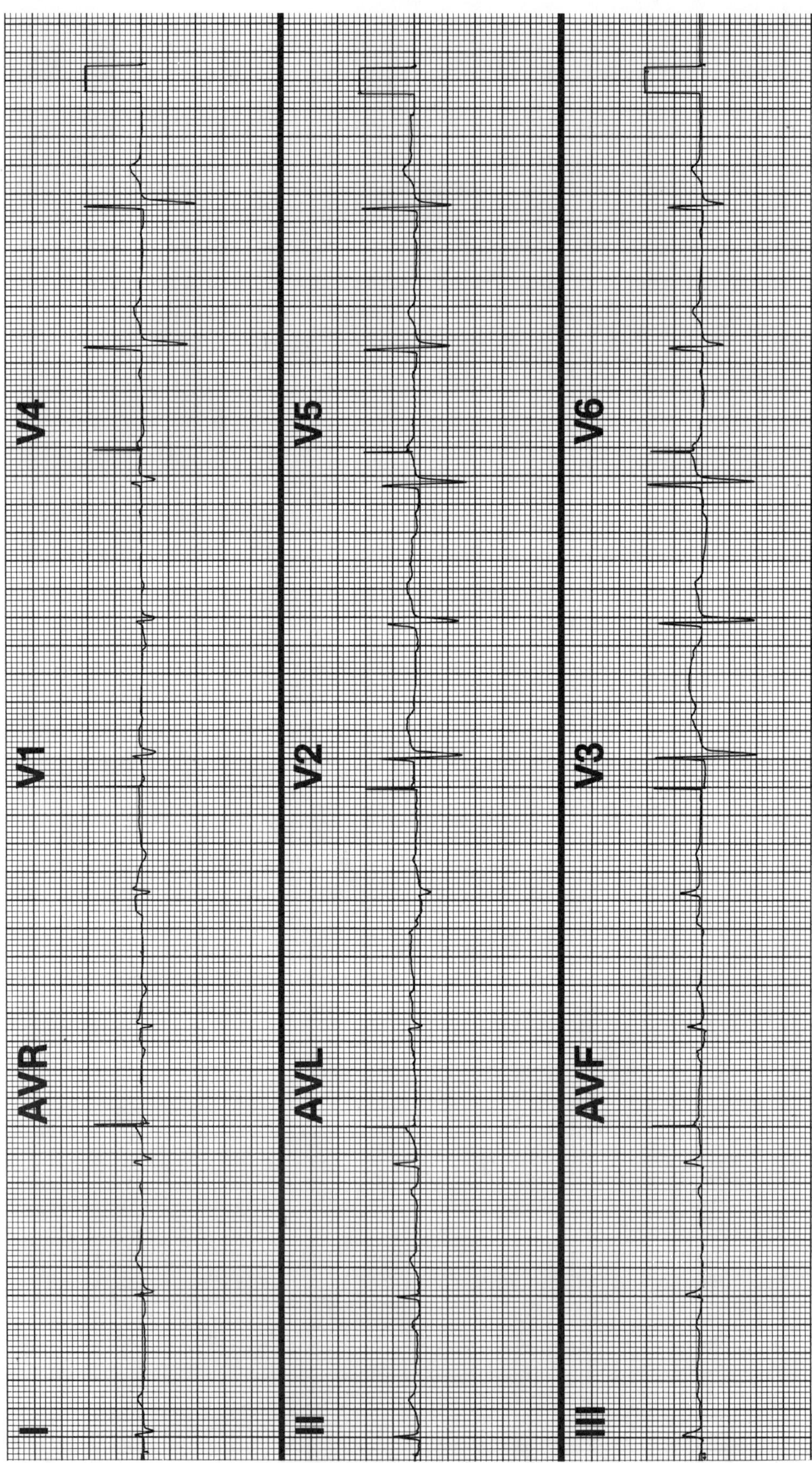
I
AVR
V1
V4
II
AVL
V2
V5
III
AVF
V3
V6

Electrocardiogram #15

Atrial Rate	**64**	**Beats/Minute**
Ventricular Rate	**64**	**Beats/Minute**
PR Interval	**0.22**	**Second**
QRS Duration	**0.09**	**Second**
QT-QTc	**0.41–0.40**	**Second**
QRS Complex Axis	**90**	**Degrees**

Rate: The atrial and ventricular rates are 64 beats per minute.

Rhythm: The PR interval is 0.22 second. The diagnosis is normal sinus rhythm (borderline sinus bradycardia).

Conduction Abnormalities: Since the PR interval is prolonged and constant, the diagnosis of first degree atrioventricular block should be made.

QRS Complex Axis: The mean QRS complex axis is perpendicular to lead I; therefore, it is 90°.

Chamber Enlargement: No criteria present in this electrocardiogram.

Infarction: No criteria present in this electrocardiogram.

ST Segment and T Wave Abnormalities: No criteria present in this electrocardiogram.

Other Findings: Although the voltages in the standard leads are low, this electrocardiogram does not meet criteria for low voltage. The term low voltage is used to describe an electrocardiogram in which the amplitude of each QRS complex is less than 10 mm in all leads. In this tracing there is an RS complex in lead V4 in which the R wave is 10 mm. In addition, there is a Rs complex in lead V5 in which the R wave is 10 mm.

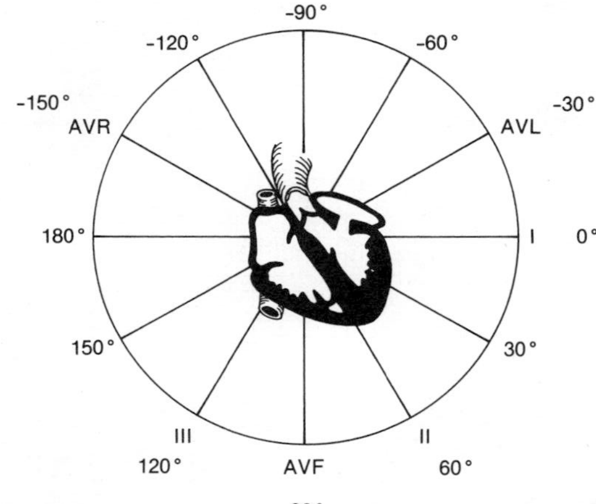

Summary

Sinus bradycardia with first degree atrioventricular block

Borderline low voltage

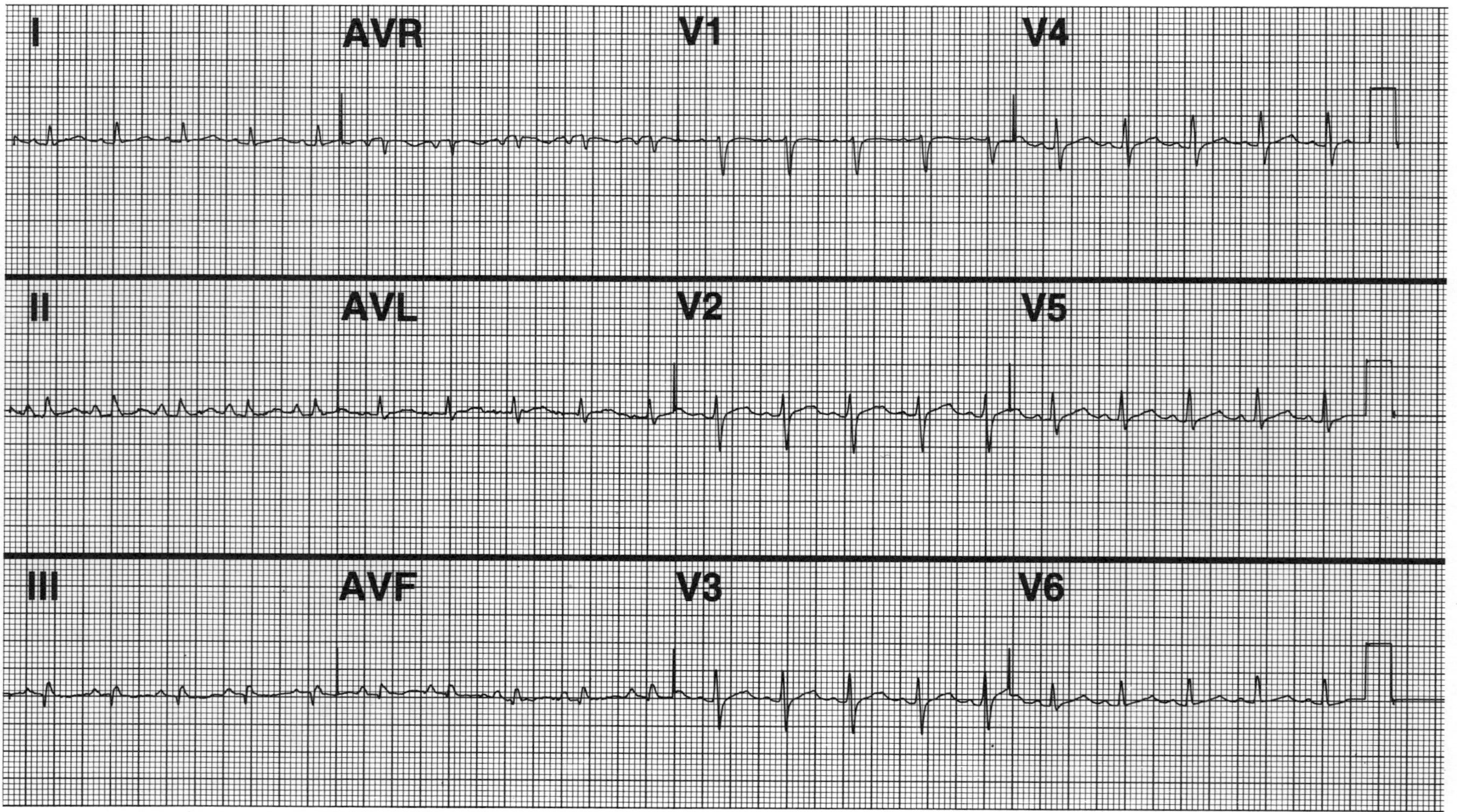
I
AVR
V1
V4
II
AVL
V2
V5
III
AVF
V3
V6

Electrocardiogram #16

Atrial Rate	**125**	**Beats/Minute**
Ventricular Rate	**125**	**Beats/Minute**
PR Interval	**0.14**	**Second**
QRS Duration	**0.09**	**Second**
QT-QTc	**0.32–0.45**	**Second**
QRS Complex Axis	**20**	**Degrees**

Rate: The atrial and ventricular rates are 125 beats per minute.

Rhythm: The PR interval is 0.14 second and constant. The diagnosis is sinus tachycardia.

Conduction Abnormalities: No criteria present in this electrocardiogram.

QRS Complex Axis: The mean QRS complex axis is 20°.

Chamber Enlargement: No criteria present in this electrocardiogram.

Infarction: No criteria present in this electrocardiogram.

ST Segment and T Wave Abnormalities: No criteria present in this electrocardiogram.

Other Findings: The striking feature of this electrocardiogram is the generalized low voltage of the QRS complex. As was noted in the previous tracing, the term low voltage is used to describe an electrocardiogram in which every lead has a QRS complex amplitude of less than 10 mm. There are many causes of reduced voltage of the electrocardiogram. Chronic obstructive lung disease and mitral stenosis are two major causes. In addition, diffuse myocardial disease as well as cardiomegaly and congestive heart failure is a known cause of reduced QRS complex voltage. Obesity and myxedema are also common causes. One of the most common causes of reduced voltage in the precordial leads alone, in the absence of chronic obstructive lung disease, myocardial or pericardial disease, is obesity. It is important to indicate that obesity generally does not diminish the limb lead voltage to the same extent as it reduces the voltage in the precordial leads.

Summary

Sinus tachycardia

Low voltage

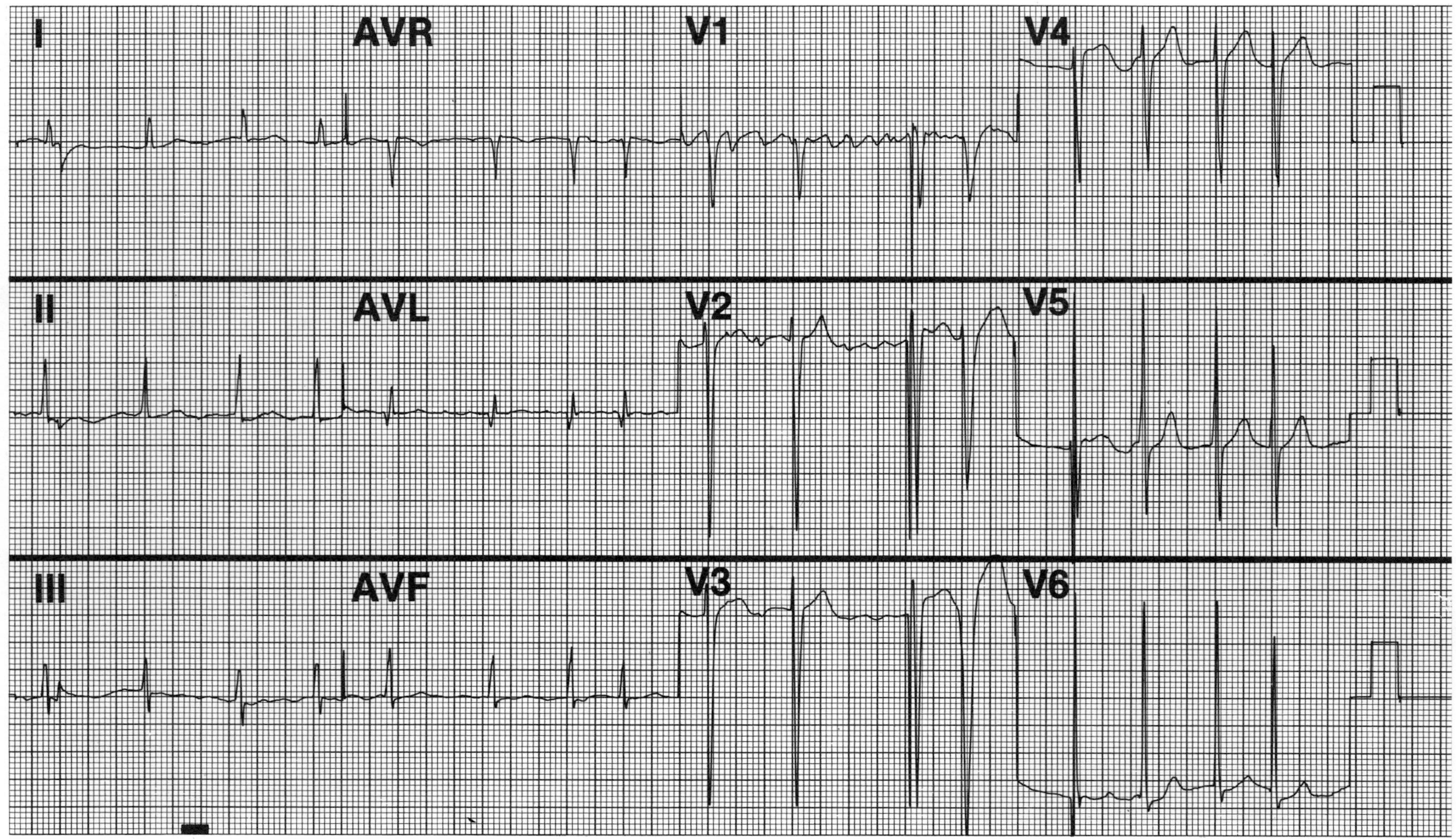
I
AVR
V1
V4
II
AVL
V2
V5
III
AVF
V3
V6

Electrocardiogram #17

Atrial Rate	—	**Beats/Minute**
Ventricular Rate	100	**Beats/Minute**
PR Interval	—	**Second**
QRS Duration	0.10	**Second**
QT-QTc	0.33–0.42	**Second**
QRS Complex Axis	50	**Degrees**

Rate: The average ventricular rate is 100 beats per minute.

Rhythm: The rhythm is grossly irregular and is said to be "irregularly irregular." This means the timing of the R-R complexes is irregular, and there is no regularity to the irregularity. This rhythm is therefore atrial fibrillation.

Conduction Abnormalities: No criteria present in this electrocardiogram.

QRS Complex Axis: The mean QRS complex axis is 50°.

Chamber Enlargement: One notices immediately the striking high voltage seen in the precordial leads. The R wave in lead V6 measures 35 mm, and the S waves in lead V2 measures 35 mm. Therefore, voltage criteria for left ventricular enlargement is present.

Infarction: No criteria present in this electrocardiogram.

ST Segment and T Wave Abnormalities: There is ST segment depression seen in the lateral precordial leads. These are secondary ST segment changes (strain pattern) seen in association with left ventricular hypertrophy. These changes provide additional evidence for left ventricular hypertrophy.

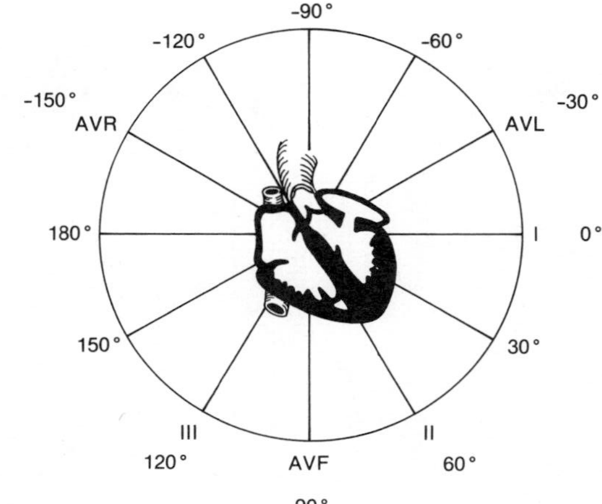

Summary

Atrial fibrillation

Left ventricular hypertrophy

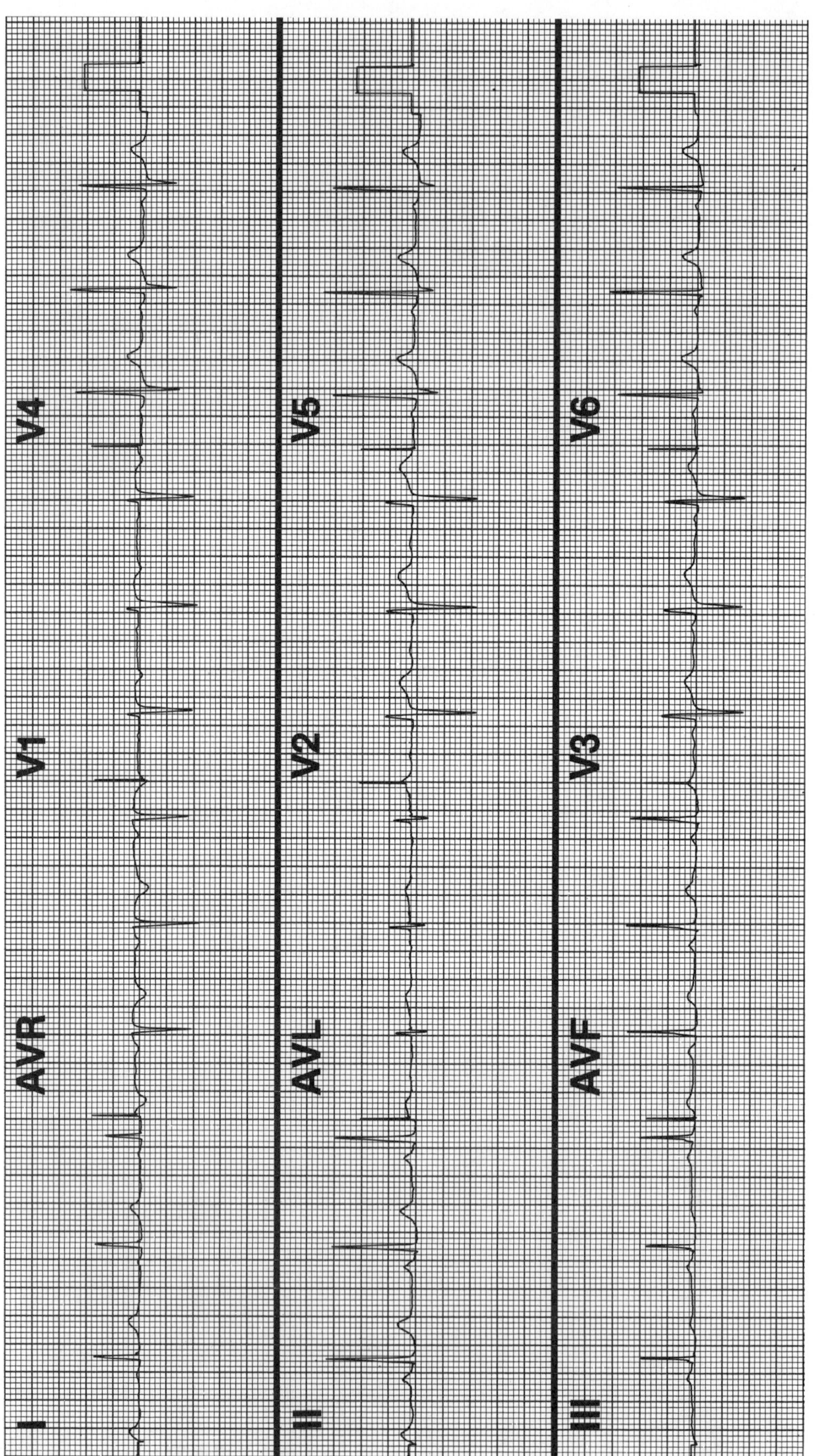
I
AVR
V1
V4
II
AVL
V2
V5
III
AVF
V3
V6

Electrocardiogram #18

Atrial Rate	**79**	**Beats/Minute**
Ventricular Rate	**79**	**Beats/Minute**
PR Interval	**0.16**	**Second**
QRS Duration	**0.09**	**Second**
QT-QTc	**0.39–0.44**	**Second**
QRS Complex Axis	**60**	**Degrees**

Rate: The atrial and ventricular rates are 79 beats per minute.

Rhythm: The PR interval is 0.16 second and constant. The rhythm is normal sinus rhythm.

Conduction Abnormalities: No criteria present in this electrocardiogram.

QRS Complex Axis: The mean QRS complex axis is 60°.

Chamber Enlargement: No criteria present in this electrocardiogram.

Infarction: No criteria present in this electrocardiogram.

ST Segment and T Wave Abnormalities: No criteria present in this electrocardiogram.

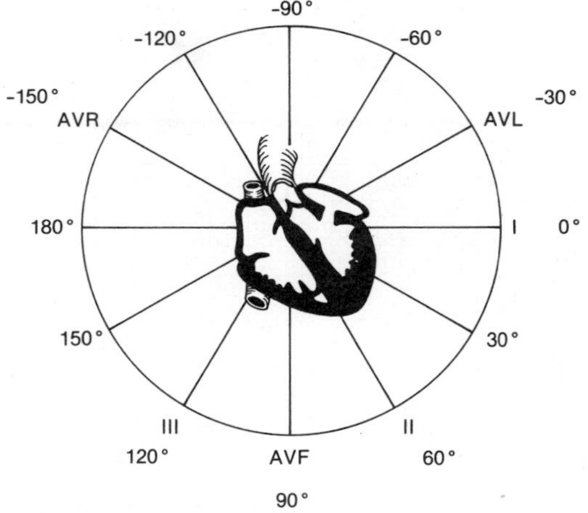

Summary

Normal sinus rhythm

Normal electrocardiogram

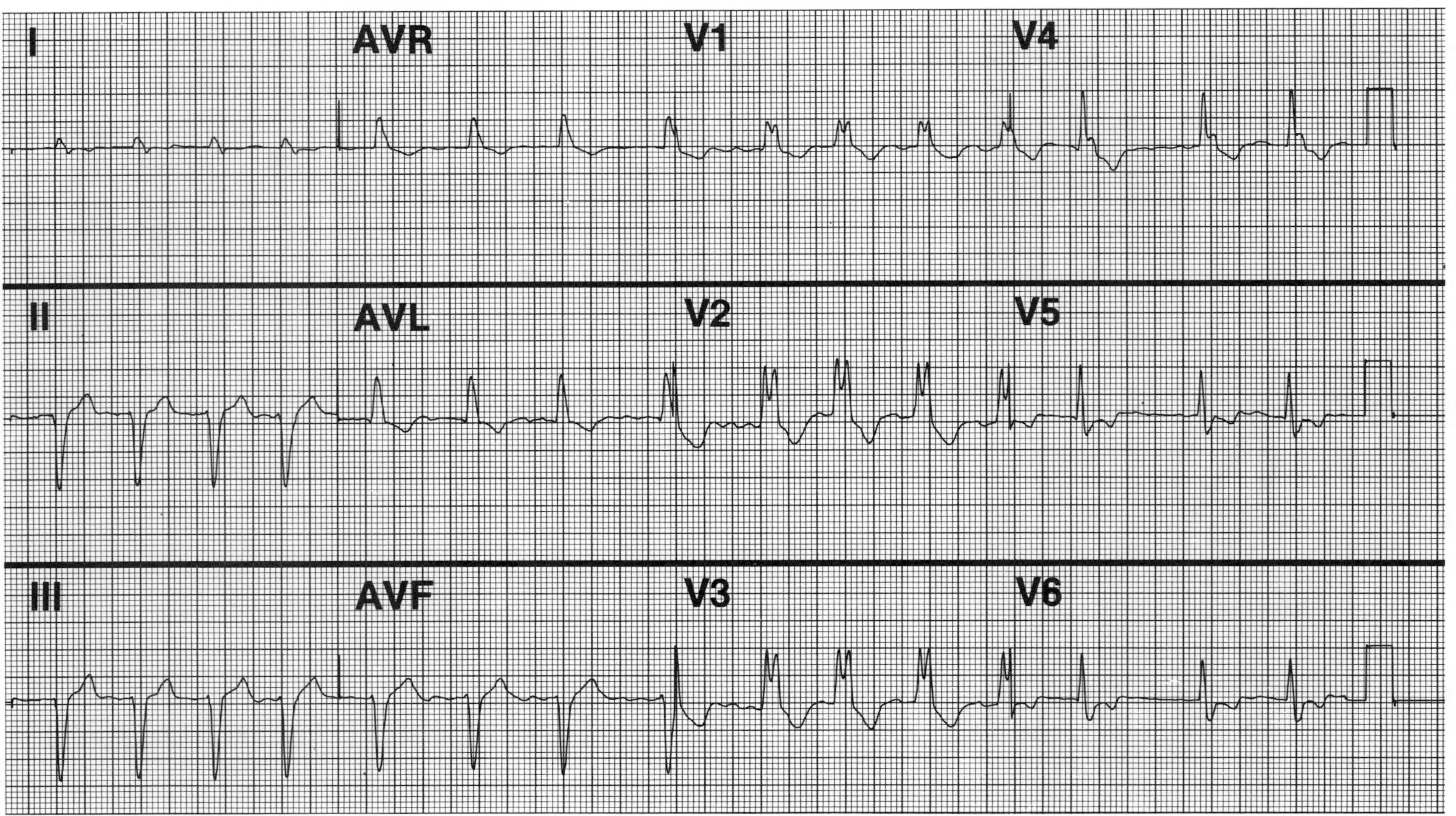

I
AVR
V1
V4
II
AVL
V2
V5
III
AVF
V3
V6

Electrocardiogram #19

Atrial Rate	**—**	**Beats/Minute**
Ventricular Rate	**90**	**Beats/Minute**
PR Interval	**—**	**Second**
QRS Duration	**0.16**	**Second**
QT-QTc	**0.38–0.46**	**Second**
QRS Complex Axis	**−80**	**Degrees**

Rate: The average ventricular rate is 90 beats per minute.

Rhythm: Notice that the P waves are absent, and the rhythm is irregular. There is also no regularity to this irregular rhythm. Therefore, the rhythm is atrial fibrillation.

Conduction Abnormalities: The QRS complex duration is 0.16 second. A notched R complex is seen in leads V1 to V3, and slurring of the S wave is seen in leads V5 and V6. These findings are indicative of a right bundle branch block. In addition, there is significant abnormal left axis deviation (−80°) seen in this electrocardiogram. This axis is the result of the large Rs complex seen in lead I and the rS complex in leads II, III and AVF, which are diagnostic of a left anterior hemiblock. This patient has a right bundle branch block and a left anterior fascicular block. This is termed bifascicular block.

QRS Complex Axis: The mean QRS complex axis is approximately −80°.

Chamber Enlargement: No criteria present in this electrocardiogram.

Infarction: No criteria present in this electrocardiogram.

ST Segment and T Wave Abnormalities: The ST segment and T wave abnormalities seen in the precordial leads are secondary changes to the right bundle branch block.

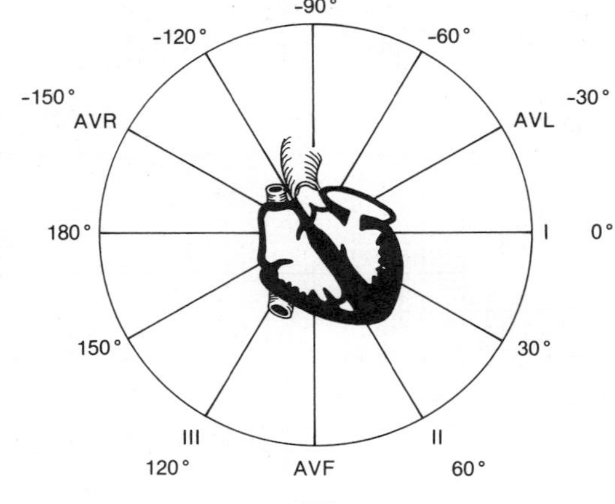

Summary

Atrial fibrillation

Right bundle branch block

Left anterior hemiblock

Bifascicular block

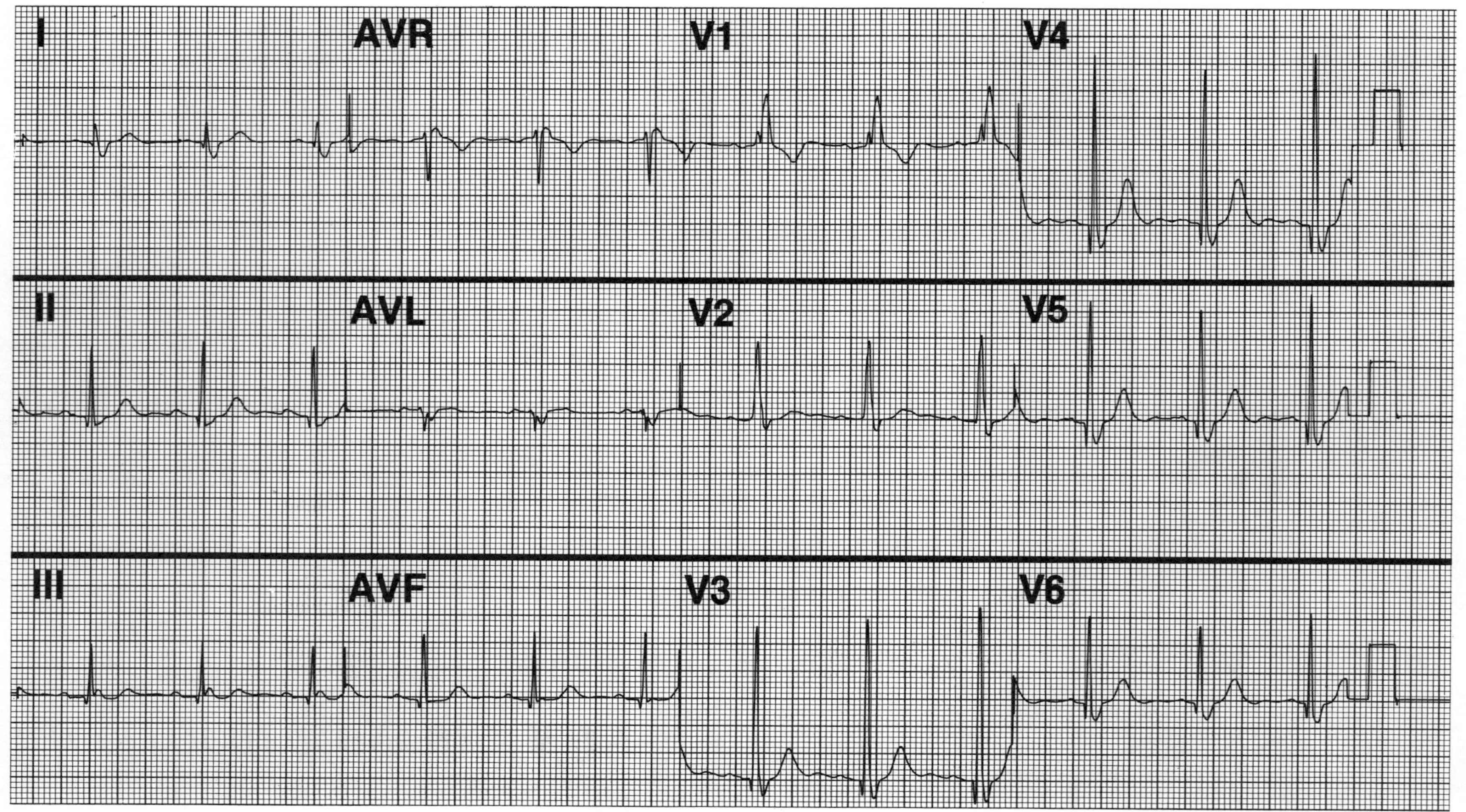
I
AVR
V1
V4
II
AVL
V2
V5
III
AVF
V3
V6

Electrocardiogram #20

Atrial Rate	75	**Beats/Minute**
Ventricular Rate	75	**Beats/Minute**
PR Interval	0.18	**Second**
QRS Duration	0.14	**Second**
QT-QTc	0.40–0.45	**Second**
QRS Complex Axis	80	**Degrees**

Rate: The atrial and ventricular rates are 75 beats per minute.

Rhythm: The PR interval is 0.18 second and constant. Therefore, the rhythm is normal sinus rhythm.

Conduction Abnormalities: There is an rsR′ complex seen in lead V1 and a slurring of the S waves in leads I and V6. These changes are indicative of a right bundle branch block. A right bundle branch block produces an abnormality of the terminal portion of the mean QRS vector and is associated with secondary ST segment and T wave changes.

QRS Complex Axis: The QRS axis is 80°.

Chamber Enlargement: No criteria present in this electrocardiogram.

Infarction: No criteria present in this electrocardiogram.

ST Segment and T Wave Abnormalities: The ST segment and T wave abnormalities seen in leads V1 and V2 are secondary changes related to the conduction abnormality.

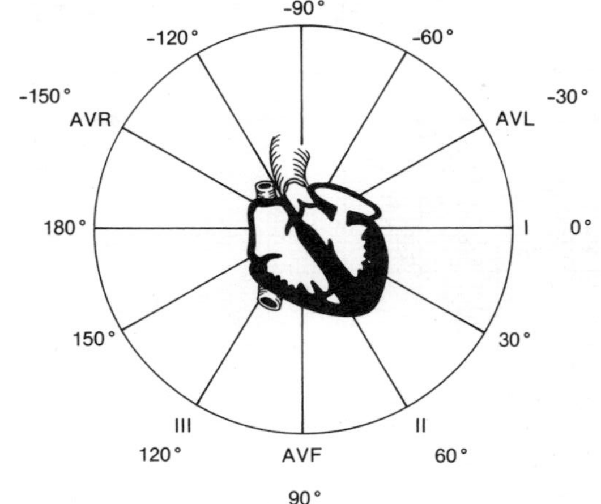

Summary

Normal sinus rhythm

Right bundle branch block

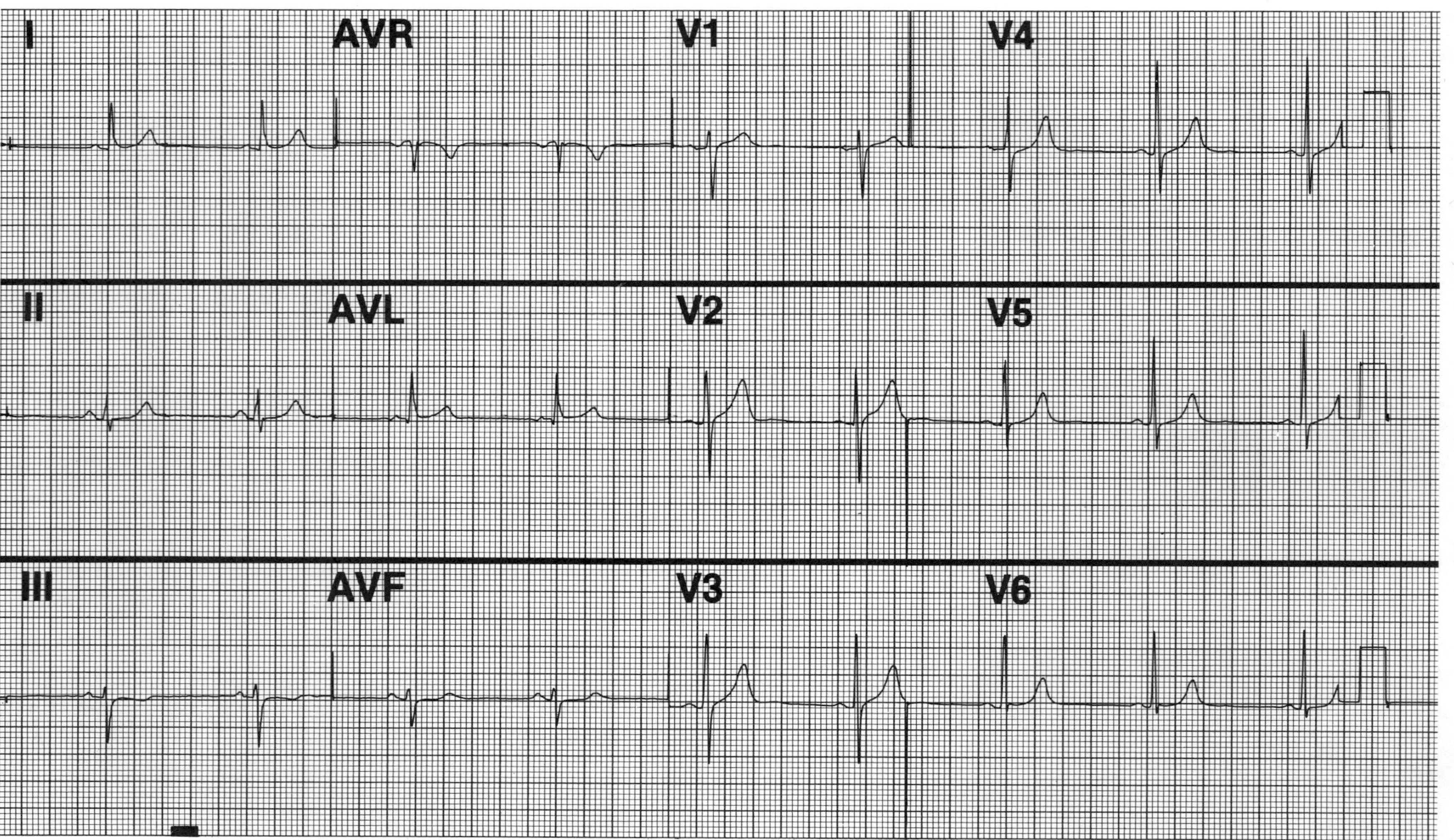
I
AVR
V1
V4
II
AVL
V2
V5
III
AVF
V3
V6

Electrocardiogram #21

Atrial Rate	57	**Beats/Minute**
Ventricular Rate	57	**Beats/Minute**
PR Interval	0.16	**Second**
QRS Duration	0.08	**Second**
QT-QTc	0.40–0.38	**Second**
QRS Complex Axis	−20	**Degrees**

Rate: The atrial and ventricular rates are 57 beats per minute.

Rhythm: The PR interval is 0.16 second and constant. The rhythm is therefore sinus bradycardia.

Conduction Abnormalities: No criteria present in this electrocardiogram.

QRS Complex Axis: The QRS complex is positive in lead I and negative in lead AVF. This places the mean QRS complex axis between 0 and −90°. The complex is most equiphasic in lead II. If the complex were equiphasic in lead II, the mean QRS complex axis would be −30°. However, since it is slightly positive in lead II, by vector resolution one would determine that the QRS axis is less negative; therefore, the mean QRS complex axis is −20°. Some of the more common causes of left axis deviation include left bundle branch block, left anterior hemiblock and left ventricular hypertrophy. It is also seen in normal individuals, especially those who are obese.

Chamber Enlargement: No criteria present in this electrocardiogram.

Infarction: No criteria present in this electrocardiogram.

ST Segment and T Wave Abnormalities: No criteria present in this electrocardiogram.

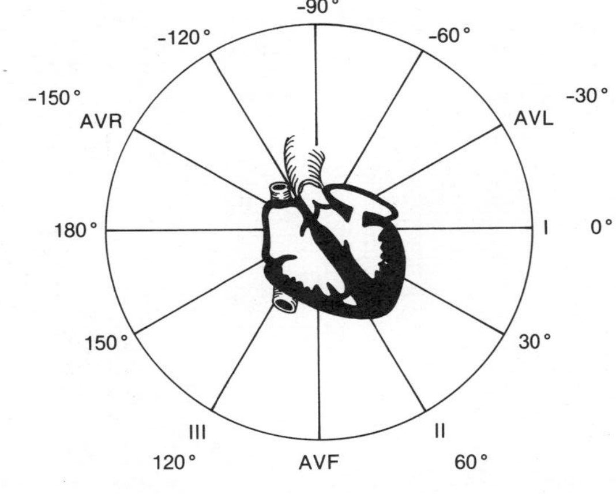

Summary

Sinus bradycardia

Leftward axis, otherwise normal electrocardiogram

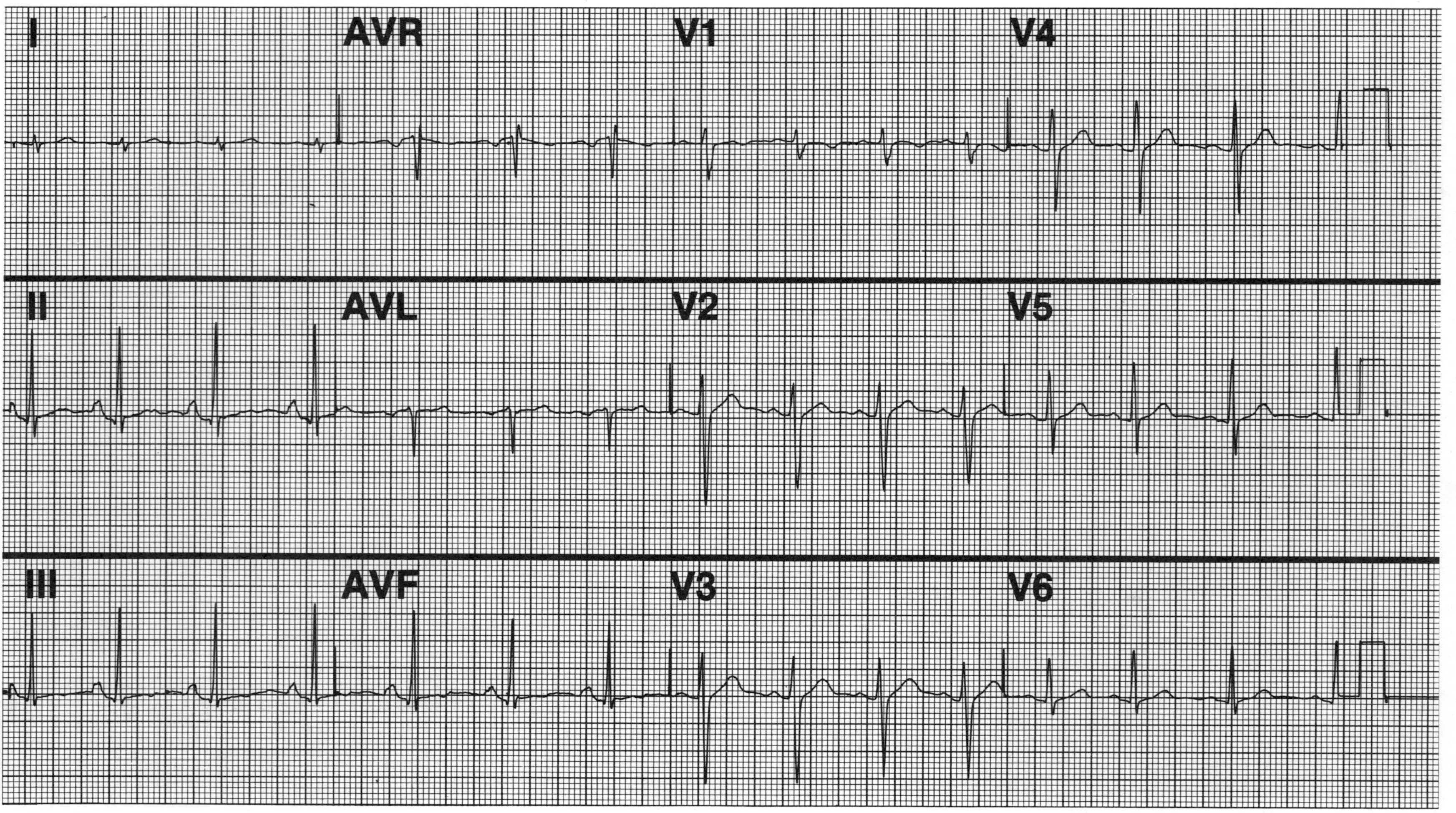
I
AVR
V1
V4
II
AVL
V2
V5
III
AVF
V3
V6

Electrocardiogram #22

Atrial Rate	**88**	**Beats/Minute**
Ventricular Rate	**88**	**Beats/Minute**
PR Interval	**0.16**	**Second**
QRS Duration	**0.09**	**Second**
QT-QTc	**0.35–0.41**	**Second**
QRS Complex Axis	**90**	**Degrees**

Rate: The atrial and ventricular rates are 88 beats per minute.

Rhythm: The PR interval is 0.16 second. The rhythm is normal sinus rhythm.

Conduction Abnormalities: No criteria present in this electrocardiogram.

QRS Complex Axis: Since the complex is equiphasic in lead I and positive in lead AVF, the mean QRS complex is +90°.

Chamber Enlargement: No criteria present in this electrocardiogram.

Infarction: No criteria present in this electrocardiogram.

ST Segment and T Wave Abnormalities: The ST segment and T waves in leads III and AVF are relatively flat; however, they appear normal in all other leads.

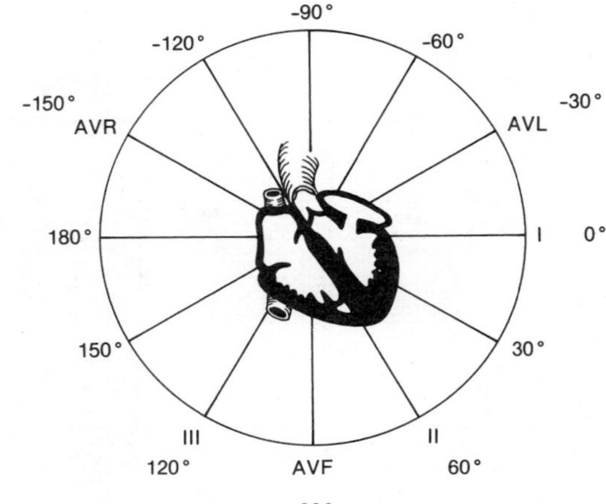

Summary

Normal sinus rhythm

Normal electrocardiogram

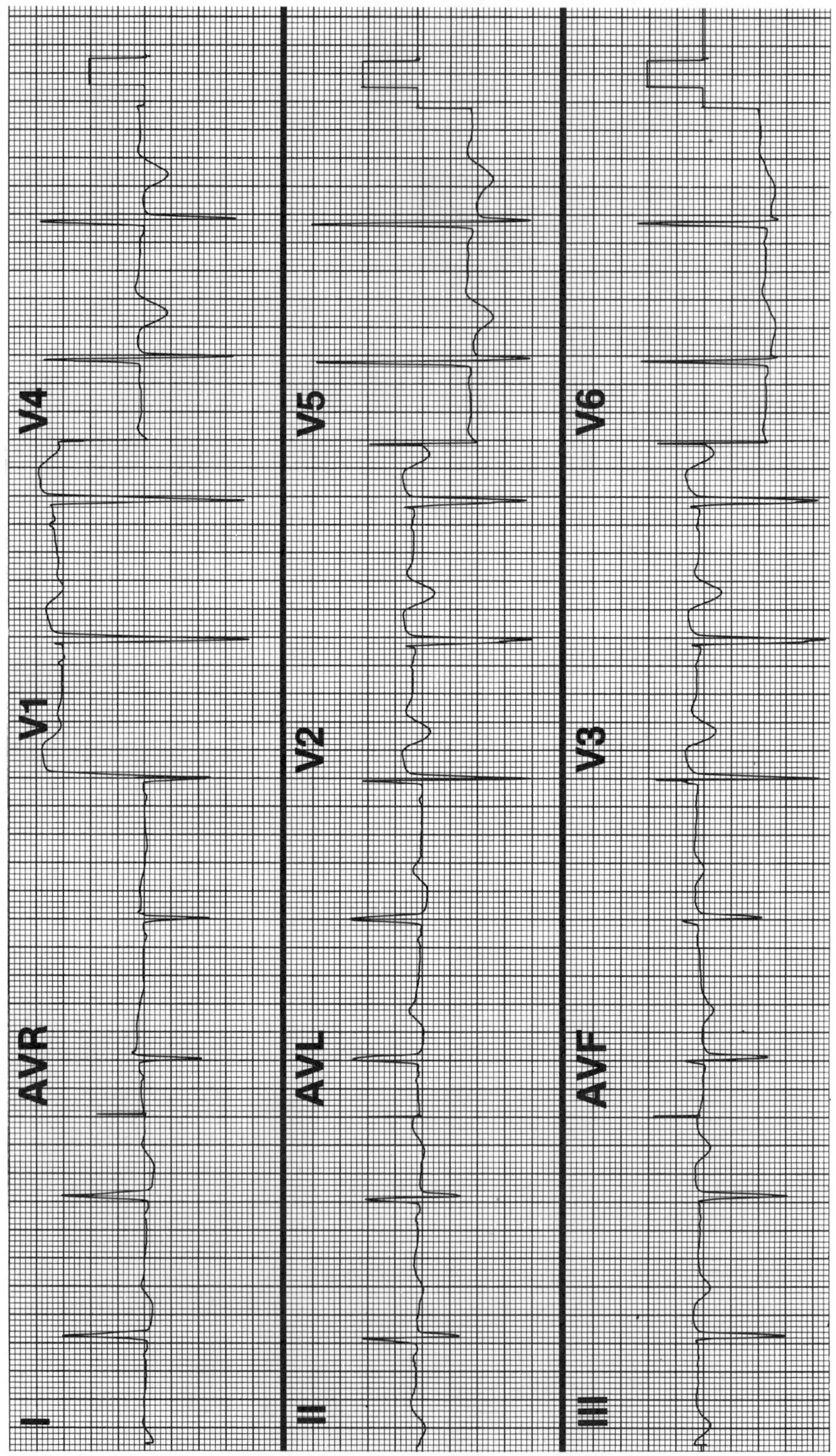
I
AVR
V1
V4
II
AVL
V2
V5
III
AVF
V3
V6

Electrocardiogram #23

Atrial Rate	**63**	**Beats/Minute**
Ventricular Rate	**63**	**Beats/Minute**
PR Interval	**0.17**	**Second**
QRS Duration	**0.10**	**Second**
QT-QTc	**0.52–0.53**	**Second**
QRS Complex Axis	**−25**	**Degrees**

Rate: The atrial and ventricular rates are 63 beats per minute.

Rhythm: The PR interval is 0.17 second and constant. The rhythm is sinus bradycardia.

Conduction Abnormalities: No criteria present in this electrocardiogram.

QRS Complex Axis: The QRS complex axis is −25°. As you note, the QRS complex is positive in lead I and negative in lead AVF. It is, however, slightly more positive in lead II, which would make the complex slightly less negative than −30°. The mean QRS complex axis is therefore −25°.

Chamber Enlargement: One should note that the QRS complex in lead AVL is 13 mm. The diagnosis of left ventricular hypertrophy should be made, as the criterion in lead AVL is the most specific criterion. In addition, secondary repolarization changes are also present in this tracing.

Infarction: No criteria present in this electrocardiogram.

ST Segment and T Wave Abnormalities: There are also diffuse ST segment and T wave abnormalities throughout the precordium.

Other Findings: When one measures the QT interval and compares it with the ventricular rate, one will note that the QT interval is prolonged. When one notices a prolonged QT interval is detected, one should consider myocardial disease, electrolyte imbalance or drug effects. The QT interval is determined from the beginning of the QRS complex to the end of the T wave. The corrected QT interval (QTc) is the QT interval corrected for heart rate. Since the QT interval becomes longer with lower heart rates, dividing this by the square root of the R-R interval corrects the QT for heart rate. The QTc should never exceed 0.42 second in men and 0.43 second in women. The QT interval is prolonged with myocardial damage as well as with many commonly used drugs such as quinidine, procainamide, lidocaine and phenothiazine. In addition, hypocalcemia will prolong the QT interval. One should be careful to determine the precise QT interval and not a QU interval. The U wave is any wave that occurs just after the T wave and prior to the next P wave. The U wave generally has the same configuration as the P wave. It is generally seen in the midprecordial leads. The specific cause of the U wave is unknown, but its presence is commonly associated with bradycardia and hypokalemia.

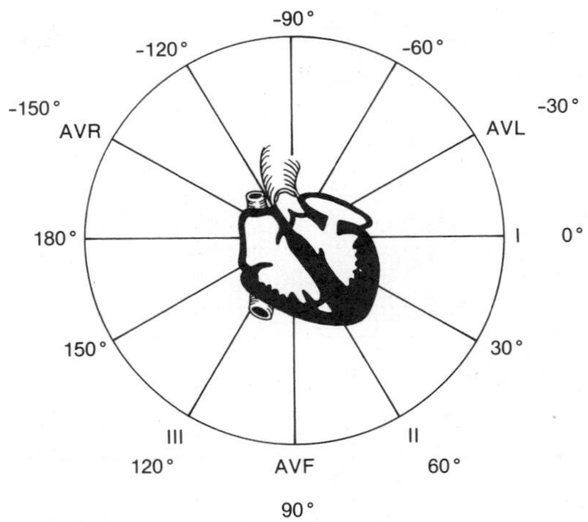

Summary

Sinus bradycardia

Left ventricular hypertrophy

Prolonged QTc interval

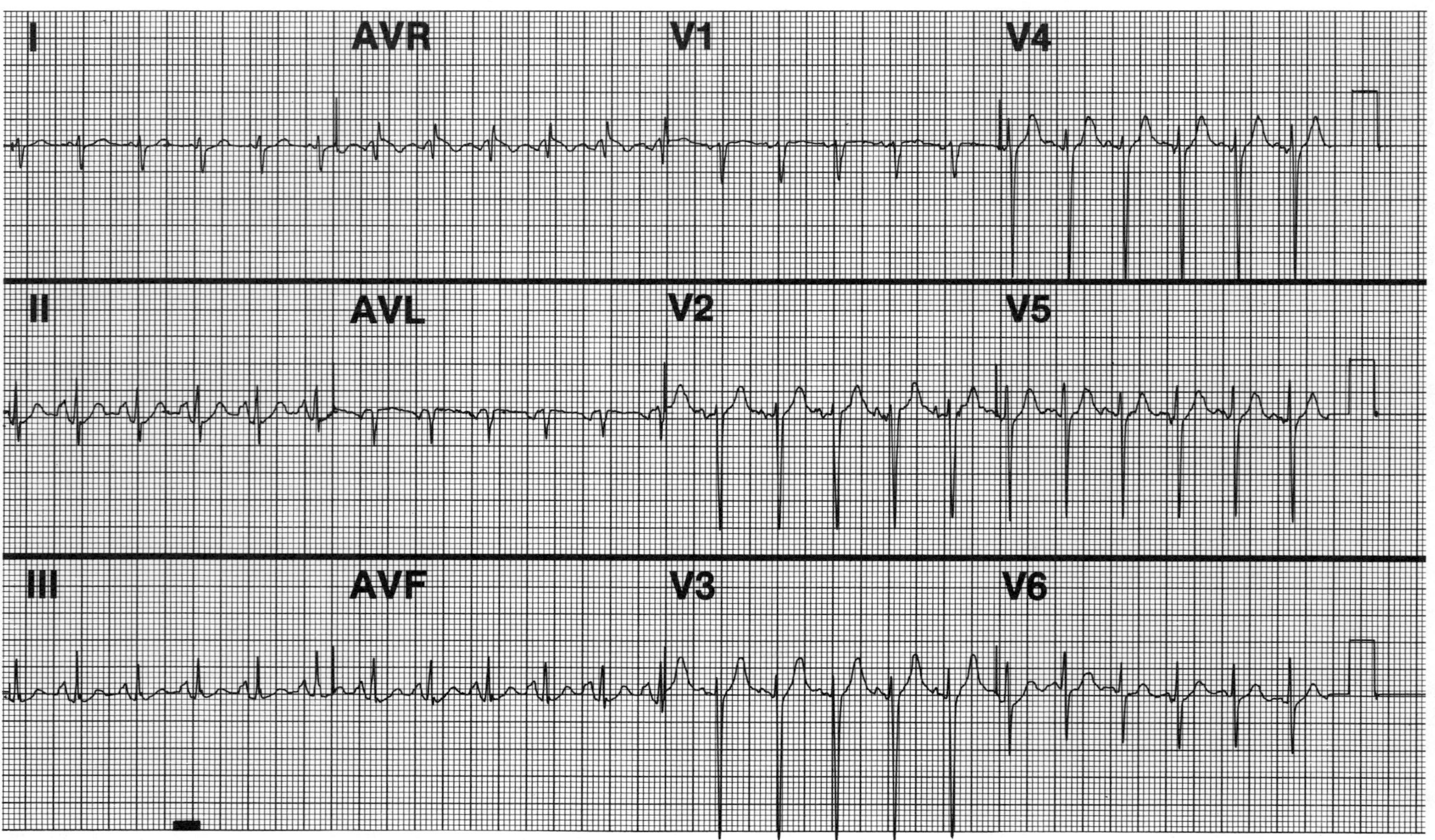
I
AVR
V1
V4
II
AVL
V2
V5
III
AVF
V3
V6

Electrocardiogram #24

Atrial Rate	**143**	**Beats/Minute**
Ventricular Rate	**143**	**Beats/Minute**
PR Interval	**0.12**	**Second**
QRS Duration	**0.07**	**Second**
QT-QTc	**0.29–0.43**	**Second**
QRS Complex Axis	**110**	**Degrees**

Rate: The atrial and ventricular rates are 143 beats per minute.

Rhythm: The PR interval is 0.12 second and constant. The rhythm is sinus tachycardia.

Conduction Abnormalities: No criteria present in this electrocardiogram.

QRS Complex Axis: The mean QRS complex axis is 110°.

Chamber Enlargement: One should note the very large P waves seen in the inferior leads, II, III and AVF. The P waves measure 3 mm in lead II. In addition to being peaked, the P waves appear notched in these leads. In addition, if one looks at the P wave in leads V1 and V2, there is a significant negative component to the P wave that is greater than one box in duration and one box in depth. This finding together with the peaking of the P waves in lead II is diagnostic of biatrial enlargement. Biatrial enlargement in association with abnormal right axis deviation is suggestive of the diagnosis of pulmonary disease.

Infarction: No criteria present in this electrocardiogram.

ST Segment and T Wave Abnormalities: No criteria present in this electrocardiogram.

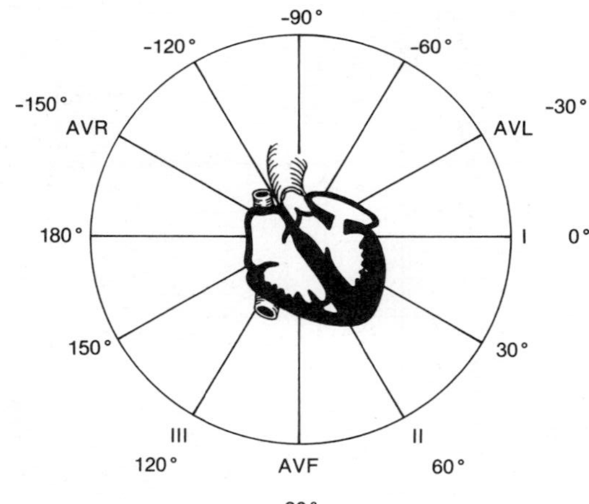

Summary

Sinus tachycardia

Biatrial enlargement

Abnormal right axis deviation

Findings suggestive of pulmonary disease

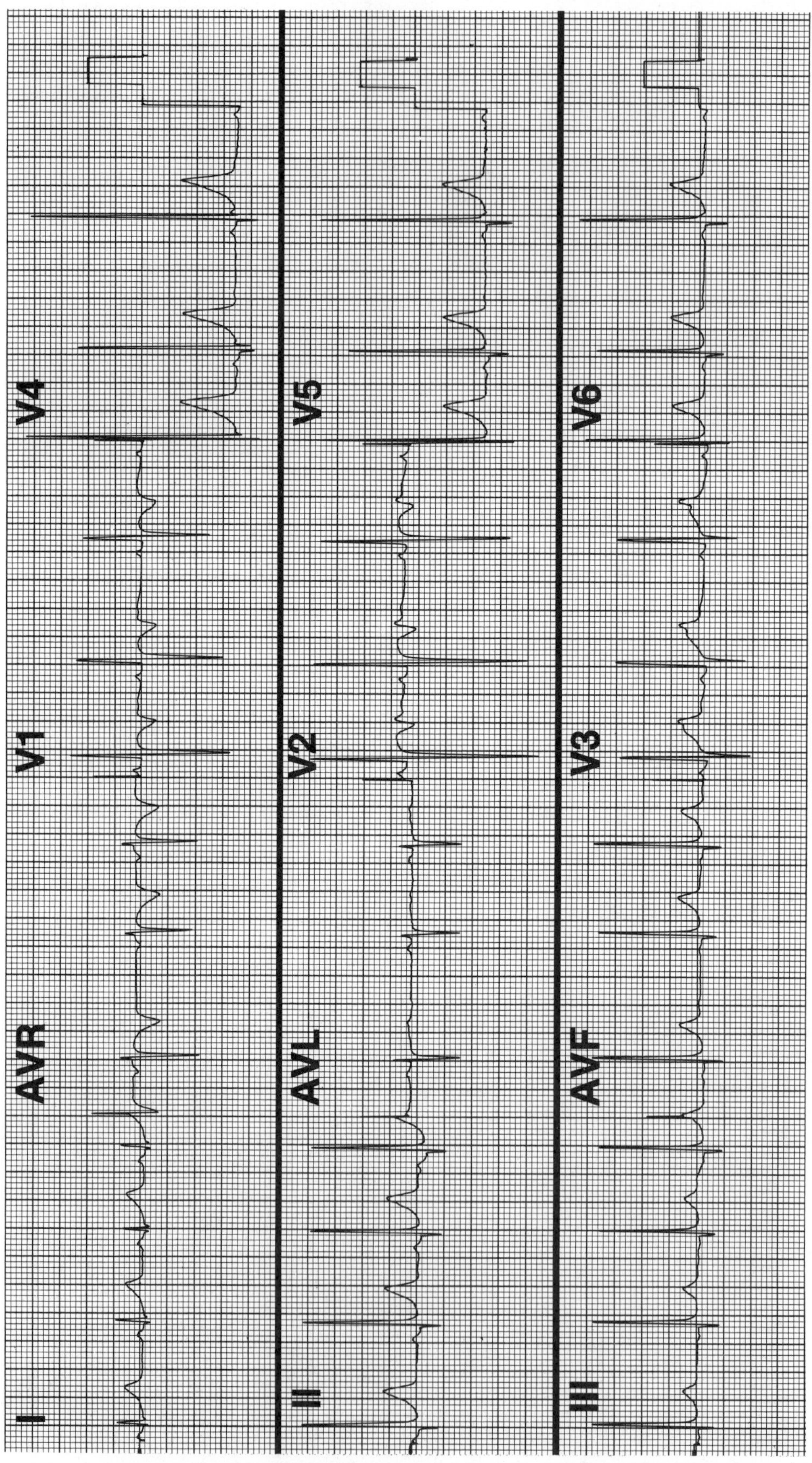
I
AVR
V1
V4
II
AVL
V2
V5
III
AVF
V3
V6

Electrocardiogram #25

Atrial Rate	80	**Beats/Minute**
Ventricular Rate	80	**Beats/Minute**
PR Interval	0.13	**Second**
QRS Duration	0.08	**Second**
QT-QTc	0.37–0.43	**Second**
QRS Complex Axis	80	**Degrees**

Rate: The atrial and ventricular rates are 80 beats per minute.

Rhythm: The PR interval is 0.13 second. Normal sinus rhythm exists, but there is a marked sinus arrhythmia present. This is best seen in leads AVR, AVL and AVF. There is a fixed PR interval, but the R-R intervals change based on the varying P-P period. The P-P intervals shorten with inspiration (rate increases) and prolong with expiration (rate decreases).

Conduction Abnormalities: No criteria present in this electrocardiogram.

QRS Complex Axis: The mean QRS complex axis is 80°.

Chamber Enlargement: No criteria present in this electrocardiogram.

Infarction: No criteria present in this electrocardiogram.

ST Segment and T Wave Abnormalities: No criteria present in this electrocardiogram.

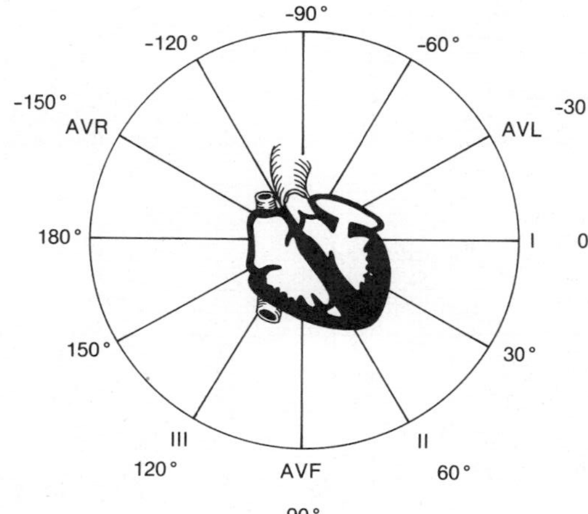

Summary

Normal sinus rhythm with marked sinus arrhythmia

Otherwise normal electrocardiogram

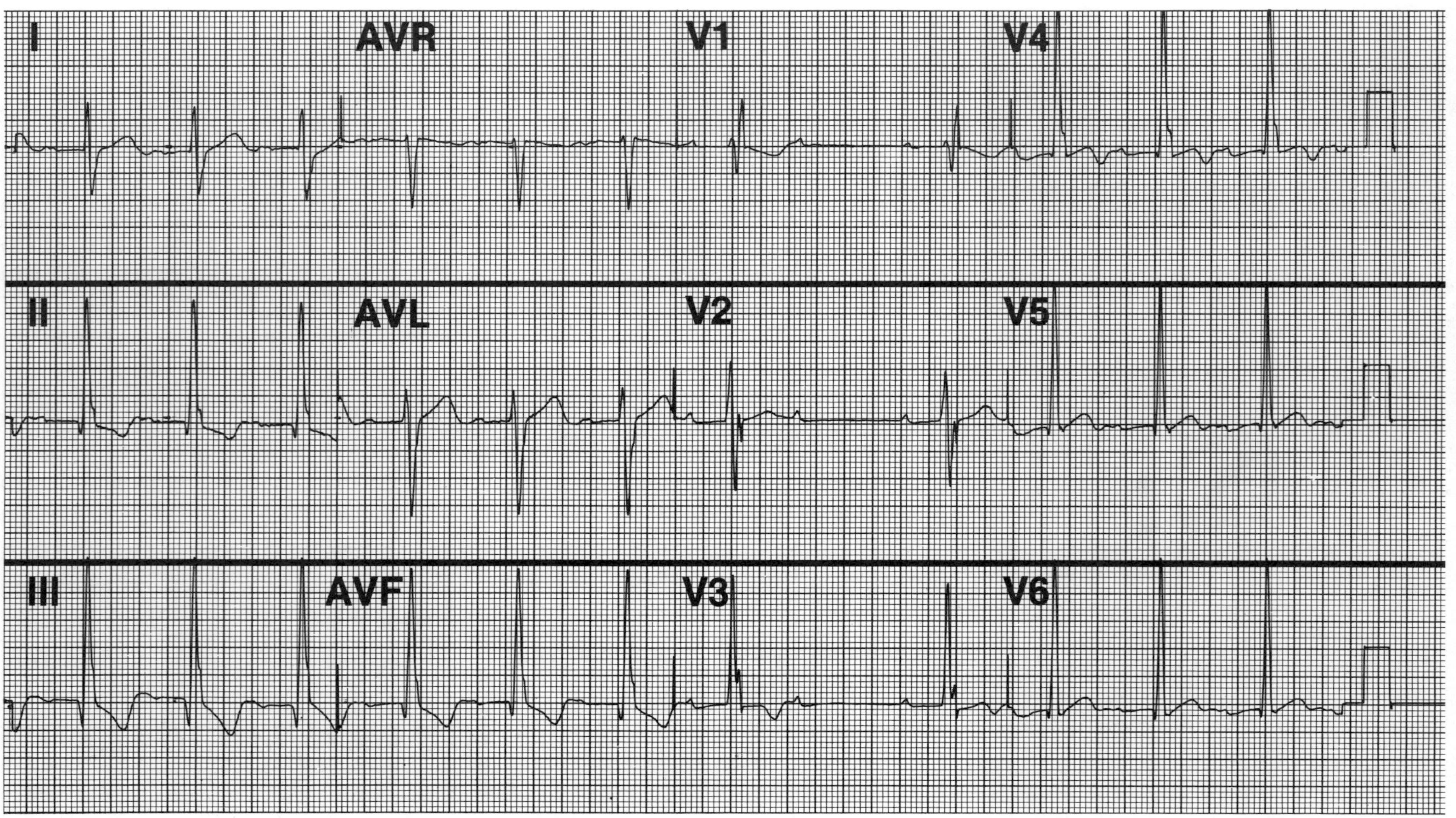
I
AVR
V1
V4
II
AVL
V2
V5
III
AVF
V3
V6

Electrocardiogram #26

Atrial Rate	**79**	**Beats/Minute**
Ventricular Rate	**79**	**Beats/Minute**
PR Interval	**0.30**	**Second**
QRS Duration	**0.14**	**Second**
QT-QTc	**0.40–0.46**	**Second**
QRS Complex Axis	**90**	**Degrees**

Rate: The atrial and ventricular rates are 79 beats per minute.

Rhythm: The PR interval is 0.30 second and constant. The rhythm is normal sinus rhythm.

Conduction Abnormalities: The striking abnormality in this electrocardiogram is the pause that takes place after the first QRS complex in leads V1, V2 and V3. One will notice that there is a P wave followed after 0.30 second by a QRS complex. This is followed by a P wave occurring on time that is not followed by a QRS complex. A P wave followed 0.30 second later by a QRS complex completes the beats seen in this lead set. Therefore, the rhythm is first degree atrioventricular block with second degree Mobitz type II atrioventricular block. In addition, there is a nonspecific intraventricular block that may be related to ventricular enlargement.

QRS Complex Axis: The mean QRS complex axis is 90°.

Chamber Enlargement: No criteria present in this electrocardiogram.

Infarction: An inferior wall myocardial infarction is present. There is a significant Q wave in leads II, III, and AVF.

ST Segment and T Wave Abnormalities: There is ST segment depression and T wave inversions in leads II, III and AVF, which are repolarization abnormalities associated with the myocardial infarction.

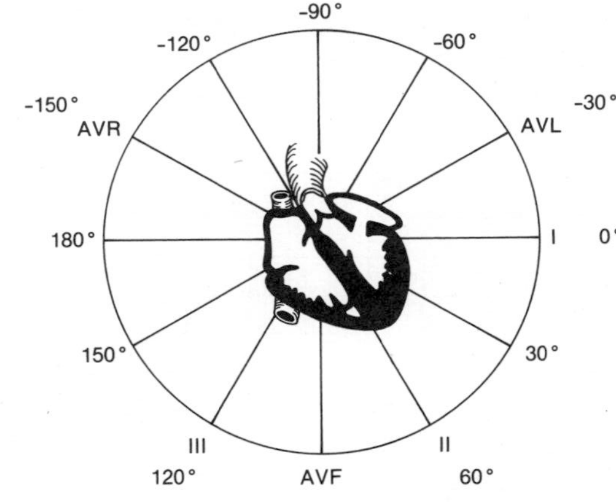

Summary

Normal sinus rhythm with first degree atrioventricular block and second degree Mobitz type II atrioventricular block

Inferior myocardial infarction, age undetermined

Left ventricular hypertrophy

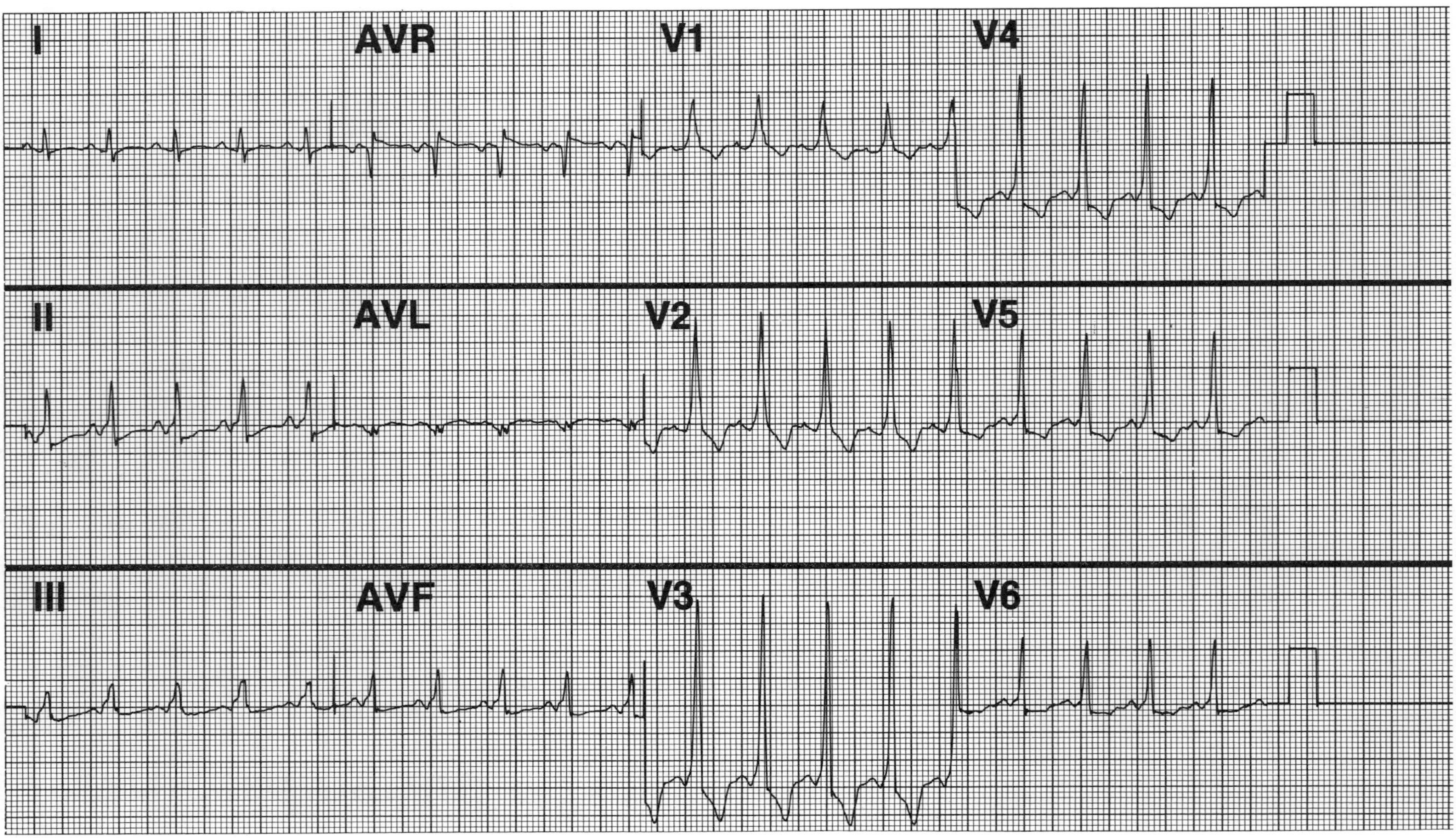
I
AVR
V1
V4
II
AVL
V2
V5
III
AVF
V3
V6

Electrocardiogram #27

Atrial Rate	**136**	**Beats/Minute**
Ventricular Rate	**136**	**Beats/Minute**
PR Interval	**0.11**	**Second**
QRS Duration	**0.12**	**Second**
QT-QTc	**0.32–0.47**	**Second**
QRS Complex Axis	**75**	**Degrees**

Rate: The atrial and ventricular rates are 136 beats per minute.

Rhythm: The PR interval is 0.11 second and constant. At first notice the QRS complex duration is prolonged at 0.12 second. In addition, upon further evaluation, one will note that the PR interval is short and measures 0.11 second. The QRS complex duration is prolonged primarily because of an initial delay in the QRS complex. There is a very prominent delta wave seen in leads II, III and AVF as well as throughout the precordial leads. This delay in ventricular activation together with the short PR interval is classical for ventricular pre-excitation. This electrocardiogram, which demonstrates Wolff-Parkinson-White syndrome (type A), should not be confused with the pattern of left bundle branch block. In left bundle branch block, the QRS complex would also be prolonged, but a delta wave would not be present, and the PR interval would be normal. In type A Wolff-Parkinson-White syndrome, there is a prominent R wave in leads V1 and V6. The delta wave is caused by a delay in ventricular activation, since the ventricles are depolarized by way of the ventricular myocardium instead of the specialized conducting pathways.

Conduction Abnormalities: No criteria present in this electrocardiogram.

QRS Complex Axis: The mean QRS complex axis is 75°.

Chamber Enlargement: No criteria present in this electrocardiogram.

Infarction: No criteria present in this electrocardiogram.

ST Segment and T Wave Abnormalities: No criteria present in this electrocardiogram.

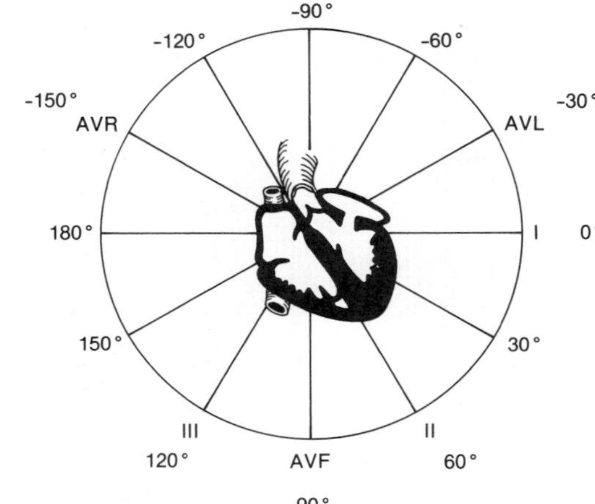

Summary

Wolff-Parkinson-White syndrome (type A)

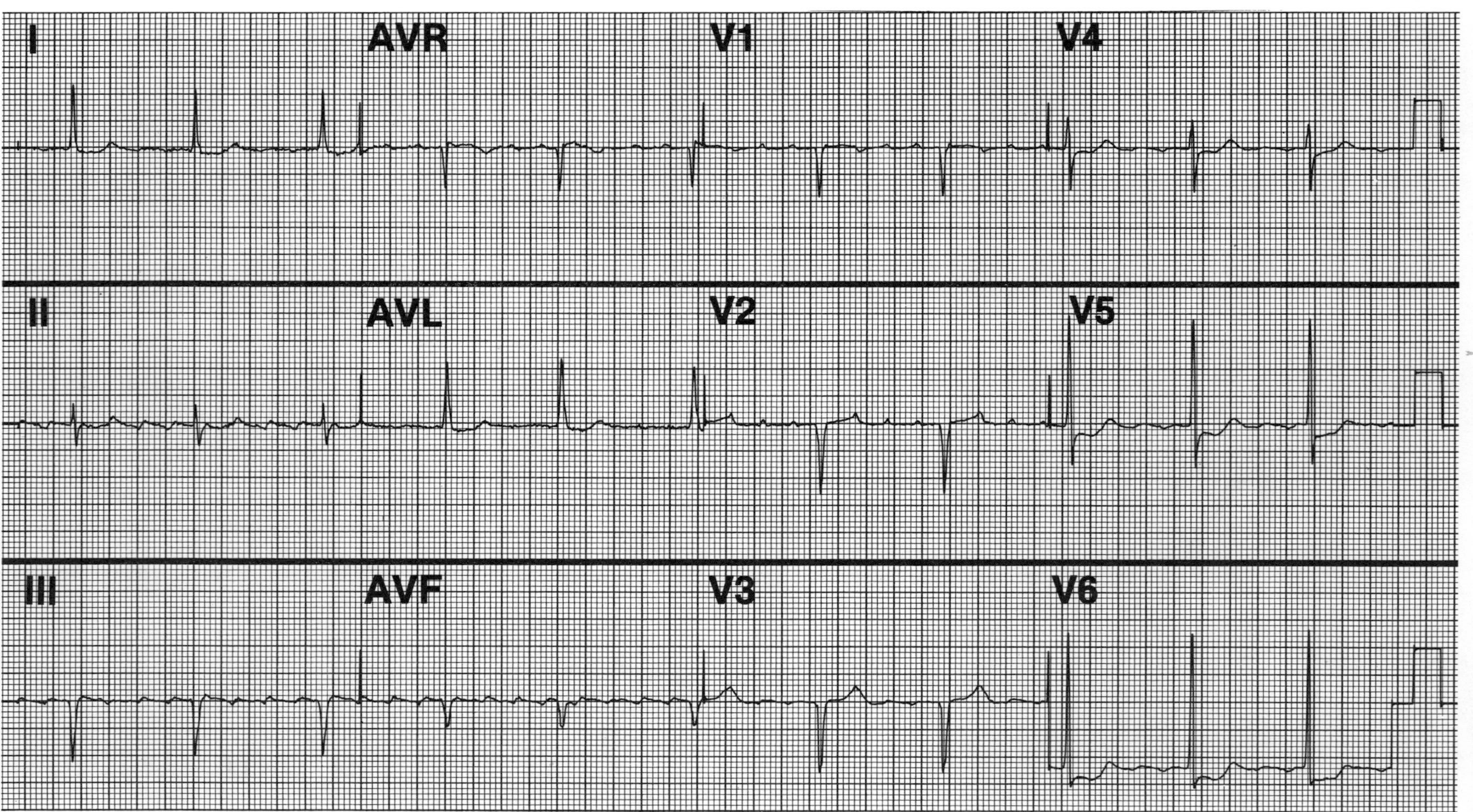
I
AVR
V1
V4
II
AVL
V2
V5
III
AVF
V3
V6

Electrocardiogram #28

Atrial Rate	300	**Beats/Minute**
Ventricular Rate	66	**Beats/Minute**
PR Interval	0.22	**Second**
QRS Duration	0.08	**Second**
QT-QTc	0.40–0.43	**Second**
QRS Complex Axis	−30	**Degrees**

Rate: The average ventricular rate is 66 beats per minute.

Rhythm: When one looks for the P waves, one will see a saw-toothed pattern, especially in leads II, III and AVF. This saw-toothed pattern of atrial activity occurs at 300 beats per minute. However, the ventricular rate is approximately one quarter of the atrial rate. Therefore, the rhythm that is atrial flutter has a 4:1 atrioventricular block.

Conduction Abnormalities: There is a 4:1 block at the atrioventricular node. This is a normal physiological block.

QRS Complex Axis: The mean QRS complex axis is −30°.

Chamber Enlargement: No criteria present in this electrocardiogram.

Infarction: In addition, there is a QS complex in leads V1 to V3 that is diagnostic of an anteroseptal infarction, age undetermined. There is also a QRS complex in leads III and AVF that is suggestive of an inferior infarction, age undetermined. One would also like to see a QS complex in lead II to confirm the diagnosis of infarction. However, in this electrocardiogram one must be suspicious that the patient has had an inferior infarction.

ST Segment and T Wave Abnormalities: In addition, there are nonspecific ST segment and T wave abnormalities. Notice the 2 mm ST segment depression and T wave inversions in lead V6. This is suggestive of ischemia.

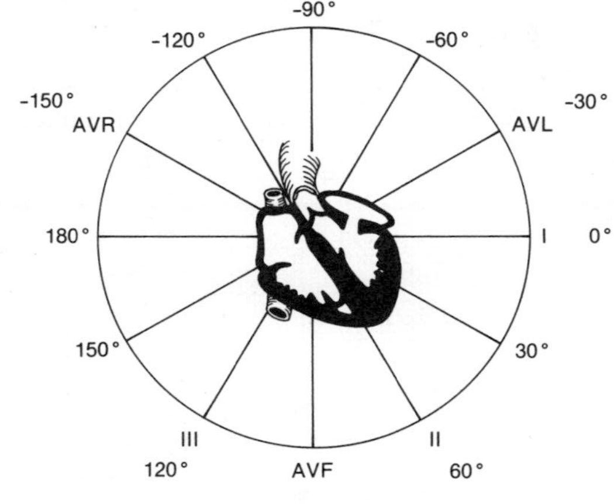

Summary

Atrial flutter with 4:1 atrioventricular block

Left ventricular hypertrophy

Anteroseptal myocardial infarction, age undetermined

Inferior myocardial infarction, age undetermined

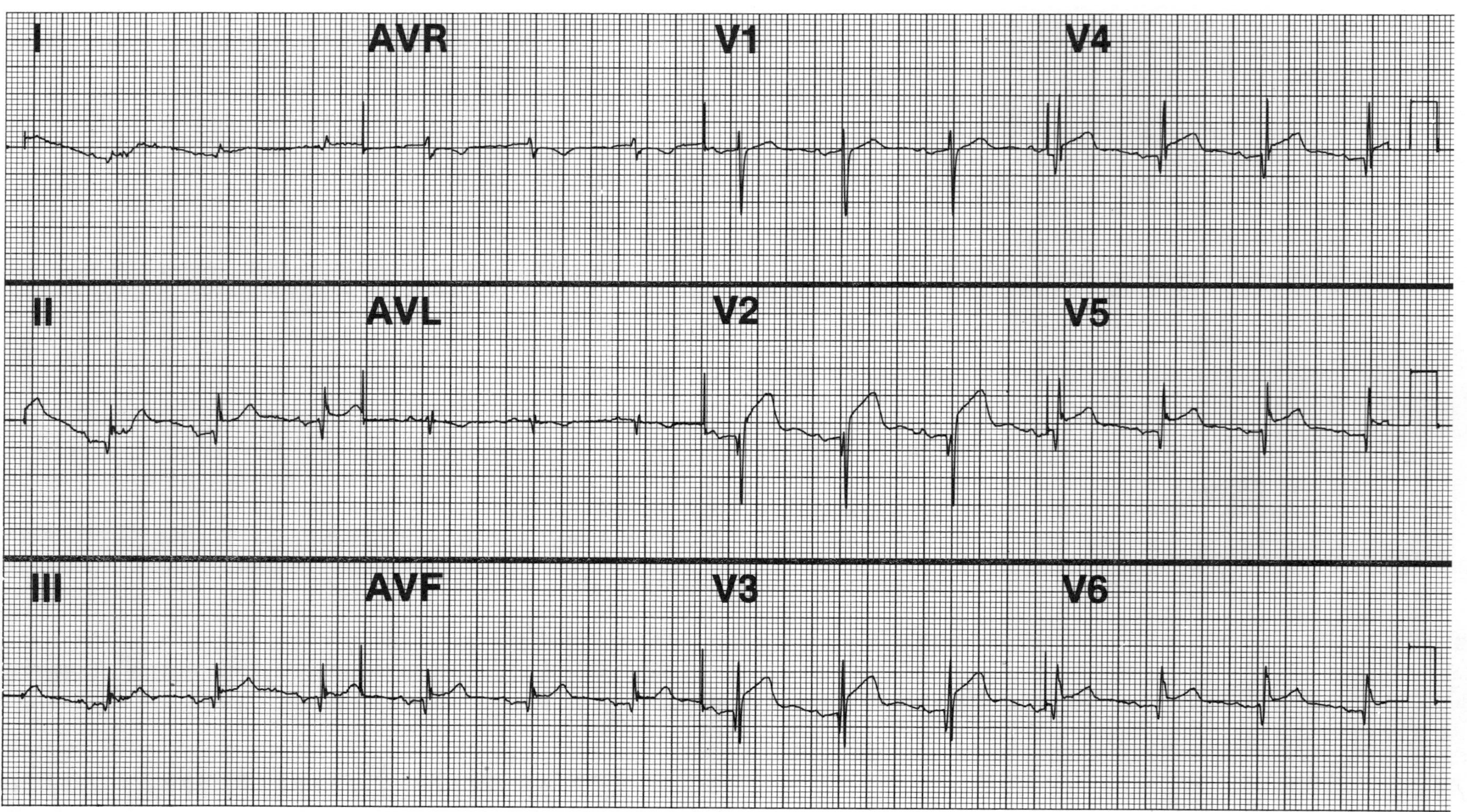
I
AVR
V1
V4
II
AVL
V2
V5
III
AVF
V3
V6

Electrocardiogram #29

Atrial Rate	78	**Beats/Minute**
Ventricular Rate	78	**Beats/Minute**
PR Interval	0.18	**Second**
QRS Duration	0.08	**Second**
QT-QTc	0.36–0.42	**Second**
QRS Complex Axis	80	**Degrees**

Rate: The atrial and ventricular rates are 78 beats per minute.

Rhythm: The PR interval is 0.18 second and constant. Therefore, the rhythm is normal sinus rhythm.

Conduction Abnormalities: No criteria present in this electrocardiogram.

QRS Complex Axis: The mean QRS complex axis is 80°.

Chamber Enlargement: Notice the ST segment elevation in leads V2 to V5 as well as elevation in leads II, III and AVF. In addition, there are significant Q waves in leads V2 and V3. The Q waves are also quite prominent in the lateral precordium and in the inferior leads. Therefore, the diagnosis of an anterior infarction and an inferior infarction should be made. The fact that there is associated ST segment elevation and peaking of T waves in these leads is suggestive that the infarction may possibly be acute.

Infarction: No criteria present in this electrocardiogram.

ST Segment and T Wave Abnormalities: No criteria present in this electrocardiogram.

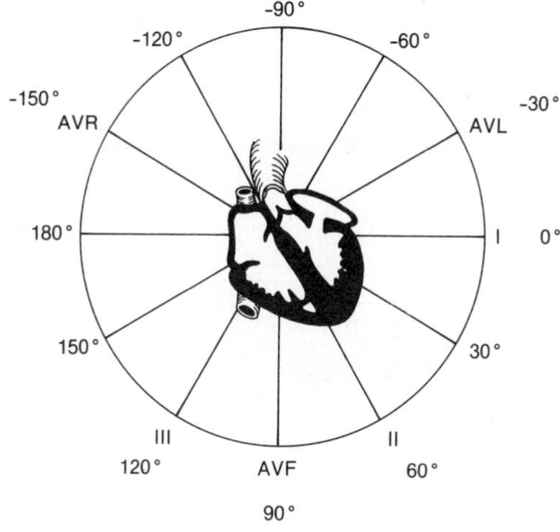

Summary

Normal sinus rhythm

Anterior myocardial infarction, possibly acute

Inferior myocardial infarction, possibly acute

I AVR V1 V4

II AVL V2 V5

III AVF V3 V6

Electrocardiogram #30

Atrial Rate	**81**	**Beats/Minute**
Ventricular Rate	**81**	**Beats/Minute**
PR Interval	**0.16**	**Second**
QRS Duration	**0.13**	**Second**
QT-QTc	**0.39–0.45**	**Second**
QRS Complex Axis	**−50**	**Degrees**

Rate: The atrial and ventricular rates are 81 beats per minute.

Rhythm: The PR interval is 0.16 second and constant. The rhythm is normal sinus rhythm.

Conduction Abnormalities: An RSR′ complex is present in lead V1 together with slurring the terminal forces (S waves in leads I, V5 and V6). The QRS complex duration is prolonged at 0.13 second. The diagnosis of right bundle branch block is, therefore, based on these findings. In addition, the extreme left axis deviation is the result of the rS complex in leads II, III and AVF. These findings make the diagnosis of left anterior hemiblock. The patient having both of these conduction abnormalities is then said to have bifascicular block. One cannot rule out, however, the presence of an inferior infarction in this tracing. Certainly, the left anterior hemiblock may mask an inferior myocardial infarction, and one should be suspicious that an inferior infarction may also be present in addition to the left anterior hemiblock.

QRS Complex Axis: The mean QRS complex axis is −50°.

Chamber Enlargement: No criteria present in this electrocardiogram.

Infarction: No criteria present in this electrocardiogram.

ST Segment and T Wave Abnormalities: The ST segment and T wave changes are the secondary repolarization changes resulting from the conduction disturbances.

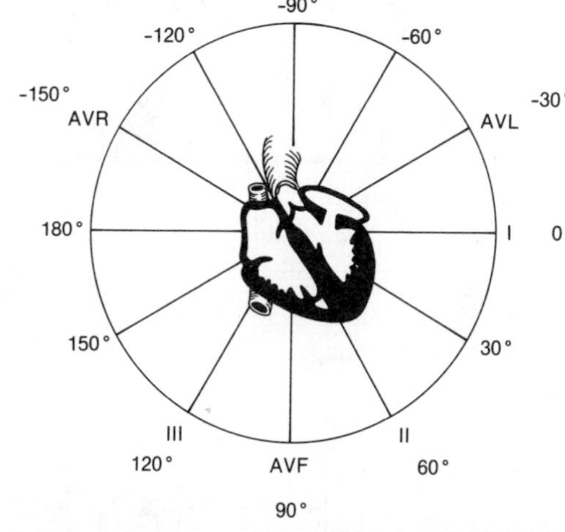

Summary

Normal sinus rhythm

Right bundle branch block

Left anterior hemiblock

Cannot rule out an inferior myocardial infarction, age undetermined

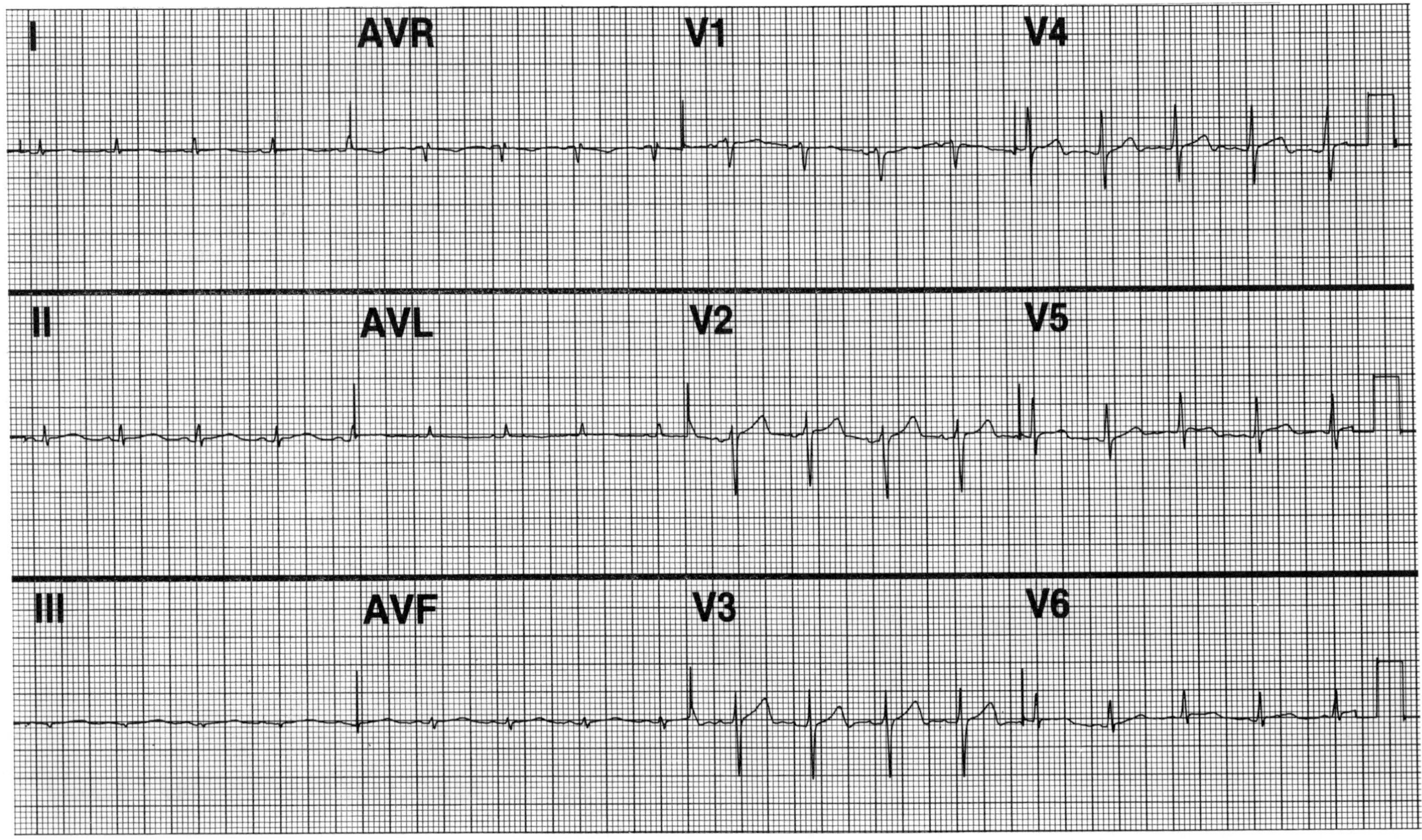
I
AVR
V1
V4
II
AVL
V2
V5
III
AVF
V3
V6

Electrocardiogram #31

Atrial Rate	**111**	**Beats/Minute**
Ventricular Rate	**111**	**Beats/Minute**
PR Interval	**0.12**	**Second**
QRS Duration	**0.08**	**Second**
QT-QTc	**0.32–0.44**	**Second**
QRS Complex Axis	**5**	**Degrees**

Rate: The atrial and ventricular rates are 111 beats per minute.

Rhythm: The PR interval is 0.12 second and constant. The rhythm is sinus tachycardia.

Conduction Abnormalities: No criteria present in this electrocardiogram.

QRS Complex Axis: The mean QRS complex axis is 5°.

Chamber Enlargement: No criteria present in this electrocardiogram.

Infarction: No criteria present in this electrocardiogram.

ST Segment and T Wave Abnormalities: There are nonspecific ST segment and T wave abnormalities seen.

Other Findings: Low voltage is present throughout on this electrocardiogram, and one should consider pulmonary disease, primary myocardial disease or pericardial effusion.

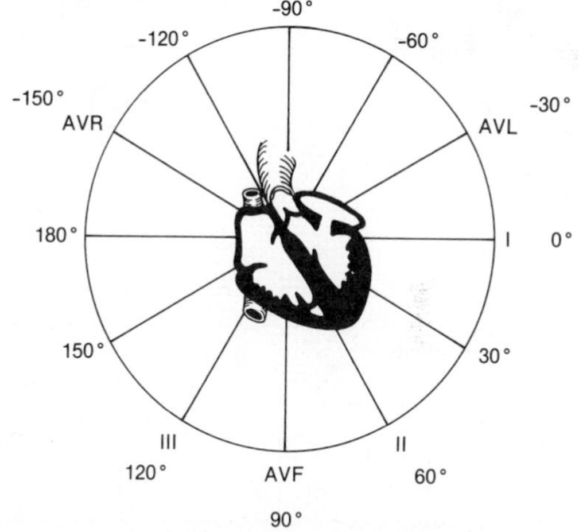

Summary

Sinus tachycardia

Low voltage

Nonspecific ST segment and T wave abnormalities

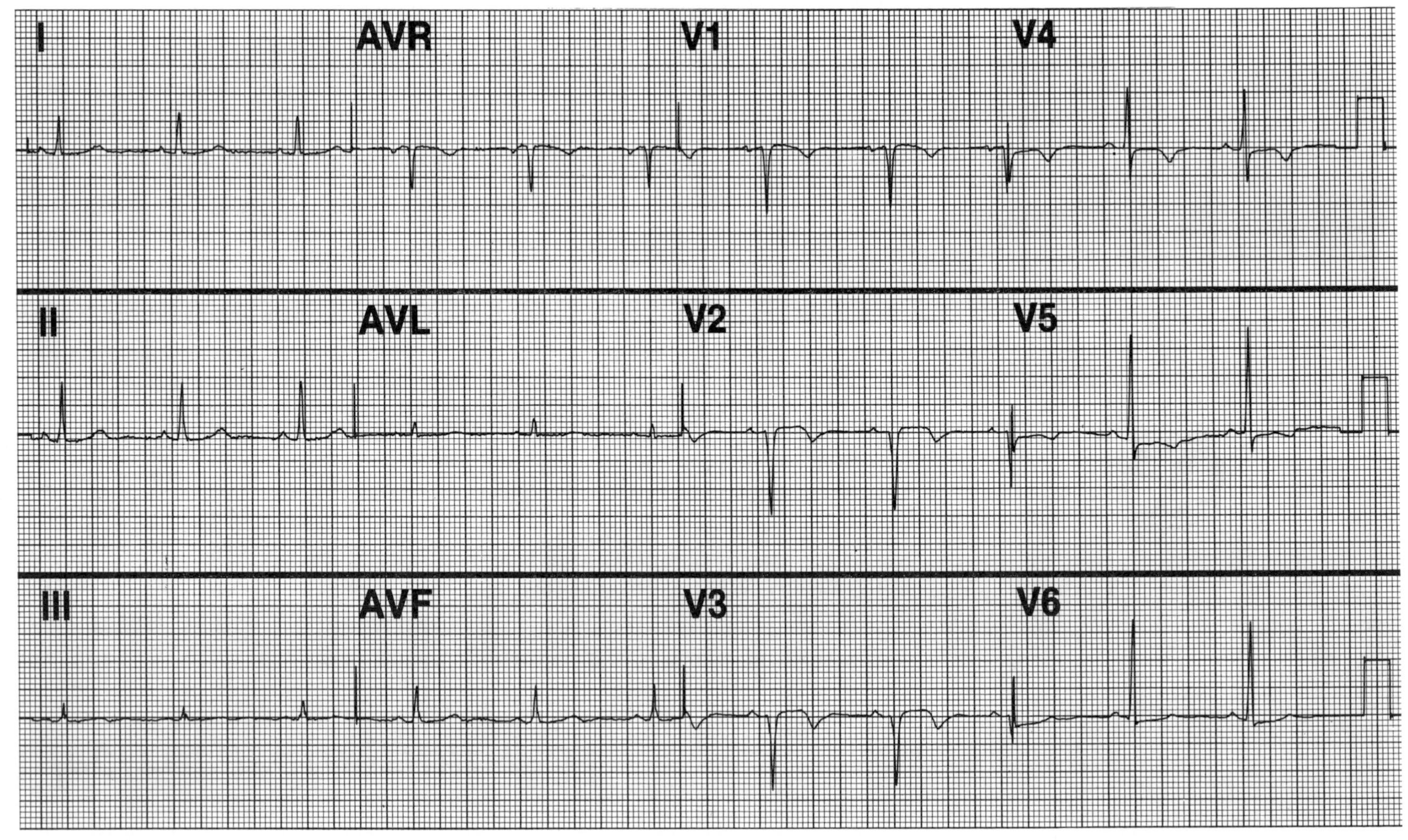
I
AVR
V1
V4
II
AVL
V2
V5
III
AVF
V3
V6

Electrocardiogram #32

Atrial Rate	**68**	**Beats/Minute**
Ventricular Rate	**68**	**Beats/Minute**
PR Interval	**0.15**	**Second**
QRS Duration	**0.08**	**Second**
QT-QTc	**0.43–0.46**	**Second**
QRS Complex Axis	**50**	**Degrees**

Rate: The atrial and ventricular rates are 68 beats per minute.

Rhythm: The PR interval is 0.15 second and constant. The rhythm is normal sinus rhythm.

Conduction Abnormalities: No criteria present in this electrocardiogram.

QRS Complex Axis: The mean QRS complex axis is 50°.

Chamber Enlargement: No criteria present in this electrocardiogram.

Infarction: There is a QS complex in leads V1 to V3 together with ST segment elevation and T wave inversions that persist through lead V5. The diagnosis, therefore, should be anteroseptal infarction, age undetermined.

ST Segment and T Wave Abnormalities: There are significant ST segment and T wave abnormalities seen especially throughout the precordium indicative of ischemia.

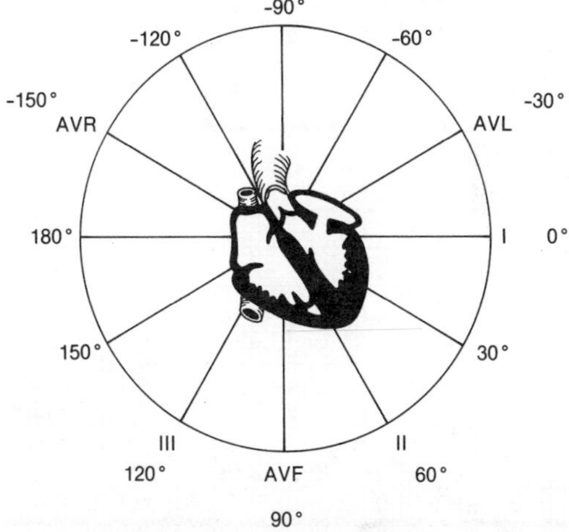

Summary

Normal sinus rhythm

Anteroseptal myocardial infarction, age undetermined

Lateral wall ischemia

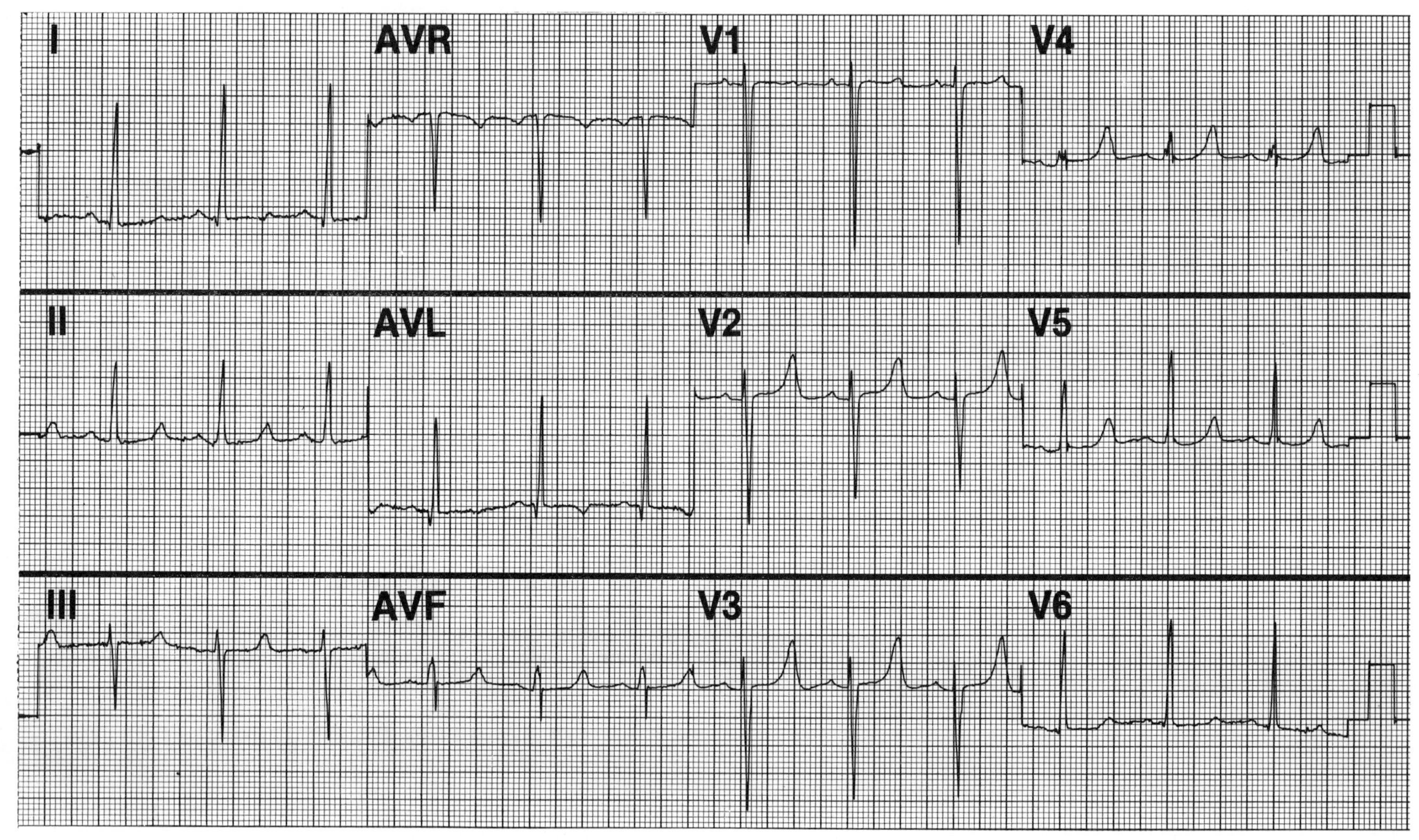
I
AVR
V1
V4
II
AVL
V2
V5
III
AVF
V3
V6

Electrocardiogram #33

Atrial Rate	75	**Beats/Minute**
Ventricular Rate	75	**Beats/Minute**
PR Interval	0.18	**Second**
QRS Duration	0.08	**Second**
QT-QTc	0.46–0.52	**Second**
QRS Complex Axis	5	**Degrees**

Rate: The atriál and ventricular rates are 75 beats per minute.

Rhythm: The PR interval is 0.18 second and constant. The rhythm is normal sinus rhythm.

Conduction Abnormalities: No criteria present in this electrocardiogram.

QRS Complex Axis: The mean QRS complex axis is 5°.

Chamber Enlargement: The QRS voltage in lead AVL is 20 mm, and this is associated with T wave inversions in the same lead. This is the most specific criterion for left ventricular hypertrophy. This data has been based on post-mortem studies.

Infarction: No criteria present in this electrocardiogram.

ST Segment and T Wave Abnormalities: No criteria present in this electrocardiogram.

Other Findings: In addition, the QT interval is 0.46 second, which when corrected for rate is 0.52 second (see Chapter 4, Review of Complexes). This prolonged QT interval should make one suspicious of myocardial disease, electrolyte imbalance or drug effects—especially antiarrhythmic agents.

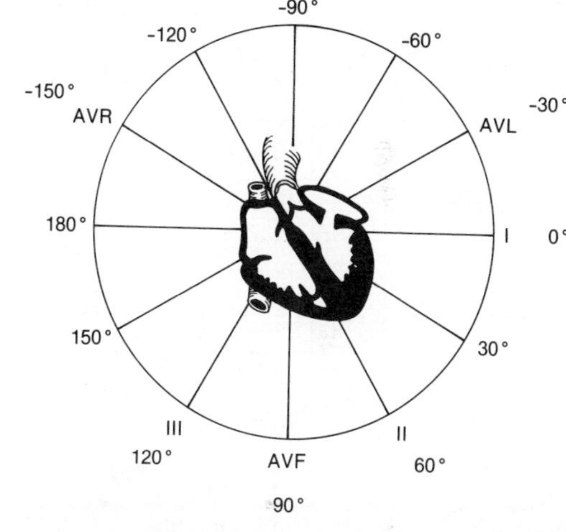

Summary

Normal sinus rhythm

Left ventricular hypertrophy

Prolonged QTc interval

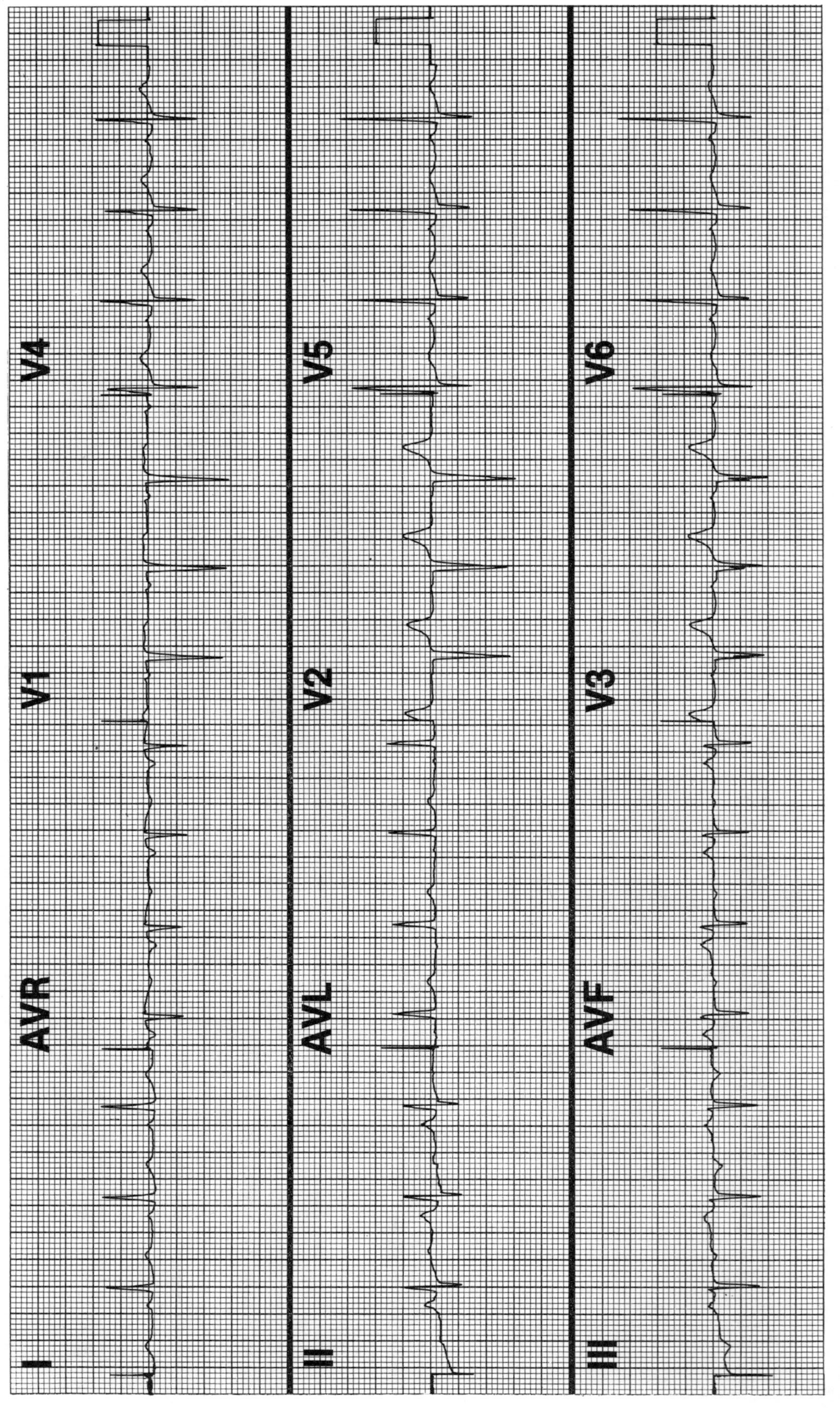
I
AVR
V1
V4
II
AVL
V2
V5
III
AVF
V3
V6

Electrocardiogram #34

Atrial Rate	88	Beats/Minute
Ventricular Rate	88	Beats/Minute
PR Interval	0.17	Second
QRS Duration	0.08	Second
QT-QTc	0.37–0.45	Second
QRS Complex Axis	−20	Degrees

Rate: The atrial and ventricular rates are 88 beats per minute.

Rhythm: The PR interval is 0.17 second and constant. The rhythm is normal sinus rhythm.

Conduction Abnormalities: No criteria present in this electrocardiogram.

QRS Complex Axis: The mean QRS complex axis is −20°.

Chamber Enlargement: No criteria present in this electrocardiogram.

Infarction: The QS complex appears in leads V1 to V3, which is diagnostic of an anteroseptal myocardial infarction, age undetermined.

ST Segment and T Wave Abnormalities: No criteria present in this electrocardiogram.

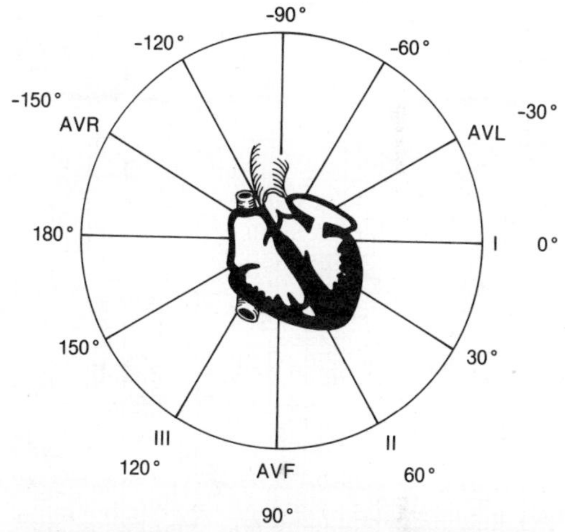

Summary

Normal sinus rhythm

Anteroseptal myocardial infarction, age undetermined

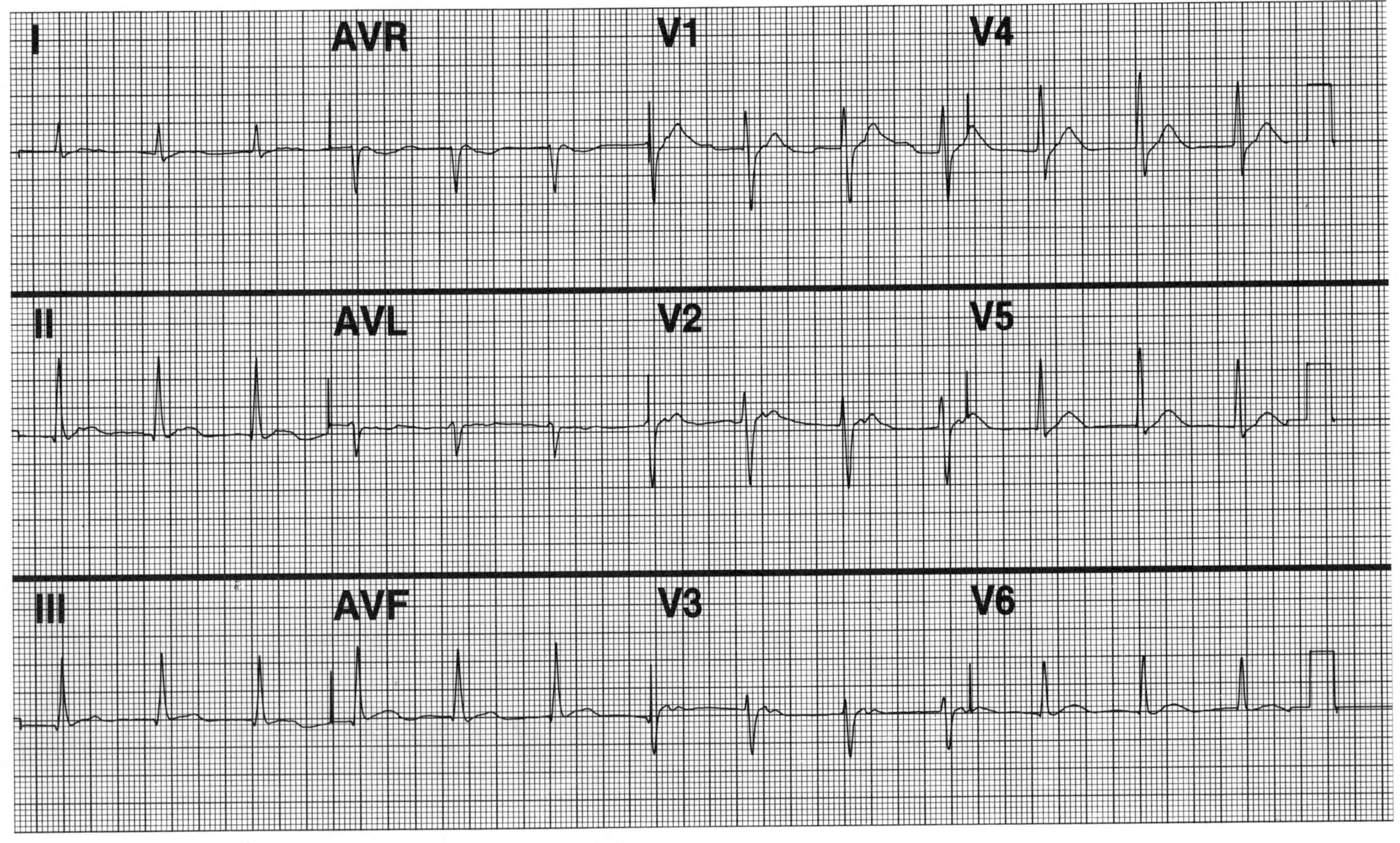
I
AVR
V1
V4
II
AVL
V2
V5
III
AVF
V3
V6

Electrocardiogram #35

Atrial Rate	82	Beats/Minute
Ventricular Rate	82	Beats/Minute
PR Interval	0.18	Second
QRS Duration	0.11	Second
QT-QTc	0.40–0.46	Second
QRS Complex Axis	80	Degrees

Rate: The atrial and ventricular rates are 82 beats per minute.

Rhythm: There are no P waves preceding the complexes. However, notice that there is a deformation of the ascending limb of the T wave that occurs at 0.18 second after the beginning of the QRS complex. This is a retrograde P wave associated with an accelerated junctional rhythm. The R wave precedes the P wave, and the interval is therefore termed the "RP interval." Since the rate is 82 beats per minute, the rhythm is nonparoxysmal junctional tachycardia (see Junctional Rhythms, page 45).

Conduction Abnormalities: The QRS complex is widened to 0.11 second. However, there are no other criteria for either right or left bundle branch block. Therefore, a nonspecific intraventricular conduction delay exists.

QRS Complex Axis: The mean QRS complex axis is 80°.

Chamber Enlargement: No criteria present in this electrocardiogram.

Infarction: No criteria present in this electrocardiogram.

ST Segment and T Wave Abnormalities: There are nonspecific T wave abnormalities seen in leads I, AVL and V6. The T wave should be larger in lead V6 than in lead V1.

Other Findings: The QT interval is prolonged.

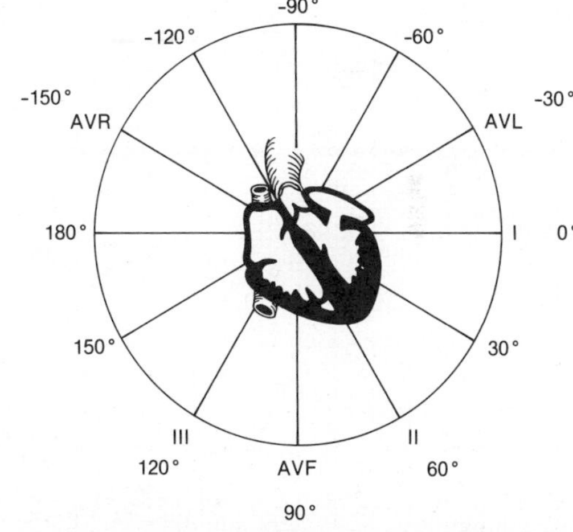

Summary

Nonparoxysmal junctional tachycardia

Nonspecific intraventricular conduction delay

Nonspecific T wave abnormality

Prolonged QTc interval

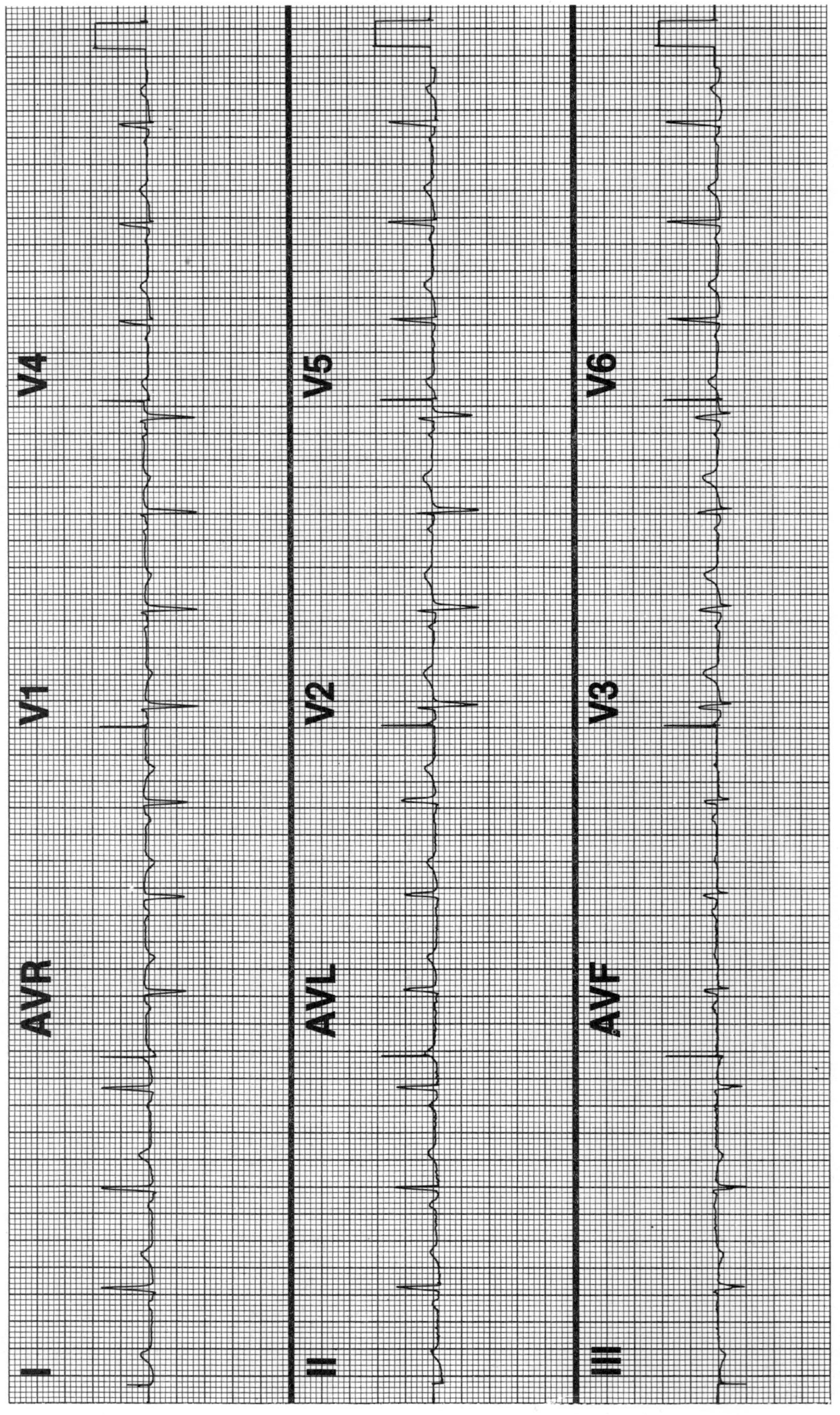
I
AVR
V1
V4
II
AVL
V2
V5
III
AVF
V3
V6

Electrocardiogram #36

Atrial Rate	83	Beats/Minute
Ventricular Rate	83	Beats/Minute
PR Interval	0.14	Second
QRS Duration	0.07	Second
QT-QTc	0.36–0.42	Second
QRS Complex Axis	10	Degrees

Rate: The atrial and ventricular rates are 83 beats per minute.

Rhythm: The PR interval is 0.14 second and constant. The rhythm is normal sinus rhythm.

Conduction Abnormalities: No criteria present in this electrocardiogram.

QRS Complex Axis: The mean QRS complex axis is 10°.

Chamber Enlargement: No criteria present in this electrocardiogram.

Infarction: No criteria present in this electrocardiogram.

ST Segment and T Wave Abnormalities: No criteria present in this electrocardiogram.

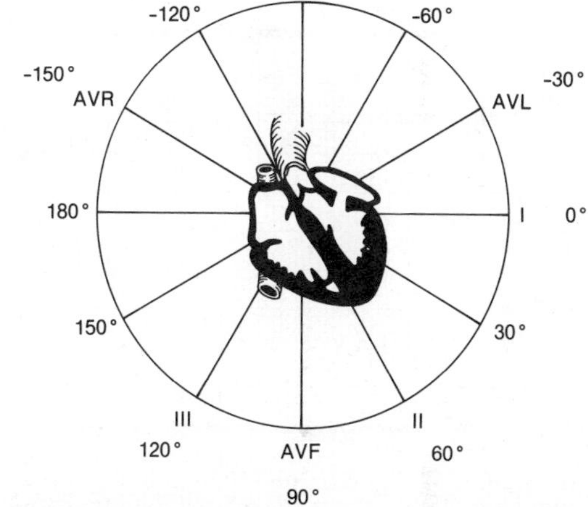

Summary

Normal sinus rhythm

Normal electrocardiogram

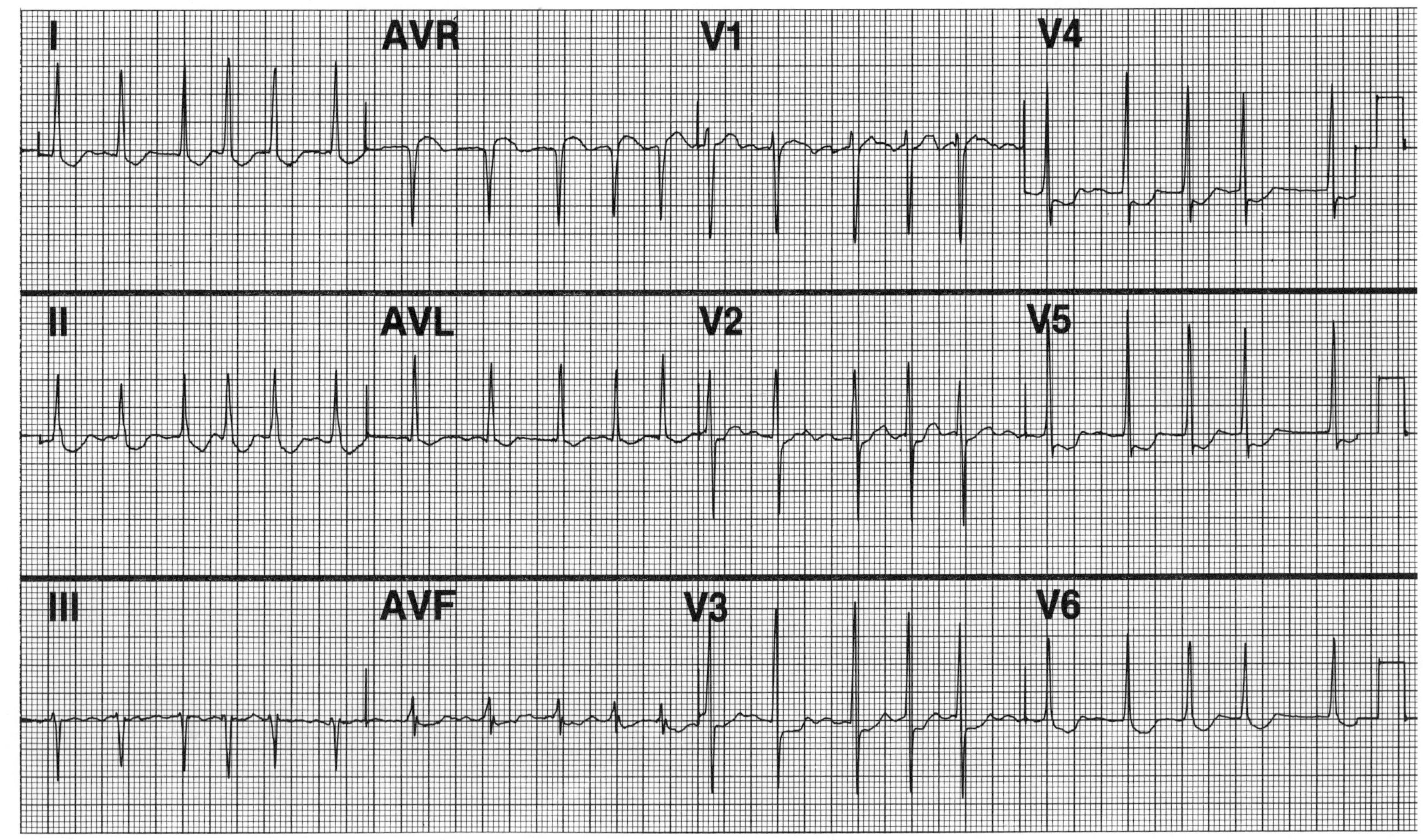
I
AVR
V1
V4
II
AVL
V2
V5
III
AVF
V3
V6

Electrocardiogram #37

Atrial Rate	—	**Beats/Minute**
Ventricular Rate	130	**Beats/Minute**
PR Interval	—	**Second**
QRS Duration	0.08	**Second**
QT-QTc	0.30–0.44	**Second**
QRS Complex Axis	5	**Degrees**

Rate: The average ventricular rate is 130 beats per minute.

Rhythm: No P waves are seen throughout this tracing. The baseline is undulating. The rhythm is atrial fibrillation with a rapid ventricular response.

Conduction Abnormalities: No criteria present in this electrocardiogram.

QRS Complex Axis: The mean QRS complex axis is 5°.

Chamber Enlargement: The voltage criteria for left ventricular hypertrophy is made by the R wave being greater than 13 mm in lead AVL. Other leads also demonstrate the increased voltage. The R wave in lead I plus the S wave in lead III is greater than 25 mm, and the S wave in lead V1 plus the R wave in lead V5 is greater than 35 mm.

Infarction: No criteria present in this electrocardiogram.

ST Segment and T Wave Abnormalities: There is significant ST segment depression of 3 mm seen in leads V5 and V6 together with T wave inversions in these same leads. This ST segment and T wave abnormality represent secondary changes to the left ventricular hypertrophy.

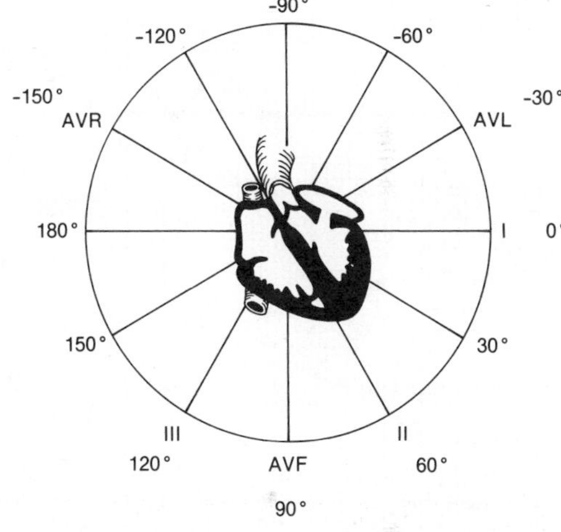

Summary

Atrial fibrillation

Left ventricular hypertrophy

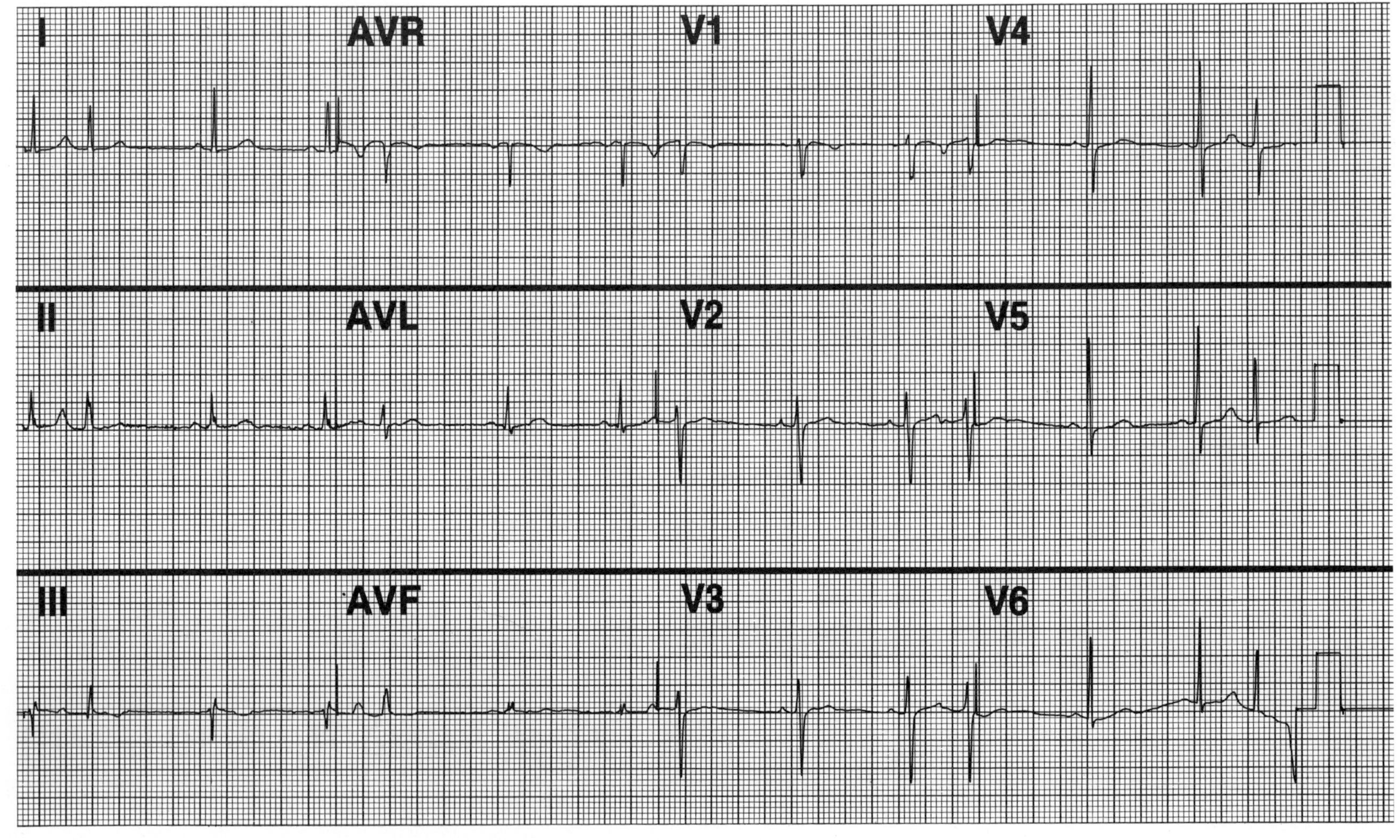
I
AVR
V1
V4
II
AVL
V2
V5
III
AVF
V3
V6

Electrocardiogram #38

Atrial Rate	**80**	**Beats/Minute**
Ventricular Rate	**80**	**Beats/Minute**
PR Interval	**0.14**	**Second**
QRS Duration	**0.08**	**Second**
QT-QTc	**0.38–0.43**	**Second**
QRS Complex Axis	**20**	**Degrees**

Rate: The atrial and ventricular rates are 80 beats per minute.

Rhythm: The PR interval is 0.14 second and constant. The rhythm is normal sinus rhythm. However, if one notices the second complex in lead I as well as the last complex in lead V4, one will notice that these are early or premature beats. All of these beats are narrow in duration and represent a supraventricular focus. Therefore, the diagnosis of normal sinus rhythm with frequent premature supraventricular complexes should be made. These complexes are clearly supraventricular, since they appear identical to the normal sinus beat. They are, however, premature.

Conduction Abnormalities: No criteria present in this electrocardiogram.

QRS Complex Axis: The mean QRS complex axis is 20°.

Chamber Enlargement: No criteria present in this electrocardiogram.

Infarction: No criteria present in this electrocardiogram.

ST Segment and T Wave Abnormalities: No criteria present in this electrocardiogram.

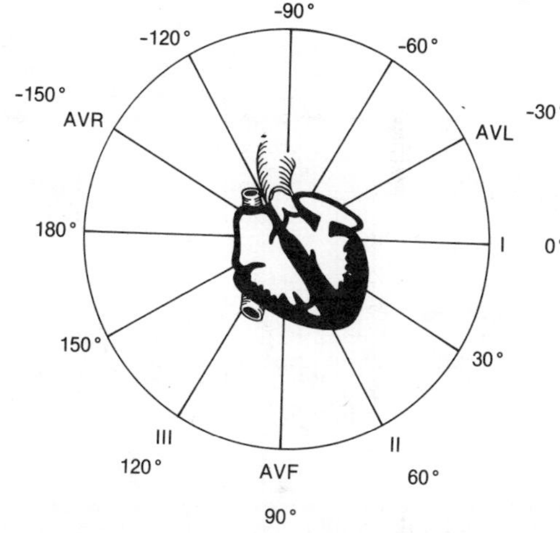

Summary

Normal sinus rhythm with frequent premature supraventricular contractions

Otherwise normal electrocardiogram

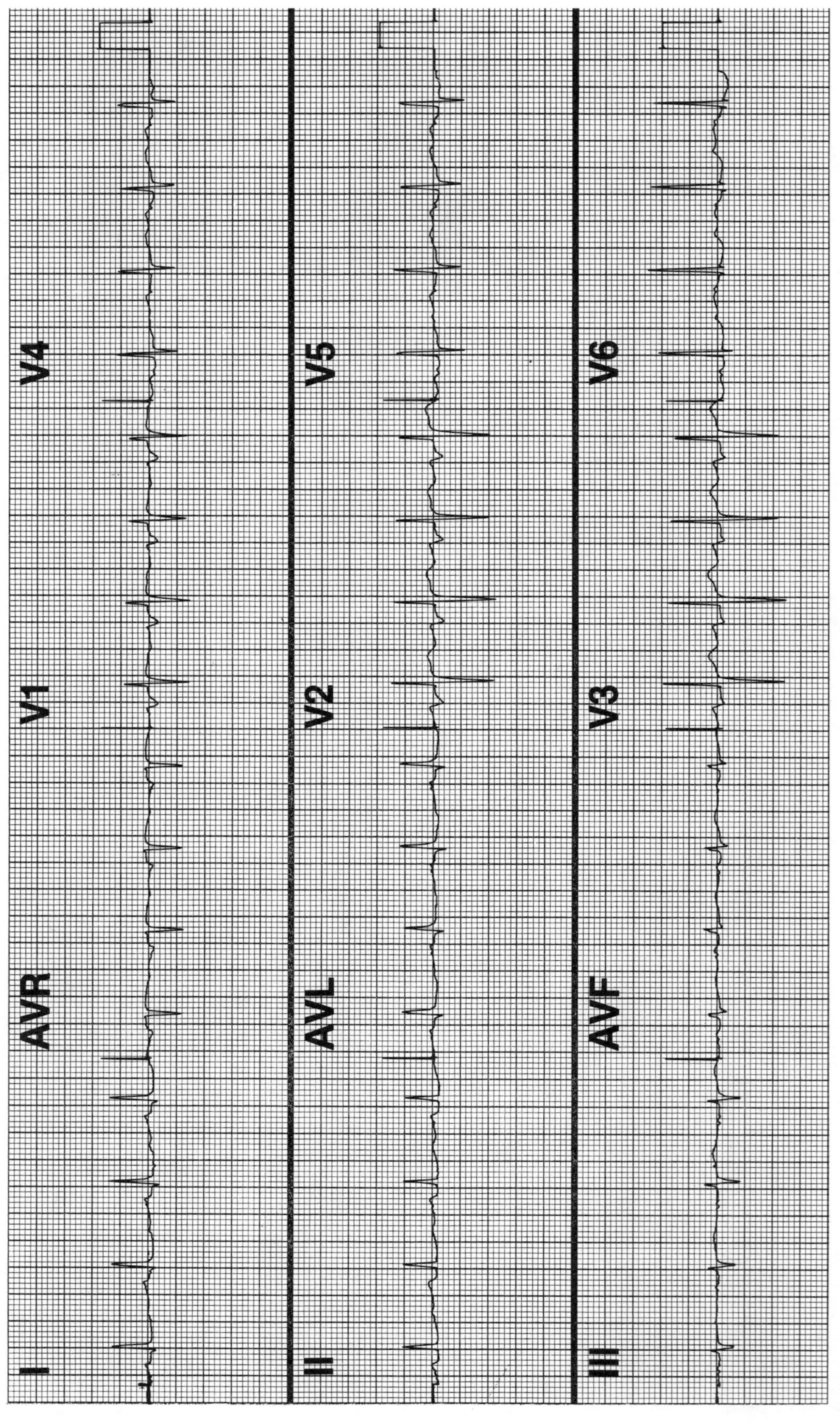
I
AVR
V1
V4
II
AVL
V2
V5
III
AVF
V3
V6

Electrocardiogram #39

Atrial Rate	**97**	**Beats/Minute**
Ventricular Rate	**97**	**Beats/Minute**
PR Interval	**0.20**	**Second**
QRS Duration	**0.09**	**Second**
QT-QTc	**0.32–0.41**	**Second**
QRS Complex Axis	**20**	**Degrees**

Rate: The atrial and ventricular rates are 97 beats per minute.

Rhythm: The PR interval is 0.20 seconds. The rhythm is normal sinus rhythm.

Conduction Abnormalities: No criteria present in this electrocardiogram.

QRS Complex Axis: The mean QRS complex axis is 20°.

Chamber Enlargement: The major abnormality is left atrial enlargement, which is best seen in lead V1. Notice the negative component of the P wave in lead V1, which measures 0.07 second in duration. This is also well seen as a notching of the P wave in leads II, III and AVF. These are all the criteria for left atrial enlargement. This wide notched P wave has been termed "p-mitrale."

Infarction: No criteria present in this electrocardiogram.

ST Segment and T Wave Abnormalities: There are minor ST segment and T wave abnormalities seen in practically all of the leads, but no specific pattern is identifiable.

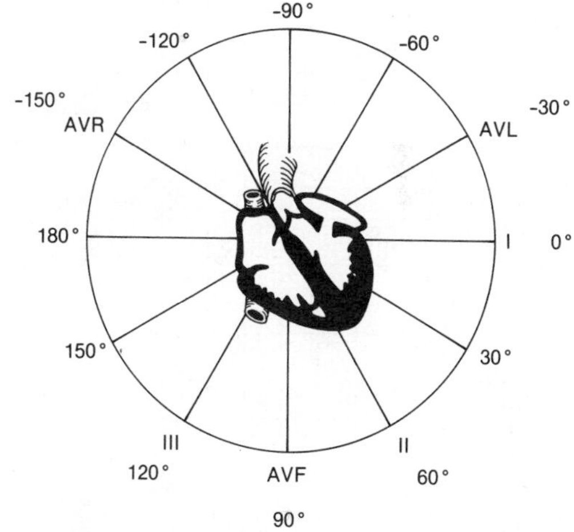

Summary

Normal sinus rhythm

Left atrial enlargement (p-mitrale)

Nonspecific ST segment and T wave abnormalities

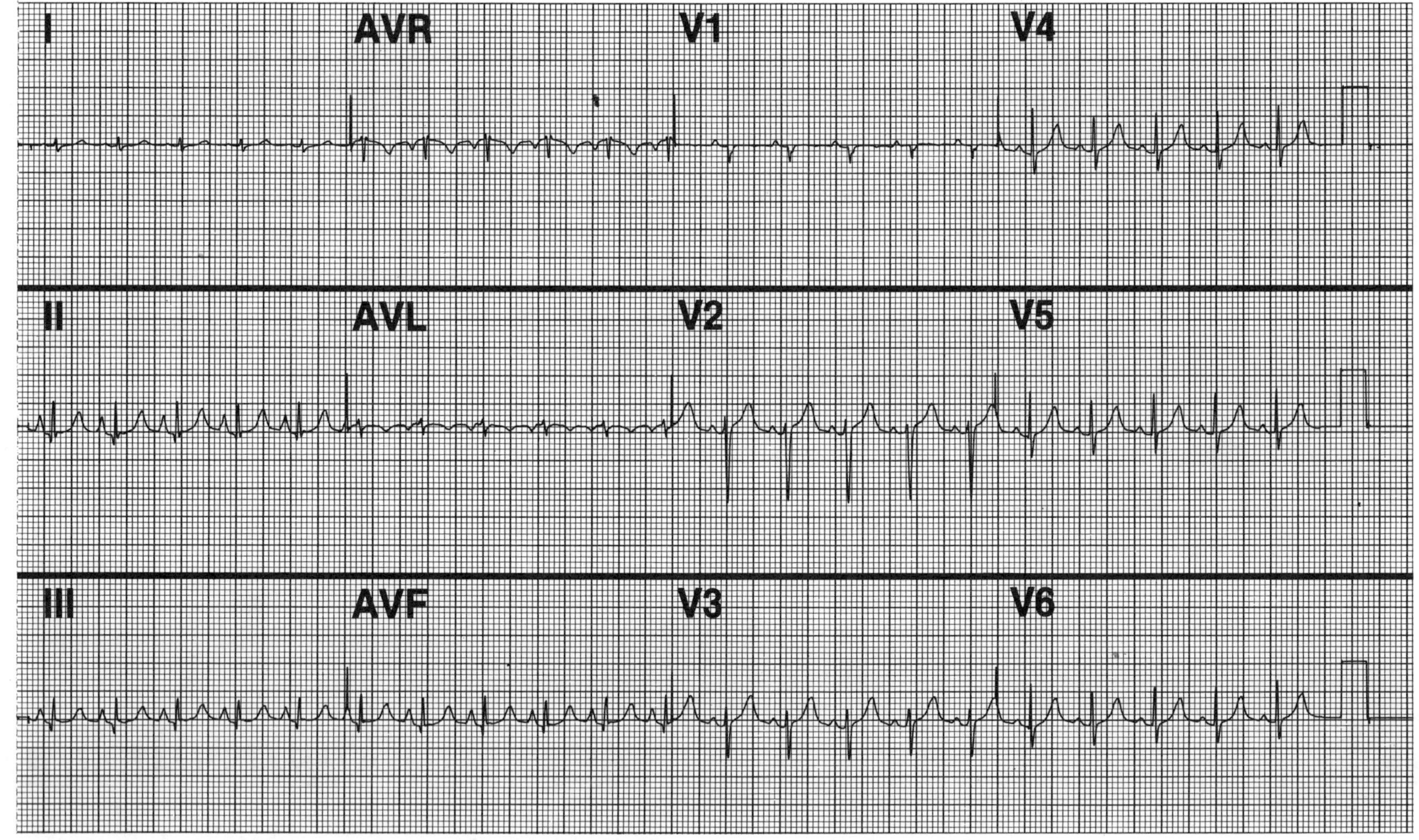
I
AVR
V1
V4
II
AVL
V2
V5
III
AVF
V3
V6

Electrocardiogram #40

Atrial Rate	130	**Beats/Minute**
Ventricular Rate	130	**Beats/Minute**
PR Interval	0.14	**Second**
QRS Duration	0.07	**Second**
QT-QTc	0.29–0.43	**Second**
QRS Complex Axis	80	**Degrees**

Rate: The atrial and ventricular rates are 130 beats per minute.

Rhythm: The PR interval is 0.14 second and constant. The rate is sinus tachycardia.

Conduction Abnormalities: No criteria present in this electrocardiogram.

QRS Complex Axis: The mean QRS complex axis is 80°.

Chamber Enlargement: The P waves are peaked in leads II, III and AVF. This peaking of the P waves in the inferior leads has been termed "p-pulmonale." This pattern is seen in right atrial enlargement.

Infarction: No criteria present in this electrocardiogram.

ST Segment and T Wave Abnormalities: No criteria present in this electrocardiogram.

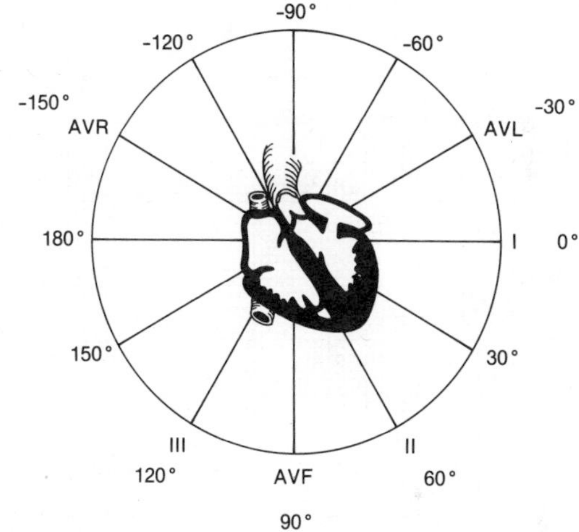

Summary

Sinus tachycardia

Right atrial enlargement (p-pulmonale)

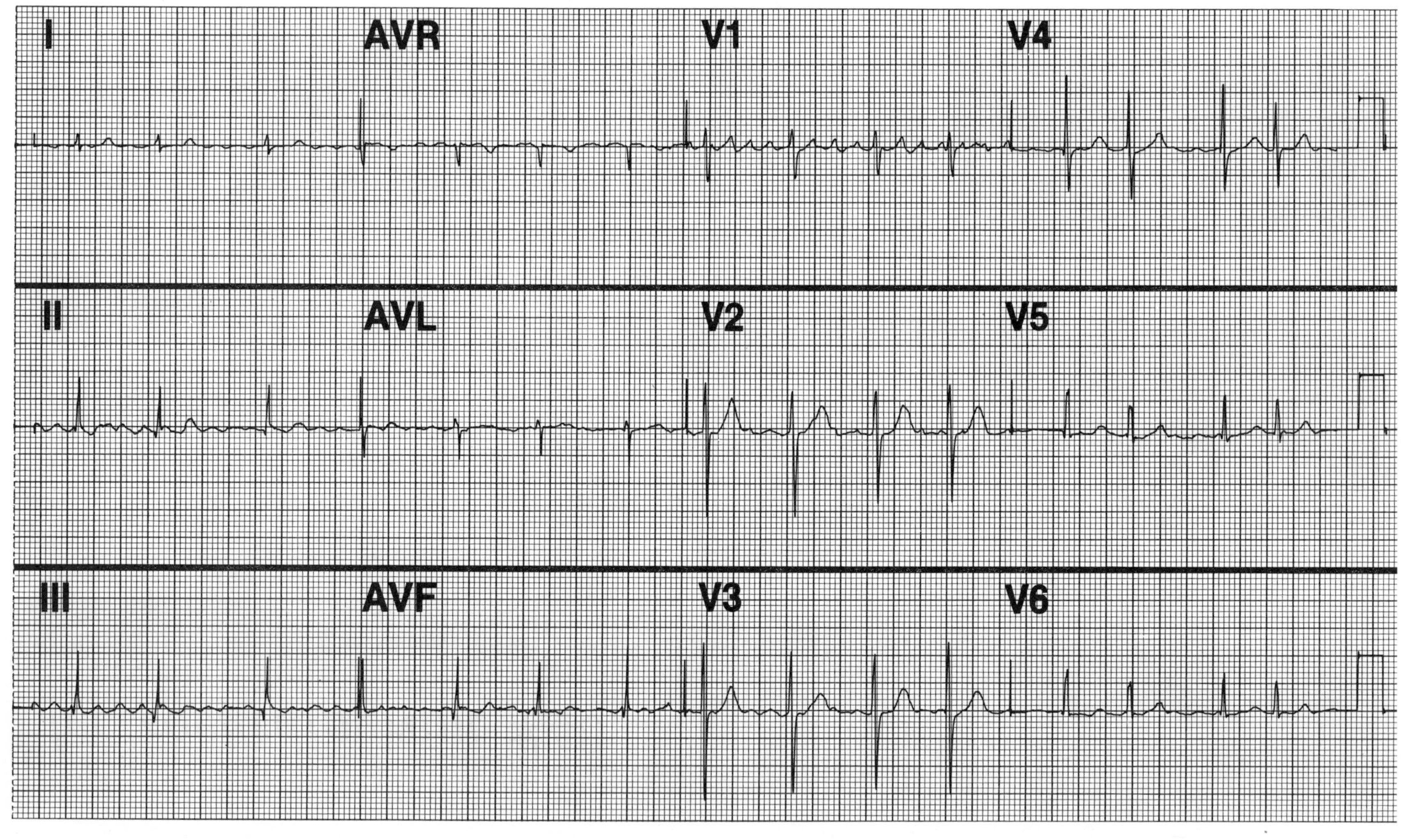
I
AVR
V1
V4
II
AVL
V2
V5
III
AVF
V3
V6

Electrocardiogram #41

Atrial Rate	**—**	**Beats/Minute**
Ventricular Rate	**90**	**Beats/Minute**
PR Interval	**—**	**Second**
QRS Duration	**0.07**	**Second**
QT-QTc	**0.33–0.41**	**Second**
QRS Complex Axis	**85**	**Degrees**

Rate: The average ventricular rate is 90 beats per minute.

Rhythm: No P waves are seen in this electrocardiogram. Instead, an undulating baseline is present. In some areas, a saw-tooth–like pattern is evident, especially in leads III and V1. The rhythm is irregularly irregular, and this would be termed a coarse atrial fibrillation. The term "fibrillation-flutter" has been applied to this type of rhythm. However, in reality this rhythm behaves much closer to that of atrial fibrillation.

Conduction Abnormalities: No criteria present in this electrocardiogram.

QRS Complex Axis: Leads I and AVF are positive, with lead I almost equiphasic. The mean QRS axis is therefore approximately 85°.

Chamber Enlargement: No criteria present in this electrocardiogram.

Infarction: No criteria present in this electrocardiogram.

ST Segment and T Wave Abnormalities: No criteria present in this electrocardiogram.

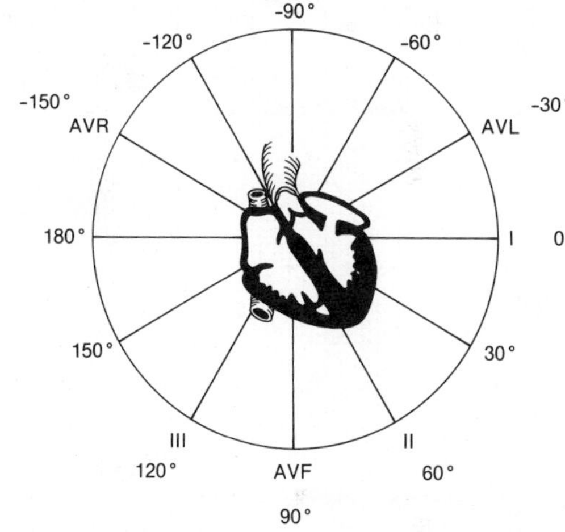

Summary

Coarse atrial fibrillation

Otherwise normal electrocardiogram

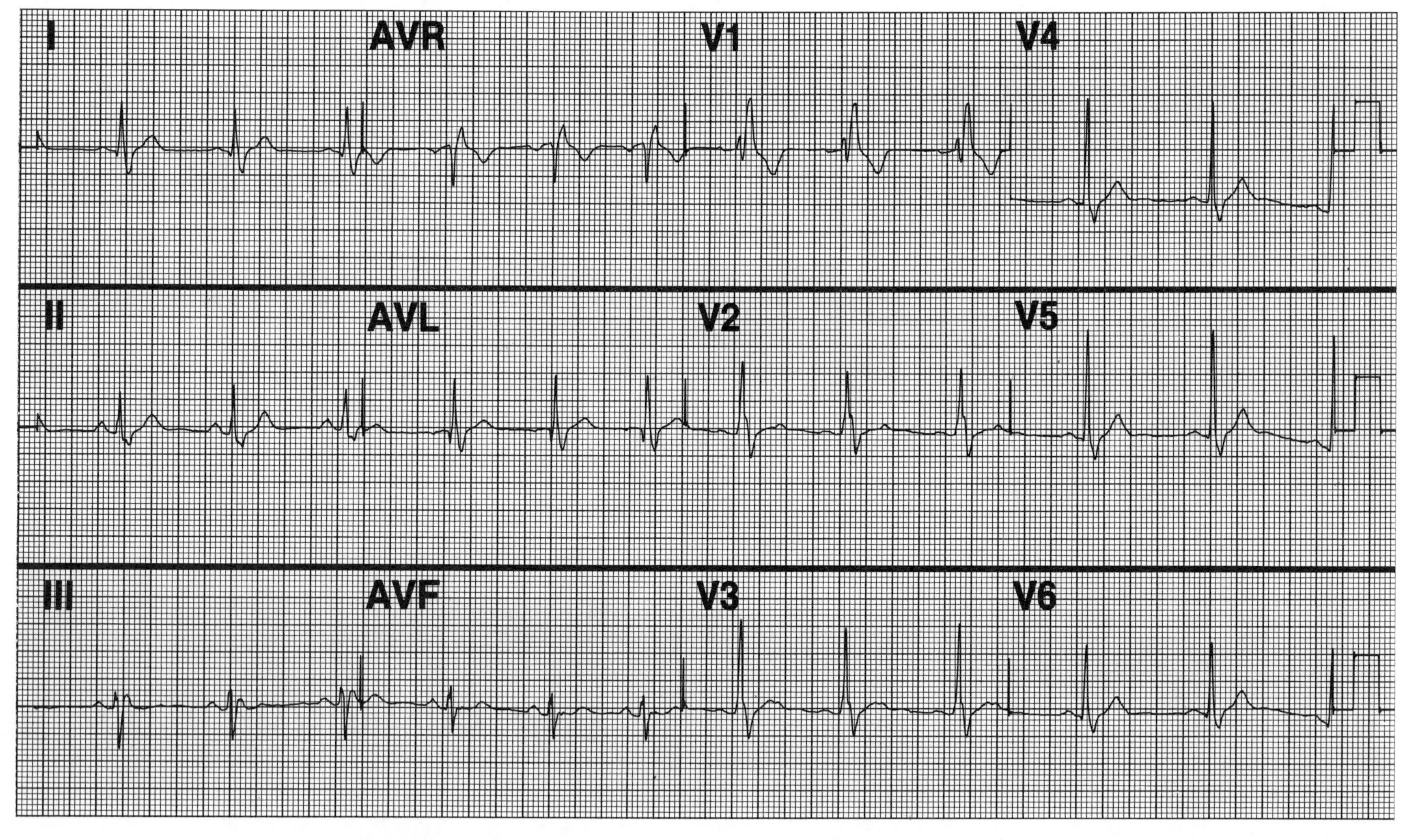
I
AVR
V1
V4
II
AVL
V2
V5
III
AVF
V3
V6

Electrocardiogram #42

Atrial Rate	**70**	**Beats/Minute**
Ventricular Rate	**70**	**Beats/Minute**
PR Interval	**0.16**	**Second**
QRS Duration	**0.07**	**Second**
QT-QTc	**0.38–0.42**	**Second**
QRS Complex Axis	**0**	**Degrees**

Rate: The atrial and ventricular rates are 70 beats per minute.

Rhythm: The PR interval is 0.16 second and constant. The rhythm is normal sinus rhythm.

Conduction Abnormalities: An rsR′ complex is clearly seen in lead V1 together with slurring of the terminal portion of the QRS complex in leads I and V5 and V6. Therefore, a right bundle branch block exists.

QRS Complex Axis: The mean QRS complex axis is 0°.

Chamber Enlargement: No criteria present in this electrocardiogram.

Infarction: No criteria present in this electrocardiogram.

ST Segment and T Wave Abnormalities: The ST segment depression and T wave inversions seen in lead V1 are a manifestation of the conduction abnormality. These are secondary repolarization changes.

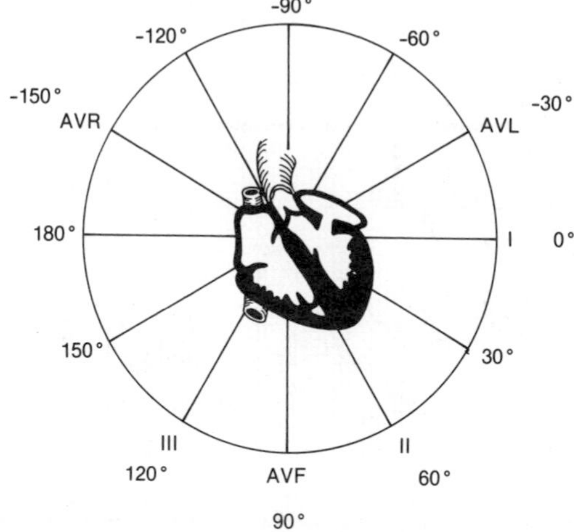

Summary

Normal sinus rhythm

Right bundle branch block

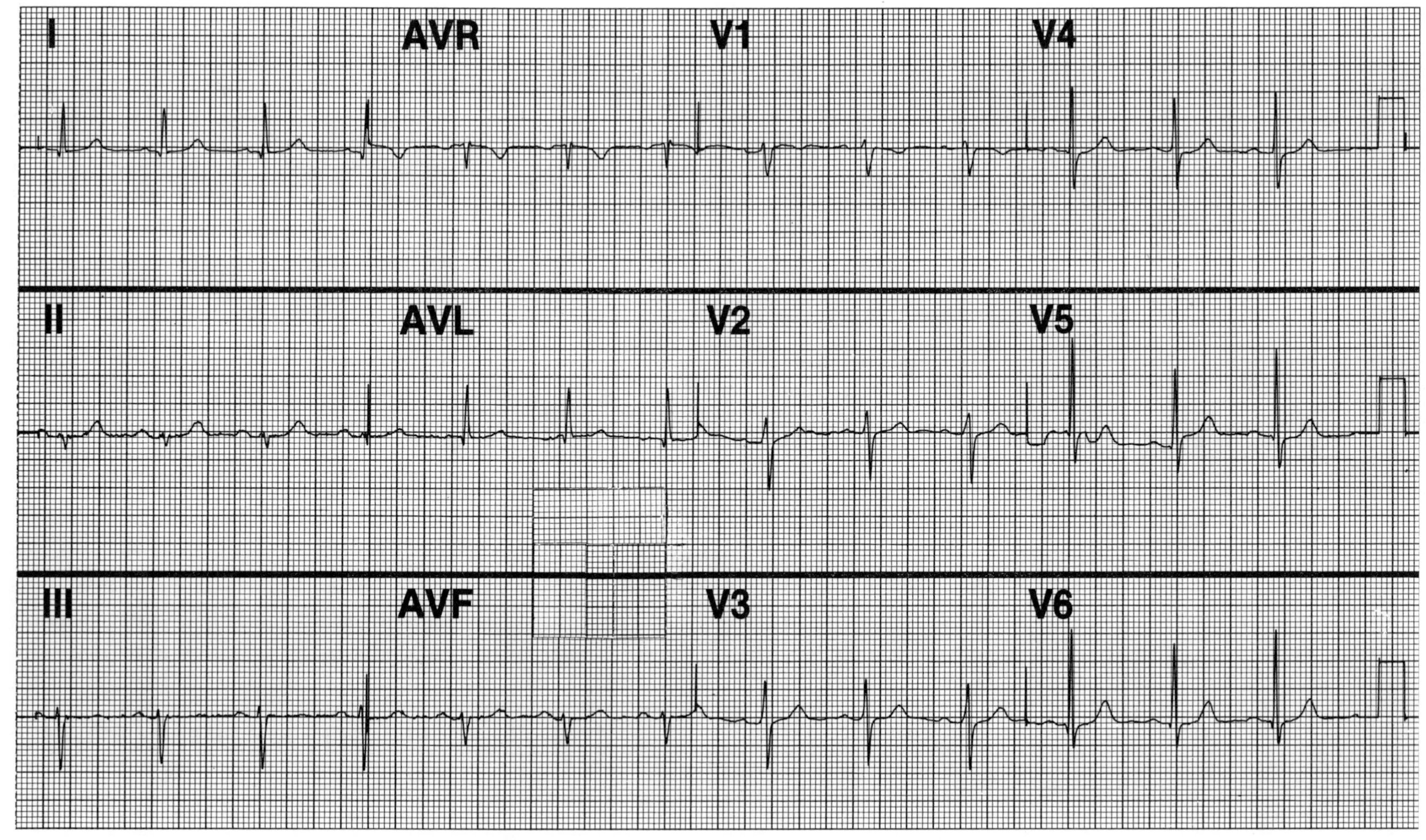
I
AVR
V1
V4
II
AVL
V2
V5
III
AVF
V3
V6

Electrocardiogram #43

Atrial Rate	79	Beats/Minute
Ventricular Rate	79	Beats/Minute
PR Interval	0.16	Second
QRS Duration	0.10	Second
QT-QTc	0.38–0.44	Second
QRS Complex Axis	−30	Degrees

Rate: The atrial and ventricular rates are 79 beats per minute.

Rhythm: The PR interval is 0.16 second and constant. The rhythm is normal sinus rhythm.

Conduction Abnormalities: No criteria present in this electrocardiogram.

QRS Complex Axis: Lead I is positive, and lead AVF is negative. Lead II is nearly equiphasic. Therefore, the mean QRS complex axis is −30°. This is left axis deviation, which is seen in left anterior hemiblock and left ventricular hypertrophy and in obese individuals. It also may be seen when the diaphragm is pushed upward, as in ascites or in pregnancy.

Chamber Enlargement: No criteria present in this electrocardiogram.

Infarction: No criteria present in this electrocardiogram.

ST Segment and T Wave Abnormalities: No criteria present in this electrocardiogram.

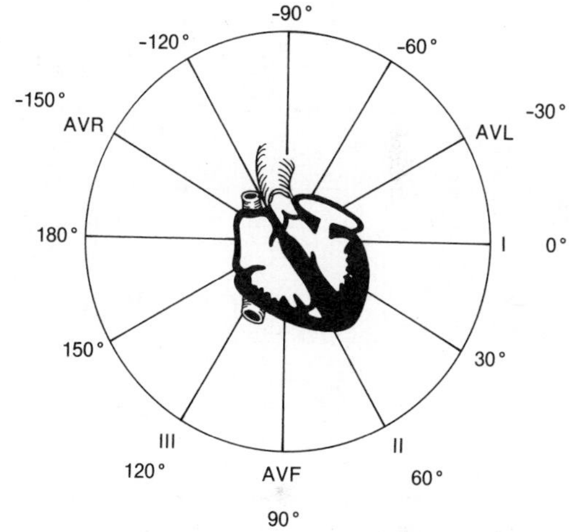

Summary

Normal sinus rhythm

Abnormal left axis deviation

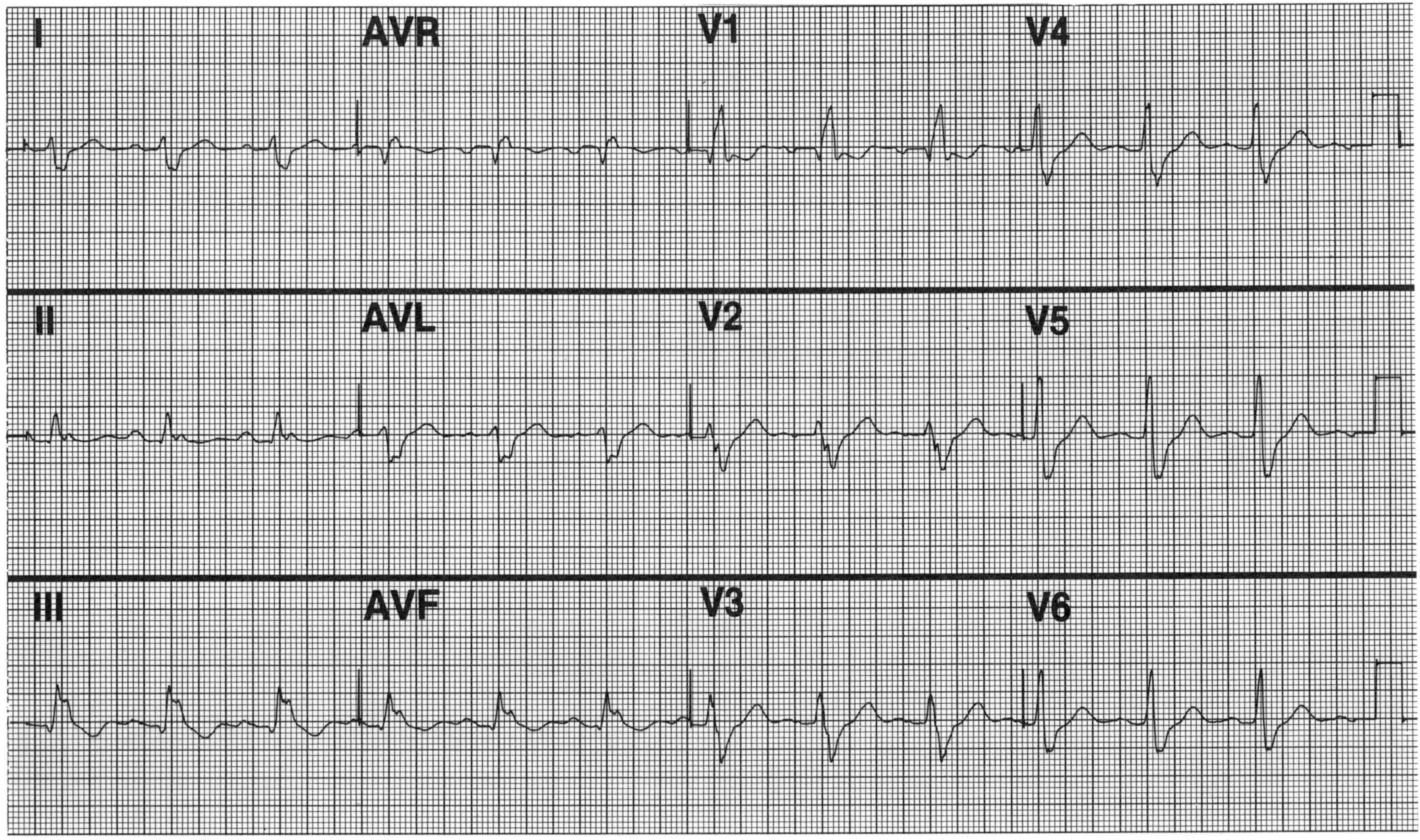
I
AVR
V1
V4
II
AVL
V2
V5
III
AVF
V3
V6

Electrocardiogram #44

Atrial Rate	75	**Beats/Minute**
Ventricular Rate	75	**Beats/Minute**
PR Interval	0.26	**Second**
QRS Duration	0.22	**Second**
QT-QTc	0.48–0.54	**Second**
QRS Complex Axis	100	**Degrees**

Rate: The atrial and ventricular rates are 75 beats per minute.

Rhythm: The PR interval is 0.26 second and constant. The rhythm is normal sinus rhythm.

Conduction Abnormalities: First degree atrioventricular block is present. In addition, a wide QRS complex of 0.22 second is seen in lead V1 together with an abnormal slope of the terminal portion of the QRS complex in leads I, V5 and V6. These changes are indicative of a right bundle branch block.

QRS Complex Axis: The mean QRS complex axis is 100°.

Chamber Enlargement: No criteria present in this electrocardiogram.

Infarction: No criteria present in this electrocardiogram.

ST Segment and T Wave Abnormalities: The ST segment and T wave abnormalities seen in lead V1 are secondary to the conduction abnormality.

Other Findings: The QTc interval is prolonged secondary to the conduction abnormality.

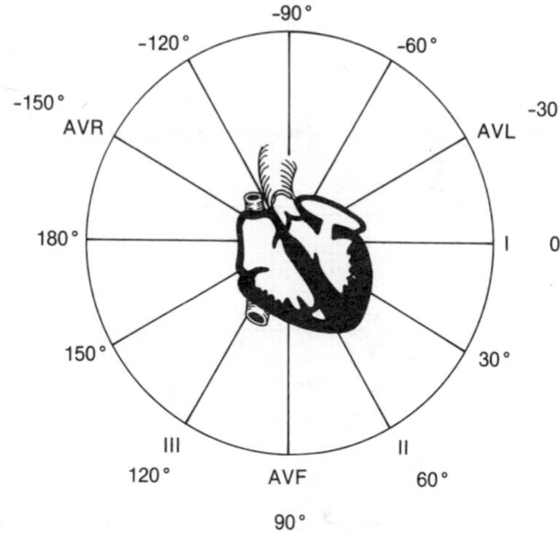

Summary

Normal sinus rhythm with first degree atrioventricular block

Right bundle branch block

I AVR V1 V4

II AVL V2 V5

III AVF V3 V6

Electrocardiogram #45

Atrial Rate	83	**Beats/Minute**
Ventricular Rate	83	**Beats/Minute**
PR Interval	0.13	**Second**
QRS Duration	0.09	**Second**
QT-QTc	0.34–0.40	**Second**
QRS Complex Axis	−15	**Degrees**

Rate: The atrial and ventricular rates are 83 beats per minute.

Rhythm: The PR interval is 0.13 second and constant. The rhythm is normal sinus rhythm.

Conduction Abnormalities: No criteria present in this electrocardiogram.

QRS Complex Axis: The mean QRS complex axis is −15°.

Chamber Enlargement: No criteria present in this electrocardiogram.

Infarction: A QS complex is seen in leads V1 to V3, with flattening of the T waves in all of the precordial leads. The diagnosis of an anteroseptal infarction, age undetermined, should be made. In addition, the QS complex in leads III and AVF together with the T wave flattening in leads II, III and AVF is indicative of an inferior infarct, age undetermined.

ST Segment and T Wave Abnormalities: No criteria present in this electrocardiogram.

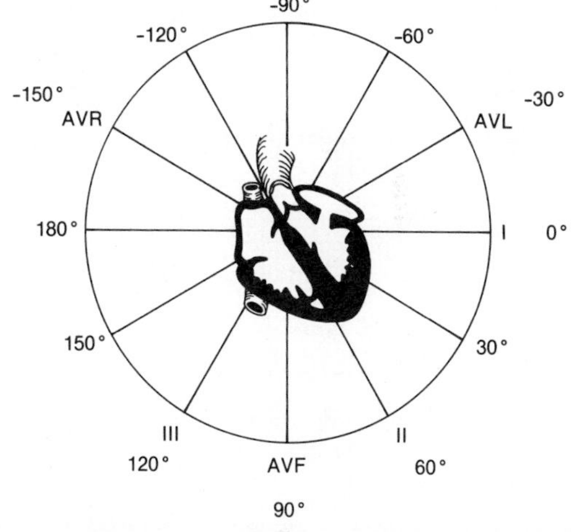

Summary

Normal sinus rhythm

Anteroseptal myocardial infarction, age undetermined

Inferior myocardial infarction, age undetermined

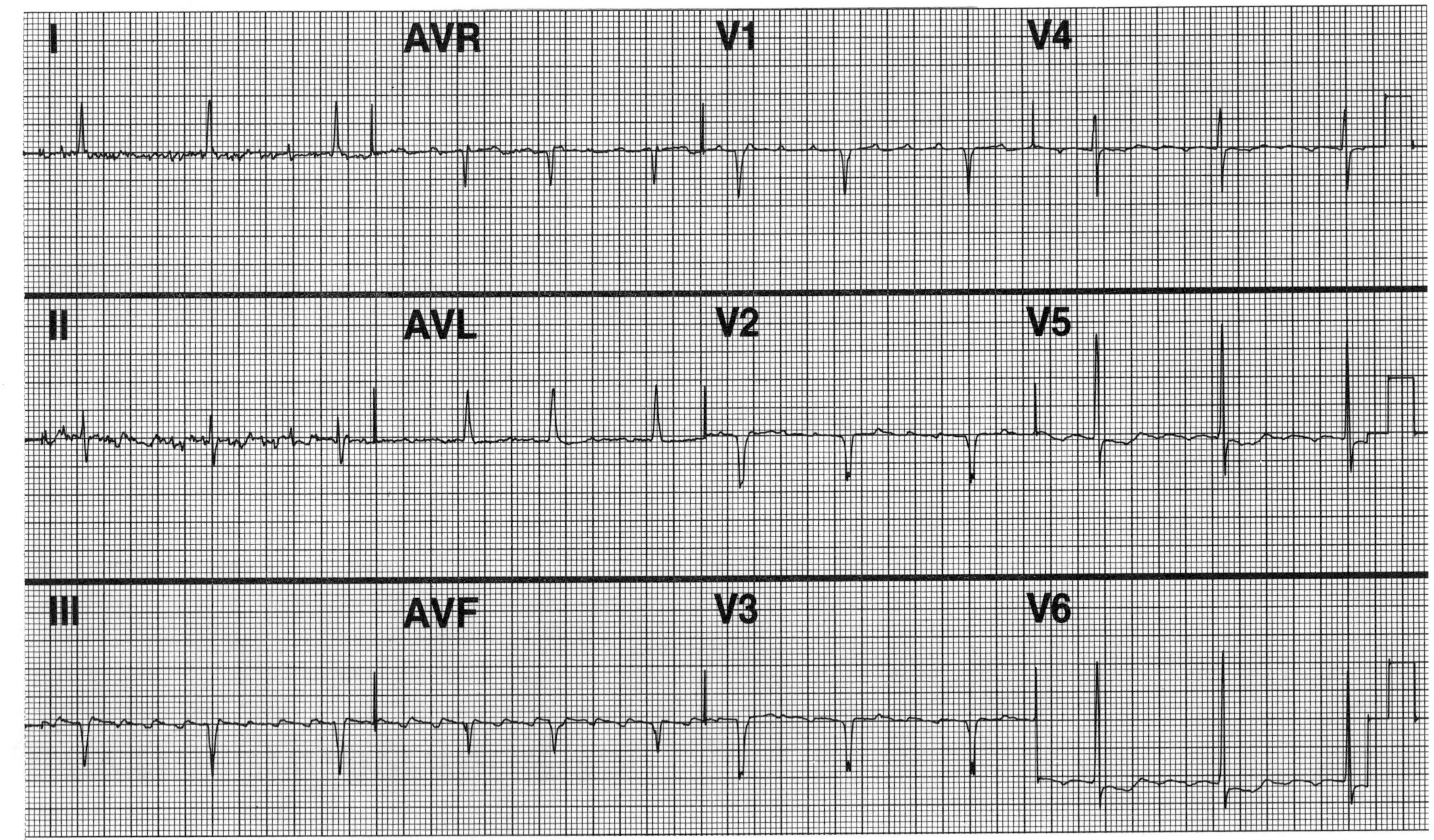
I
AVR
V1
V4
II
AVL
V2
V5
III
AVF
V3
V6

Electrocardiogram #46

Atrial Rate	**290**	**Beats/Minute**
Ventricular Rate	**70**	**Beats/Minute**
PR Interval	**—**	**Second**
QRS Duration	**0.09**	**Second**
QT-QTc	**0.36–0.40**	**Second**
QRS Complex Axis	**−30**	**Degrees**

Rate: The average ventricular rate is 70 beats per minute.

Rhythm: No P waves are seen. However, atrial activity is detected at approximately 290 beats per minute. There are approximately 4 atrial complexes to every ventricular complex. Therefore, a 4:1 atrioventricular block exists. The basic rhythm is atrial flutter.

Conduction Abnormalities: A 4:1 atrioventricular nodal block is present. This is a normal physiological block.

QRS Complex Axis: The mean QRS complex axis is −30°.

Chamber Enlargement: No criteria present in this electrocardiogram.

Infarction: A QS complex is present in leads V1 to V3 together with flattening of the T waves throughout the precordial leads. An inferior infarction is also present. This diagnosis is made from the QS complex seen in leads III and AVF.

ST Segment and T Wave Abnormalities: ST segment depression and T wave inversions are seen in the lateral leads V5 and V6.

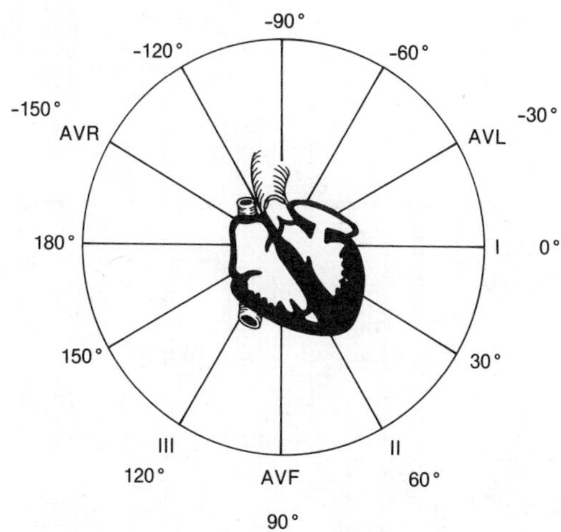

Summary

Atrial flutter with 4:1 atrioventricular block

Anteroseptal myocardial infarction, age undetermined

Inferior myocardial infarction, age undetermined

Nonspecific ST segment and T-wave abnormalities

I AVR V1 V4

II AVL V2 V5

III AVF V3 V6

Electrocardiogram #47

Atrial Rate	300	**Beats/Minute**
Ventricular Rate	75	**Beats/Minute**
PR Interval	—	**Second**
QRS Duration	0.09	**Second**
QT-QTc	0.40–0.45	**Second**
QRS Complex Axis	95	**Degrees**

Rate: The average ventricular rate is 75 beats per minute.

Rhythm: Atrial activity is detected at 300 beats per minute and has a saw-toothed configuration. Since there are approximately four atrial complexes to every ventricular complex, there is 4:1 AV block. Therefore, the rhythm is atrial flutter with 4:1 atrioventricular block.

Conduction Abnormalities: A 4:1 atrioventricular block is present. This is a normal physiological block. In addition, the rSr′ complex in lead V1 is suggestive of a right ventricular conduction delay.

QRS Complex Axis: The mean QRS complex axis is 95°.

Chamber Enlargement: No criteria present in this electrocardiogram.

Infarction: A QS complex is present in lead AVL and a qRs complex in lead I; therefore, based on this electrocardiogram one should be suspicious of lateral wall infarction.

ST Segment and T Wave Abnormalities: There are diffuse ST segment and T wave abnormalities that are suggestive of subendocardial injury.

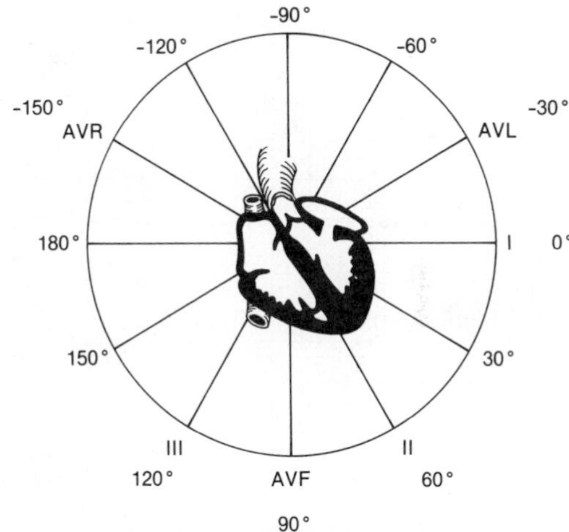

Summary

Atrial flutter with 4:1 atrioventricular block

RSR′ pattern suggestive of a right ventricular conduction delay

Lateral myocardial infarction, age undetermined

Nonspecific ST segment and T wave abnormalities

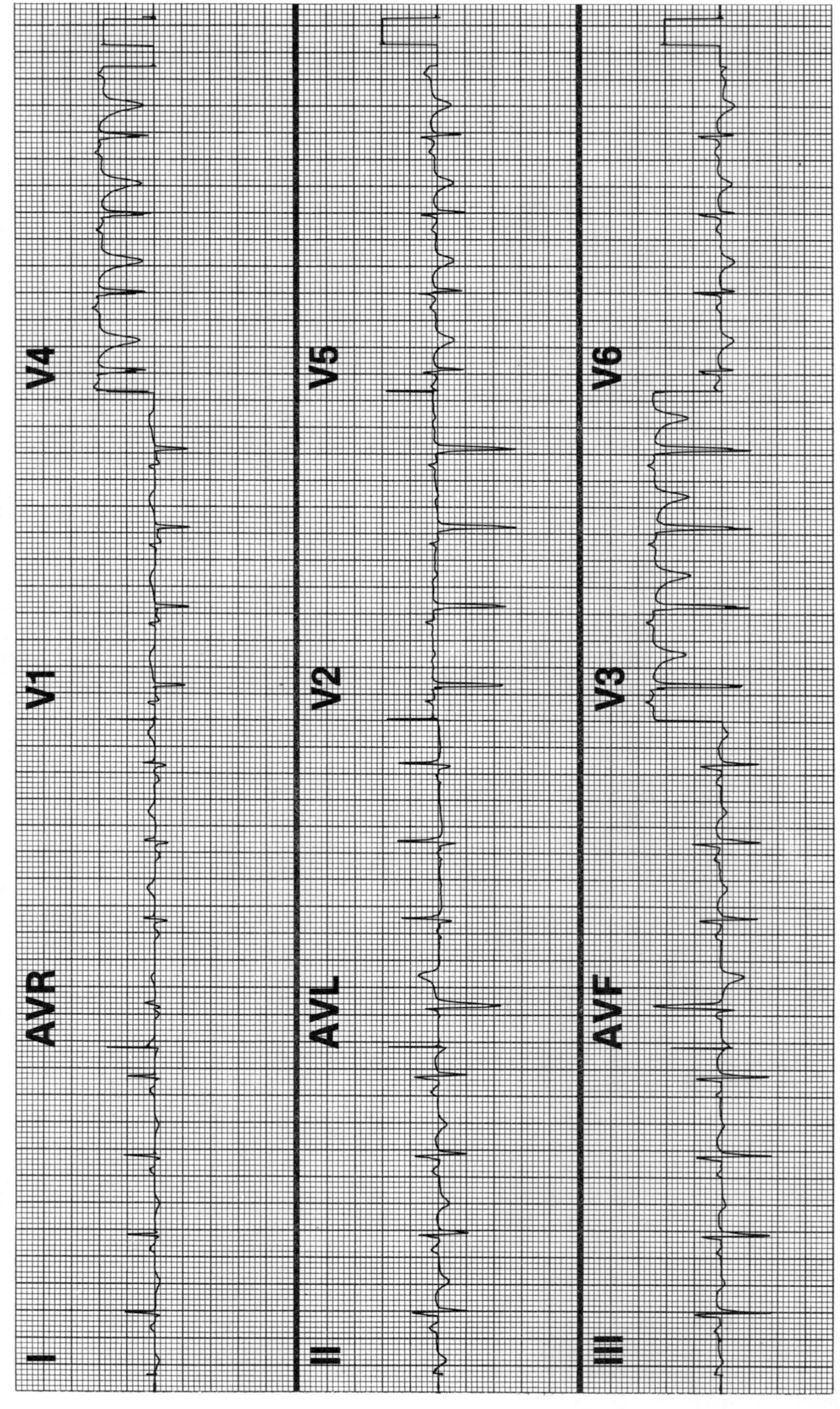
I
AVR
V1
V4
II
AVL
V2
V5
III
AVF
V3
V6

Electrocardiogram #48

Atrial Rate	**103**	**Beats/Minute**
Ventricular Rate	**103**	**Beats/Minute**
PR Interval	**0.12**	**Second**
QRS Duration	**0.08**	**Second**
QT-QTc	**0.36–0.46**	**Second**
QRS Complex Axis	**−35**	**Degrees**

Rate: The atrial and ventricular rates are 103 beats per minute.

Rhythm: The PR interval is 0.12 second and constant. The rhythm is normal sinus rhythm (borderline sinus tachycardia). One should note that the first beat clearly seen in the second lead set AVR, AVL and AVF is a premature ventricular complex.

Conduction Abnormalities: The abnormal left axis deviation is suggestive of a left anterior hemiblock. This type of conduction abnormality changes the direction of the electrical impulse. The initial wave of depolarization is posterior and to the right and produces a small q wave in lead I and a small r wave in lead II. The bulk of the depolarizaton proceeds in an upward, anterior and leftward direction. This produces the left axis deviation by inscribing a qR complex in lead I and an rS complex in lead II.

QRS Complex Axis: The mean QRS complex axis is −35°.

Chamber Enlargement: No criteria present in this electrocardiogram.

Infarction: A QS complex is seen in leads V1 to V3, with an rS complex seen in lead V4.

ST Segment and T Wave Abnormalities: There are symmetric T wave inversions throughout the precordium, especially seen in the midprecordial leads V3 and V4. There is also flattening of the T waves in leads AVL, with T wave inversions in lead I. All of these ST segment and T wave abnormalities are suggestive of ischemia.

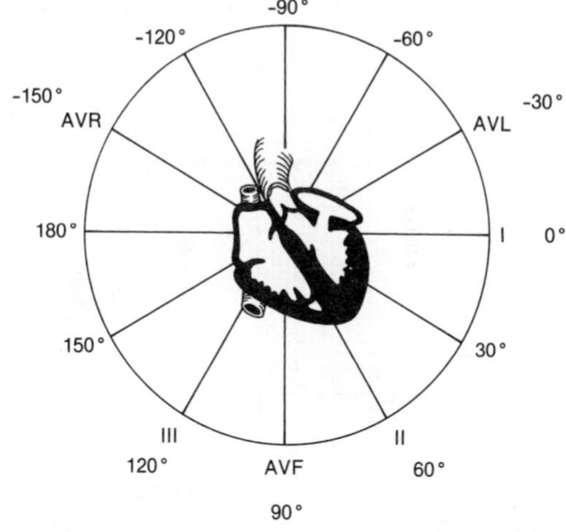

Summary

Normal sinus rhythm

Abnormal left axis deviation; consider left anterior hemiblock

Anterior myocardial infarction, age undetermined

Anterolateral ischemia

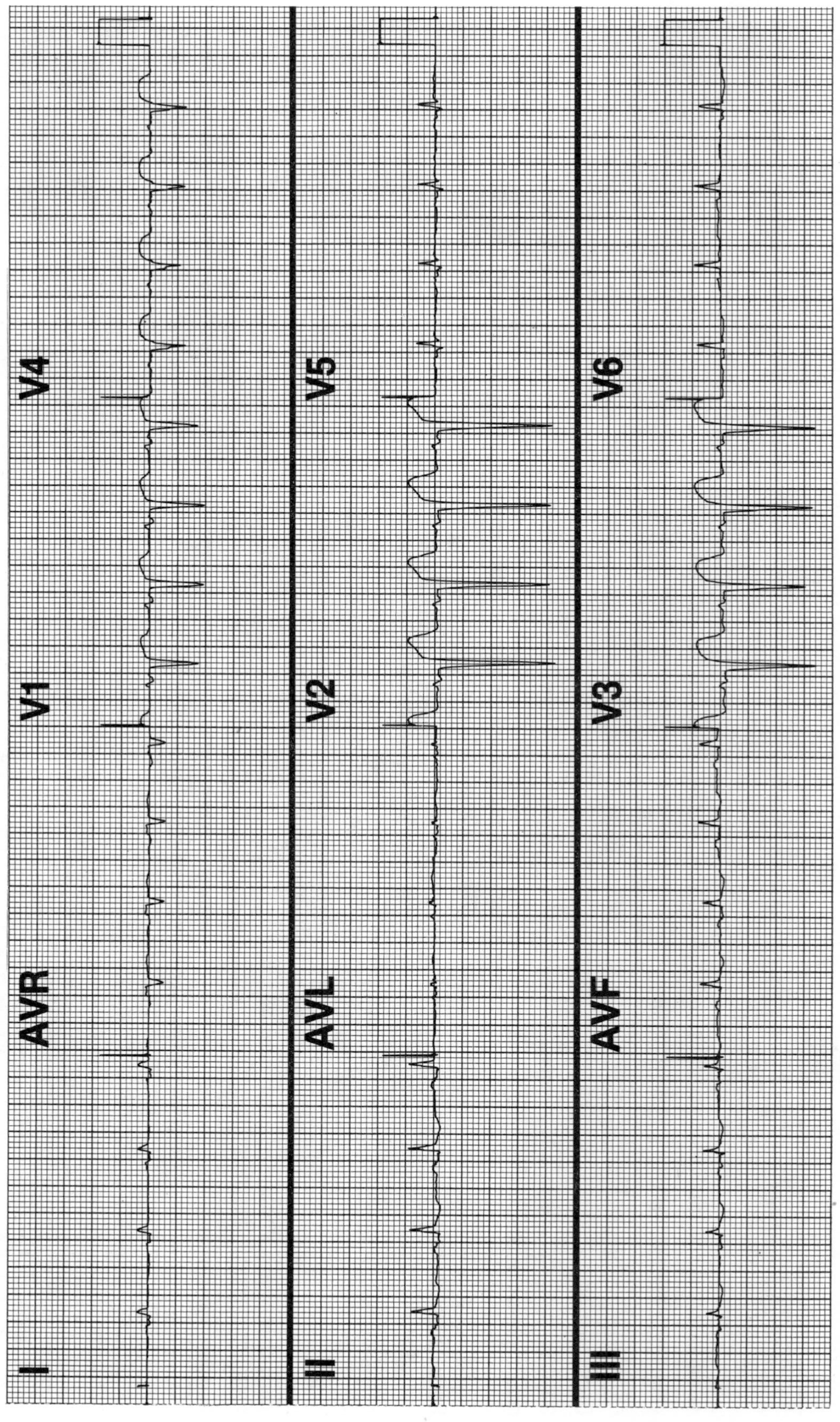
I
AVR
V1
V4
II
AVL
V2
V5
III
AVF
V3
V6

Electrocardiogram #49

Atrial Rate	**103**	**Beats/Minute**
Ventricular Rate	**103**	**Beats/Minute**
PR Interval	**0.15**	**Second**
QRS Duration	**0.09**	**Second**
QT-QTc	**0.30–0.39**	**Second**
QRS Complex Axis	**60**	**Degrees**

Rate: The atrial and ventricular rates are 103 beats per minute.

Rhythm: The PR interval is 0.15 second and constant. The rhythm is normal sinus rhythm.

Conduction Abnormalities: No criteria present in this electrocardiogram.

QRS Complex Axis: The mean QRS complex axis is 60°, since the QRS complex is most equiphasic in lead AVL.

Chamber Enlargement: No criteria present in this electrocardiogram.

Infarction: The striking abnormality of this electrocardiogram is the QS complexes present in leads V1 to V4 together with the 4-mm ST segment elevation and T wave abnormalities seen in the same leads. The diagnosis of an anteroseptal infarct, possibly acute, should be made. If one knew that this individual had a myocardial infarction 6 months earlier, an electrocardiogram such as this example with its ST segment elevations would be suggestive of anteroseptal aneurysm.

ST Segment and T Wave Abnormalities: No criteria present in this electrocardiogram.

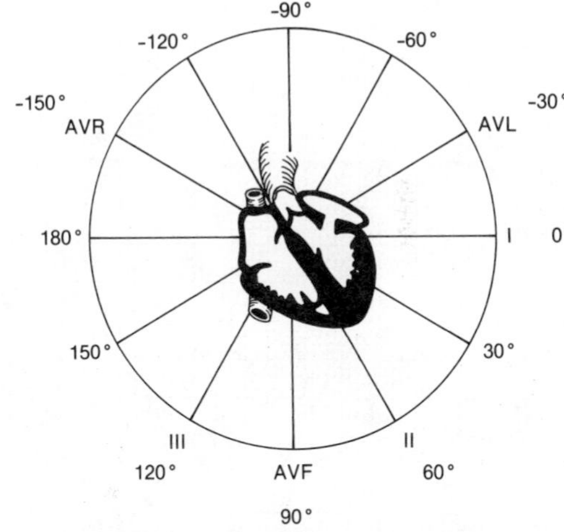

Summary

Normal sinus rhythm

Anteroseptal myocardial infarction, possibly acute

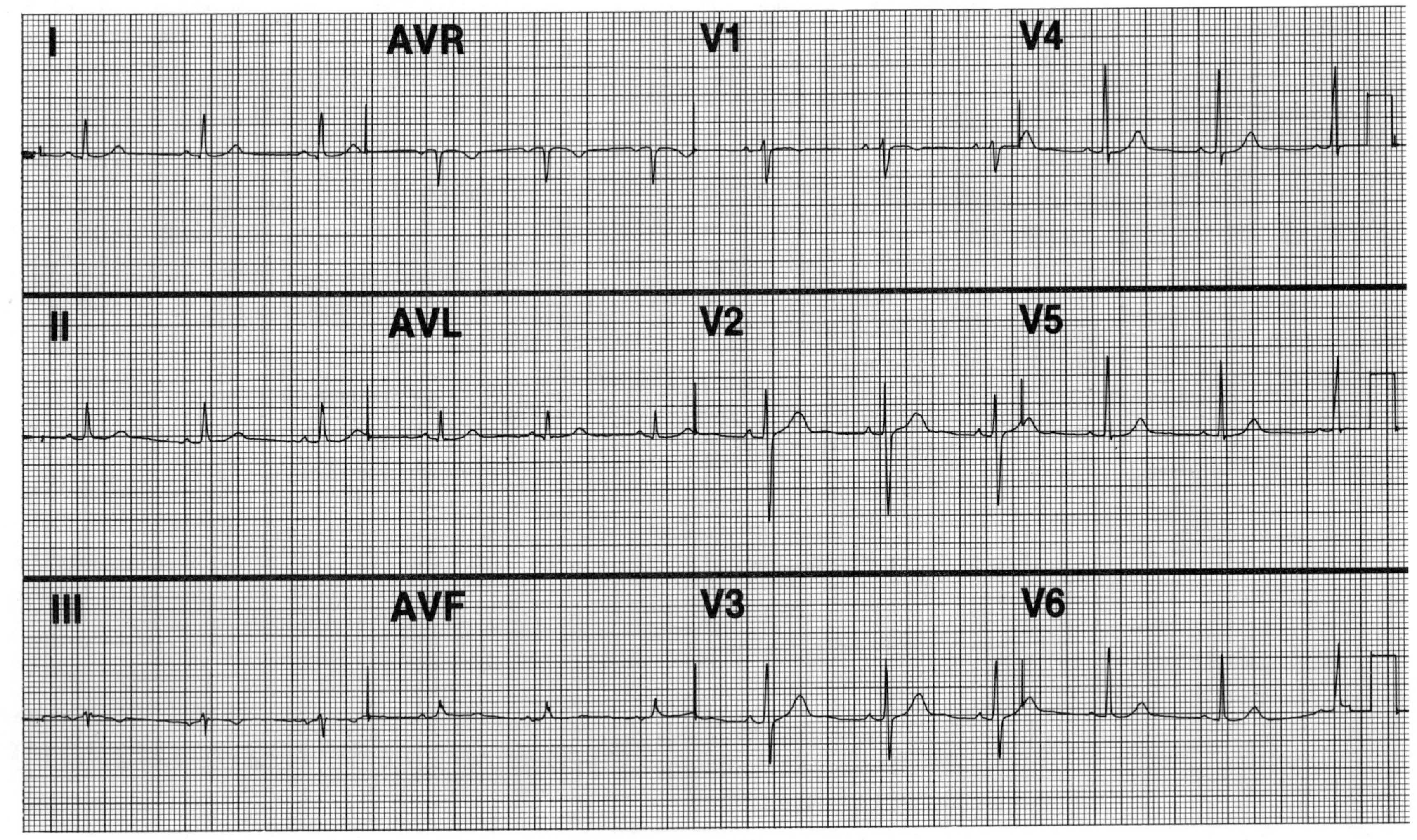
I
AVR
V1
V4
II
AVL
V2
V5
III
AVF
V3
V6

Electrocardiogram #50

Atrial Rate	70	**Beats/Minute**
Ventricular Rate	70	**Beats/Minute**
PR Interval	0.14	**Second**
QRS Duration	0.08	**Second**
QT-QTc	0.37–0.40	**Second**
QRS Complex Axis	20	**Degrees**

Rate: The atrial and ventricular rates are 70 beats per minute.

Rhythm: The PR interval is 0.14 second and constant. The rhythm is normal sinus rhythm.

Conduction Abnormalities: No criteria present in this electrocardiogram.

QRS Complex Axis: The mean QRS complex axis is 20°.

Chamber Enlargement: No criteria present in this electrocardiogram.

Infarction: No criteria present in this electrocardiogram.

ST Segment and T Wave Abnormalities: No criteria present in this electrocardiogram.

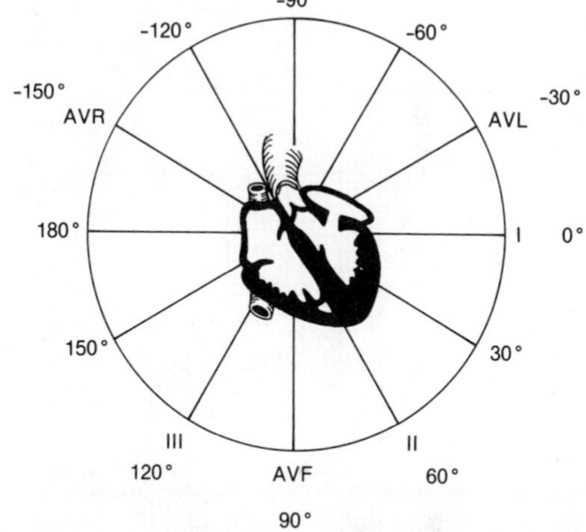

Summary

Normal sinus rhythm

Normal electrocardiogram

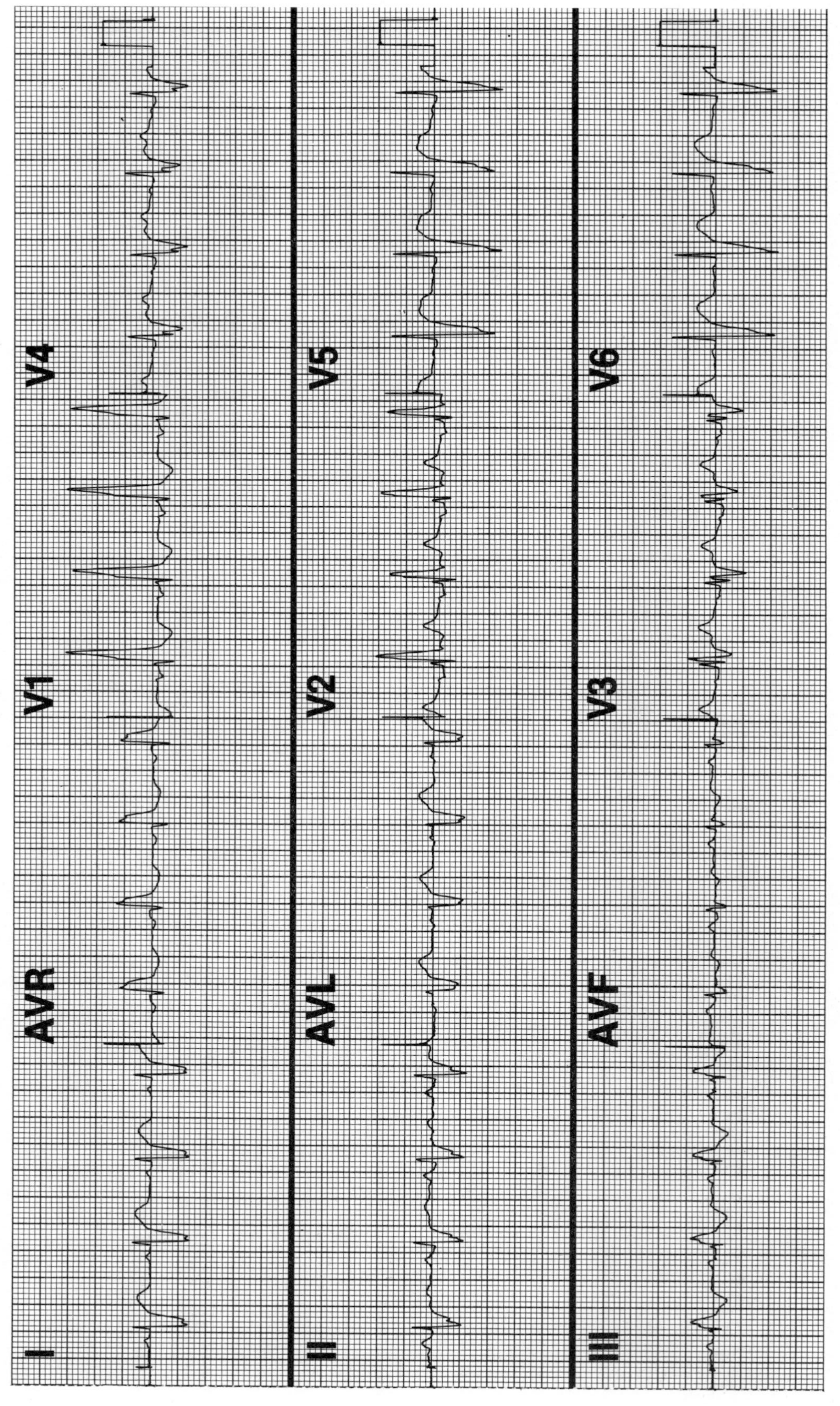
I
AVR
V1
V4
II
AVL
V2
V5
III
AVF
V3
V6

Electrocardiogram #51

Atrial Rate	97	**Beats/Minute**
Ventricular Rate	97	**Beats/Minute**
PR Interval	0.13	**Second**
QRS Duration	0.15	**Second**
QT-QTc	0.38–0.48	**Second**
QRS Complex Axis	160	**Degrees**

Rate: The atrial and ventricular rates are 97 beats per minute.

Rhythm: The PR interval is 0.13 second and constant. The rhythm is normal sinus rhythm.

Conduction Abnormalities: The QRS complex duration is prolonged at 0.15 second (>3 small boxes). An rsR′ complex ("M" pattern) is present in leads V1 and V2, which is diagnostic of a right bundle branch block.

QRS Complex Axis: The mean QRS complex axis is 160°. There is severe abnormal right axis deviation present.

Chamber Enlargement: The R wave in lead V1 is 16 mm. The rightward axis and the QRS complex in lead V1 are diagnostic of right ventricular enlargement. Another criterion for right ventricular hypertrophy is a QRS axis of +110° or more. The most specific sign for right ventricular hypertrophy is the rSR′ complex in lead V1, with the R′ greater than 10 mm. The qR complex in lead V1 is also specific for right ventricular hypertrophy.

Infarction: No criteria present in this electrocardiogram.

ST Segment and T Wave Abnormalities: The ST segment and T wave abnormalities seen in the right precordial leads are secondary changes and consistent with the right bundle branch block and right ventricular enlargement.

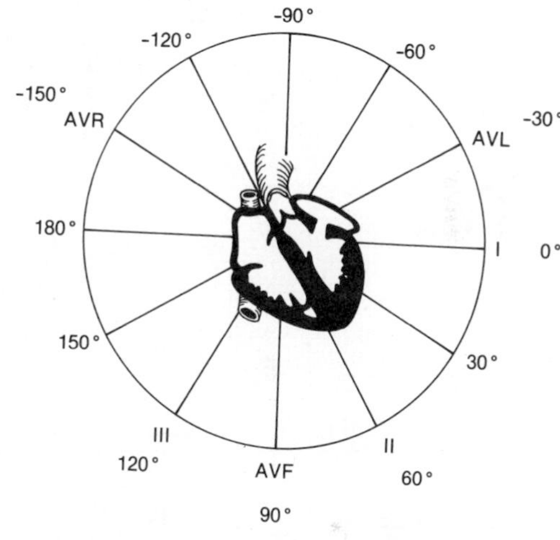

Summary

Normal sinus rhythm

Severe rightward axis

Right bundle branch block

Right ventricular hypertrophy

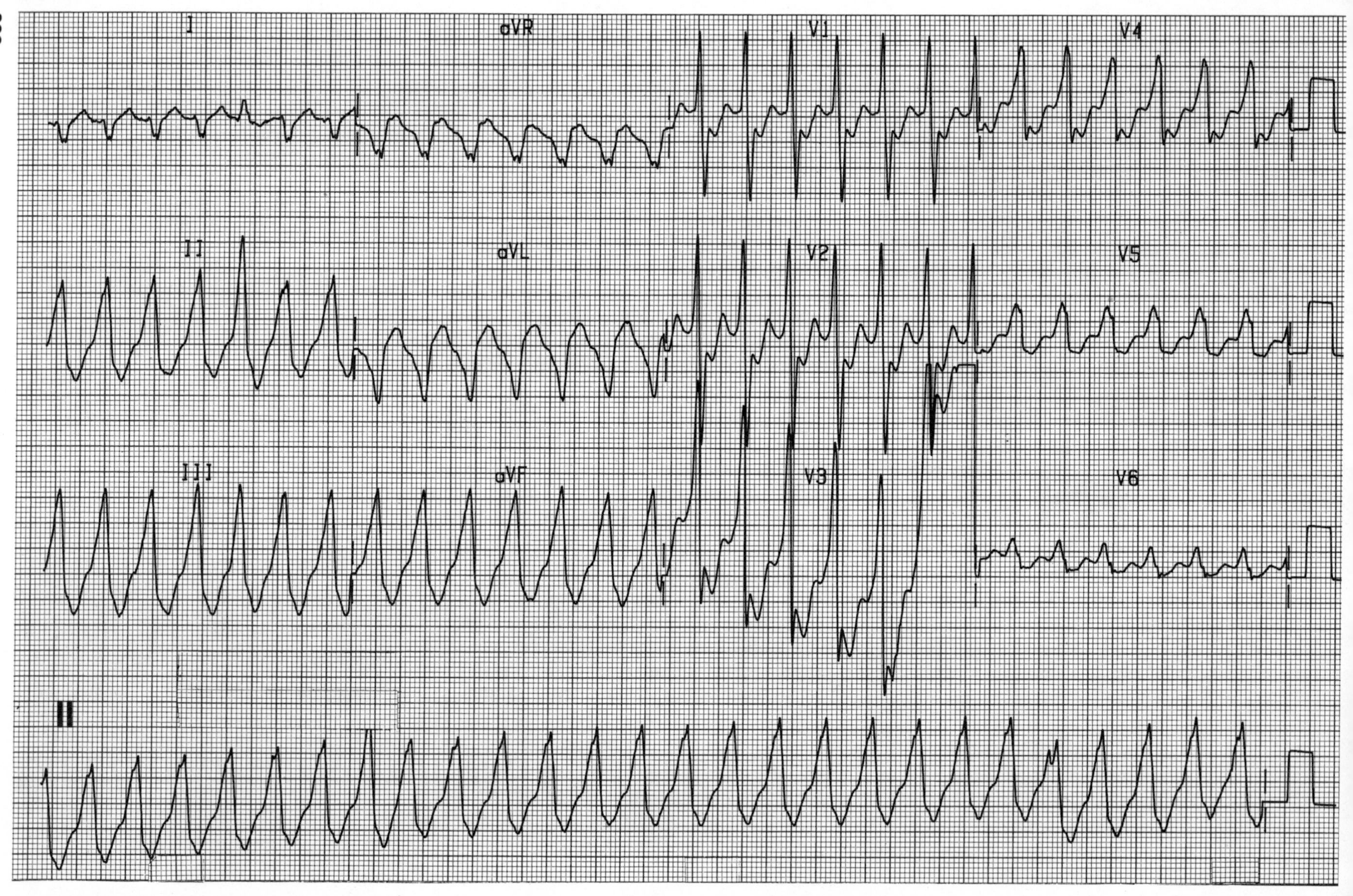
I
aVR
V1
V4
II
aVL
V2
V5
III
aVF
V3
V6
II

Electrocardiogram #52

Atrial Rate	—	**Beats/Minute**
Ventricular Rate	167	**Beats/Minute**
PR Interval	—	**Second**
QRS Duration	0.16	**Second**
QT-QTc	—	**Second**
QRS Complex Axis	110	**Degrees**

Rate: The average ventricular rate is 167 beats per minute.

Rhythm: No P waves can be seen in this very regular rhythm of a wide QRS complex measuring 0.16 second. The complex is ventricular in etiology, and the rhythm is ventricular tachycardia. The assessment of the other complexes and intervals is virtually impossible in this rhythm.

Conduction Abnormalities: No criteria present in this electrocardiogram.

QRS Complex Axis: The mean QRS complex axis is 110°.

Chamber Enlargement: No criteria present in this electrocardiogram.

Infarction: No criteria present in this electrocardiogram.

ST Segment and T Wave Abnormalities: No criteria present in this electrocardiogram.

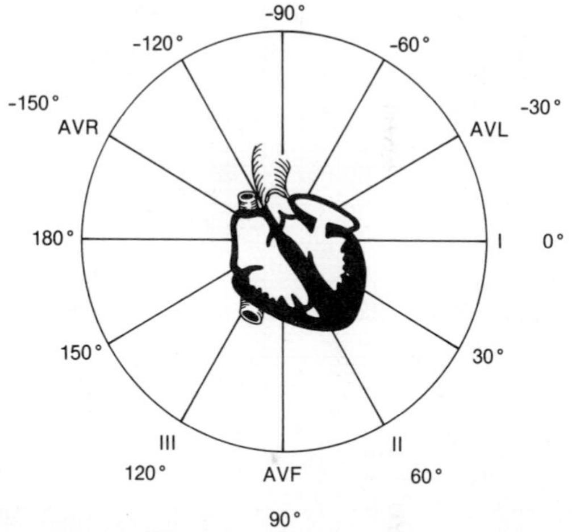

Summary

Ventricular tachycardia

Rightward axis

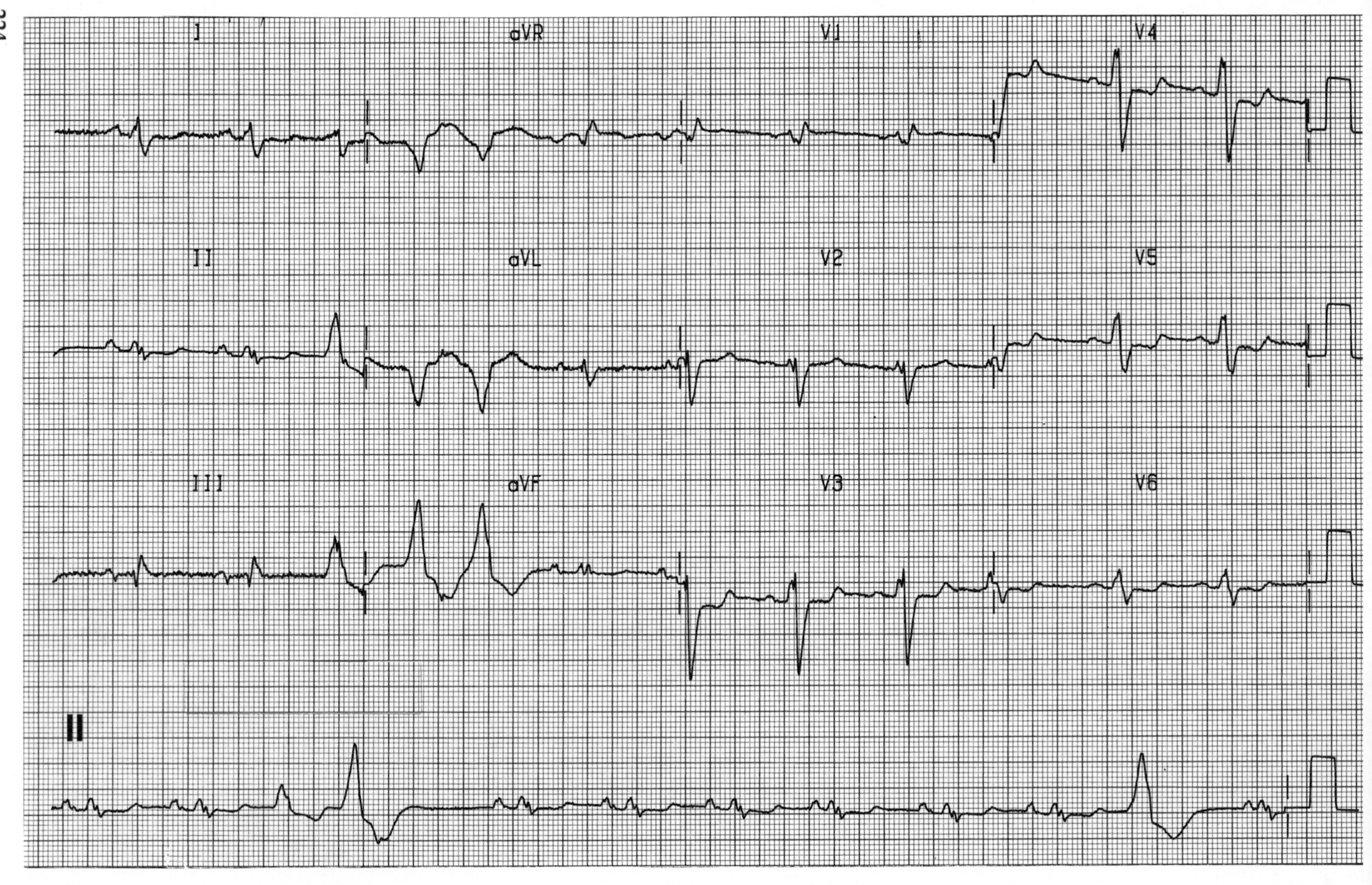
I
aVR
V1
V4
II
aVL
V2
V5
III
aVF
V3
V6
II

Electrocardiogram #53

Atrial Rate	68	Beats/Minute
Ventricular Rate	68	Beats/Minute
PR Interval	0.16	Second
QRS Duration	0.16	Second
QT-QTc	0.44–0.47	Second
QRS Complex Axis	120	Degrees

Rate: The atrial and ventricular rates are 68 beats per minute.

Rhythm: The PR interval is 0.16 second and constant. The rhythm is normal sinus rhythm. Most importantly, if one evaluates the rhythm strip at the bottom of the tracing, one notices that the third and the fourth beat are ventricular in etiology and are ventricular premature complexes. In addition, the beat prior to the last beat on the rhythm strip is also a ventricular premature complex. If one looks at leads AVR, AVL and AVF, the first two consecutive beats seen are ventricular complexes. These two complexes are called a couplet. If three ventricular complexes are together, the term ventricular tachycardia is used.

Conduction Abnormalities: The electrocardiogram shows an rSR′ complex in lead V1. The QRS complex is 0.16 second in duration; therefore, a right bundle branch block is present. Notice the slurred S waves in leads I and V6.

QRS Complex Axis: The mean QRS complex axis is +120°.

Chamber Enlargement: No criteria present in this electrocardiogram.

Infarction: No criteria present in this electrocardiogram.

ST Segment and T Wave Abnormalities: The ST segment and T wave abnormalities are secondary to the conduction abnormalities.

Other Findings: The QTc is minimally prolonged secondary to the conduction abnormality.

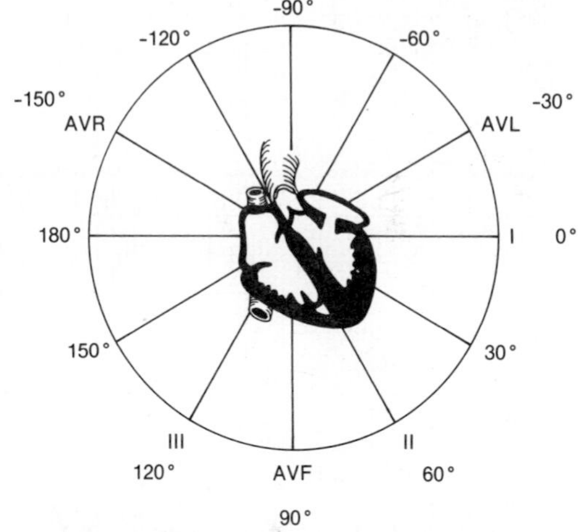

Summary

Normal sinus rhythm with frequent premature ventricular contractions forming couplets

Right bundle branch block

I AVR V1 V4

II AVL V2 V5

III AVF V3 V6

Electrocardiogram #54

Atrial Rate	65	**Beats/Minute**
Ventricular Rate	65	**Beats/Minute**
PR Interval	0.14	**Second**
QRS Duration	0.09	**Second**
QT-QTc	0.44–0.44	**Second**
QRS Complex Axis	60	**Degrees**

Rate: The atrial and ventricular rates are 65 beats per minute.

Rhythm: The PR interval is 0.14 second and constant. The rhythm is normal sinus rhythm.

Conduction Abnormalities: No criteria present in this electrocardiogram.

QRS Complex Axis: The mean QRS complex axis is 60°.

Chamber Enlargement: No criteria present in this electrocardiogram.

Infarction: The marked abnormality seen here is the presence of QS complexes in leads V1 to V4 together with 2 mm ST elevation seen in these leads. In addition, there is symmetric inversion of the T waves, which is suggestive of ischemia. The presence of the T waves and the ST elevation confirms the diagnosis of an anteroseptal myocardial infarction, age undetermined.

ST Segment and T Wave Abnormalities: No criteria present in this electrocardiogram.

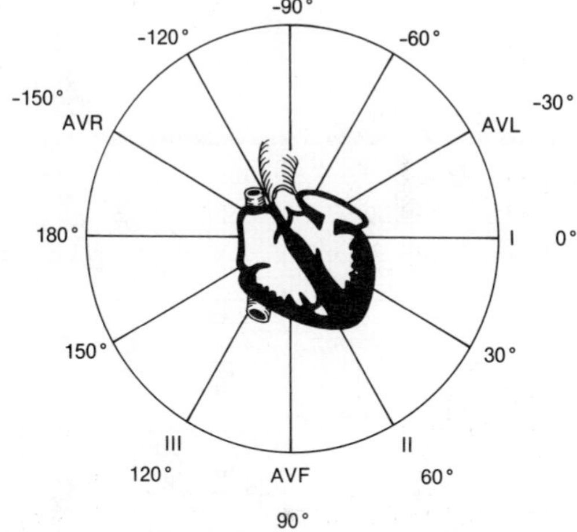

Summary

Normal sinus rhythm

Anteroseptal myocardial infarction, age undetermined

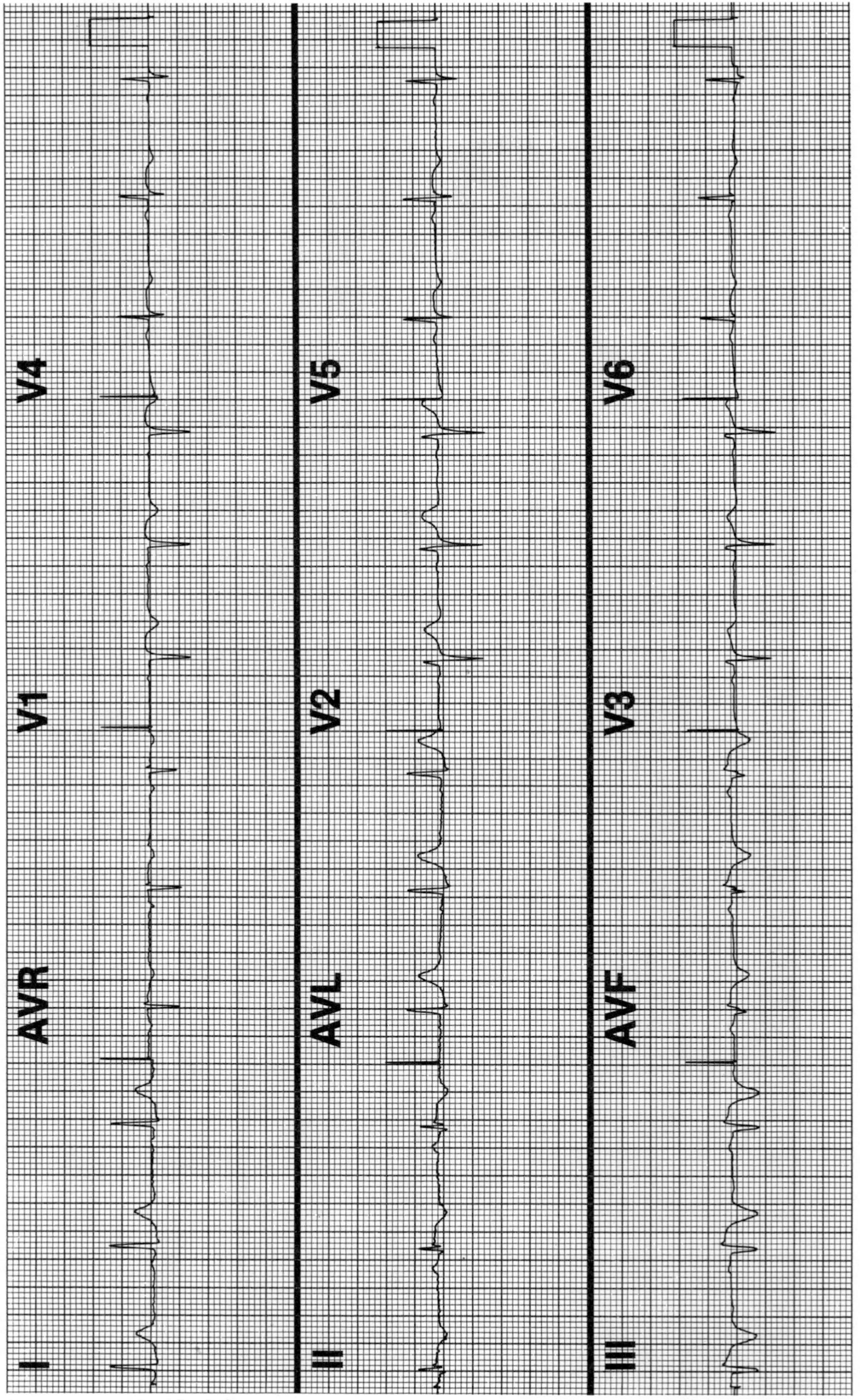
I
AVR
V1
V4
II
AVL
V2
V5
III
AVF
V3
V6

Electrocardiogram #55

Atrial Rate	71	Beats/Minute
Ventricular Rate	71	Beats/Minute
PR Interval	0.15	Second
QRS Duration	0.08	Second
QT-QTc	0.38–0.40	Second
QRS Complex Axis	0	Degrees

Rate: The atrial and ventricular rates are 71 beats per minute.

Rhythm: The PR interval is 0.15 second and constant. The rhythm is normal sinus rhythm.

Conduction Abnormalities: No criteria present in this electrocardiogram.

QRS Complex Axis: The mean QRS complex axis is 0°.

Chamber Enlargement: No criteria present in this electrocardiogram.

Infarction: There is a qR complex seen in lead II that together with the Qr complex in leads III and AVF confirms the diagnosis of an inferior infarction. In addition, there is 2 mm ST segment elevation in the same leads together with symmetric T wave inversions. Therefore, one should qualify the diagnosis of inferior infarction by stating that the age of the infarction is possibly acute. The T wave inversions seen in leads V5 and V6 are suggestive of lateral wall ischemia. This patient may be suffering from an inferolateral myocardial infarction. An occluded coronary circumflex artery will produce this event.

ST Segment and T Wave Abnormalities: See the preceding discussion under infarction.

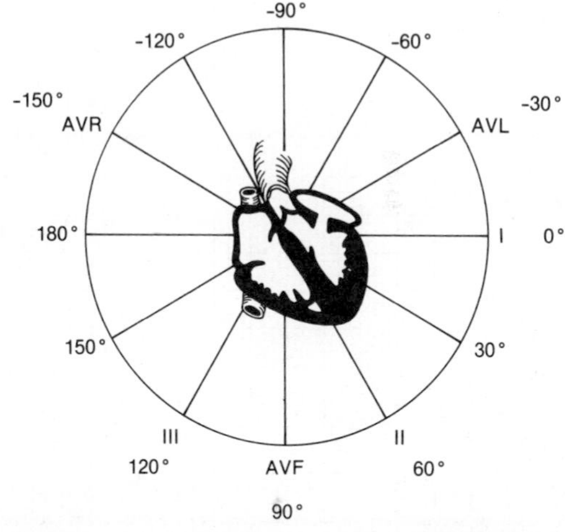

Summary

Normal sinus rhythm

Inferolateral myocardial infarction, possibly acute

Lateral wall ischemia

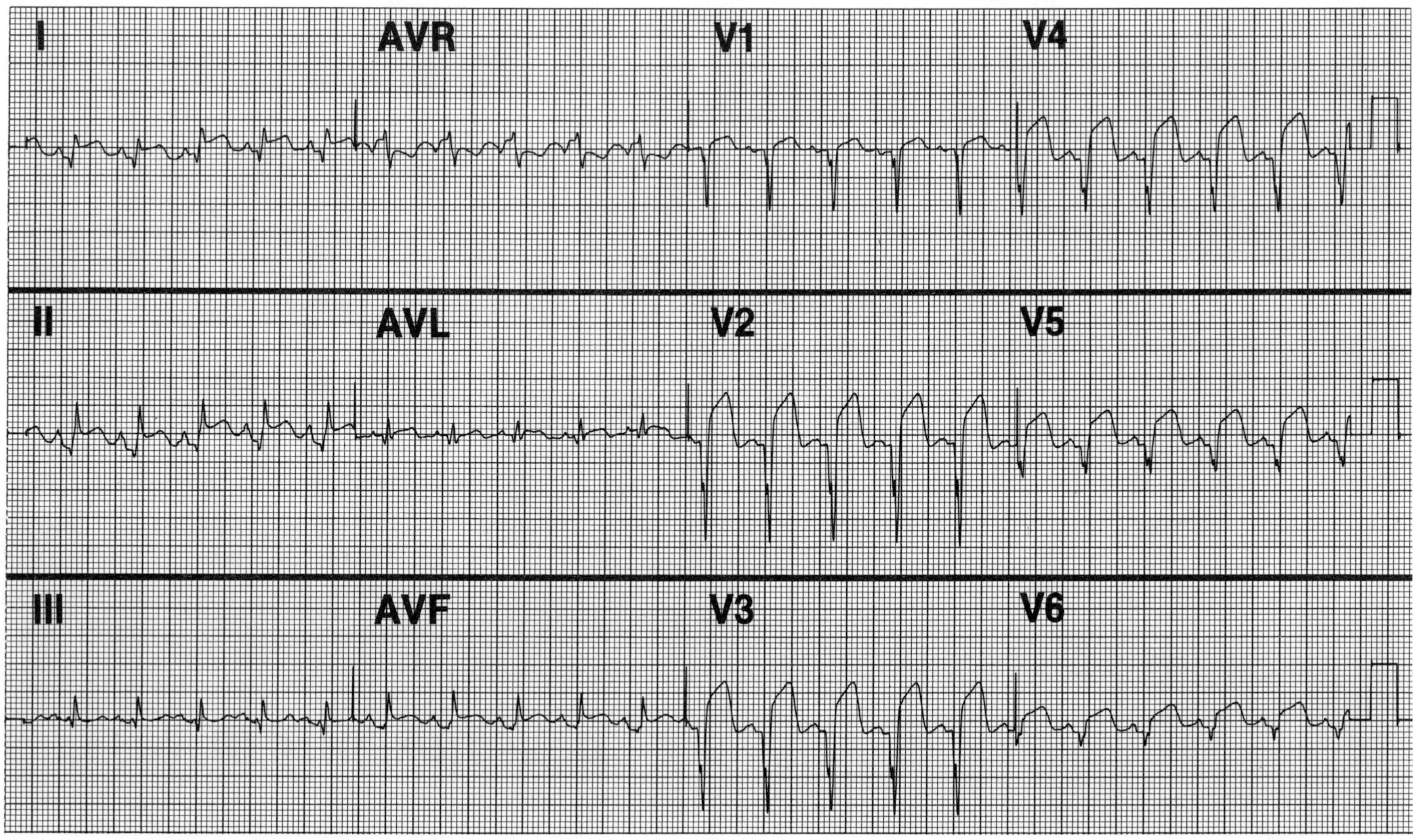
I
AVR
V1
V4
II
AVL
V2
V5
III
AVF
V3
V6

Electrocardiogram #56

Atrial Rate	125	**Beats/Minute**
Ventricular Rate	125	**Beats/Minute**
PR Interval	0.17	**Second**
QRS Duration	0.08	**Second**
QT-QTc	0.30–0.43	**Second**
QRS Complex Axis	60	**Degrees**

Rate: The atrial and ventricular rates are 125 beats per minute.

Rhythm: The PR interval is 0.17 second and constant. The diagnosis is sinus tachycardia.

Conduction Abnormalities: No criteria present in this electrocardiogram.

QRS Complex Axis: The mean QRS complex axis is 60°

Chamber Enlargement: The P waves in lead II measure 2.5 mm in height. This is suggestive of right atrial enlargement.

Infarction: There is a QS complex seen throughout all of the precordial leads. In addition, there is 6 mm ST segment elevation seen throughout the same leads with peaking of the T waves. The diagnosis of an anterior infarction, possibly acute, should be made. In addition, lead I shows a prominent Q wave with 2 mm ST segment elevation. Lead AVL shows similar changes, which are indicative of a lateral infarction, possibly acute. Finally, if one evaluates the inferior leads II, III and AVF, there is a prominent Q wave with 4 mm ST segment elevation in lead II and T wave changes suggestive of an inferior infarction, possibly acute.

ST Segment and T Wave Abnormalities: See the preceding discussion under Infarction.

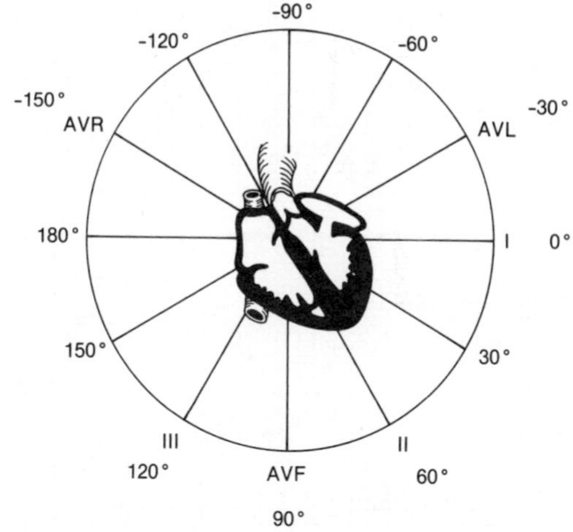

Summary

Sinus tachycardia

Right atrial enlargement

Anteroseptal myocardial infarction, possibly acute

Lateral myocardial infarction, possibly acute

Inferior myocardial infarction, possibly acute

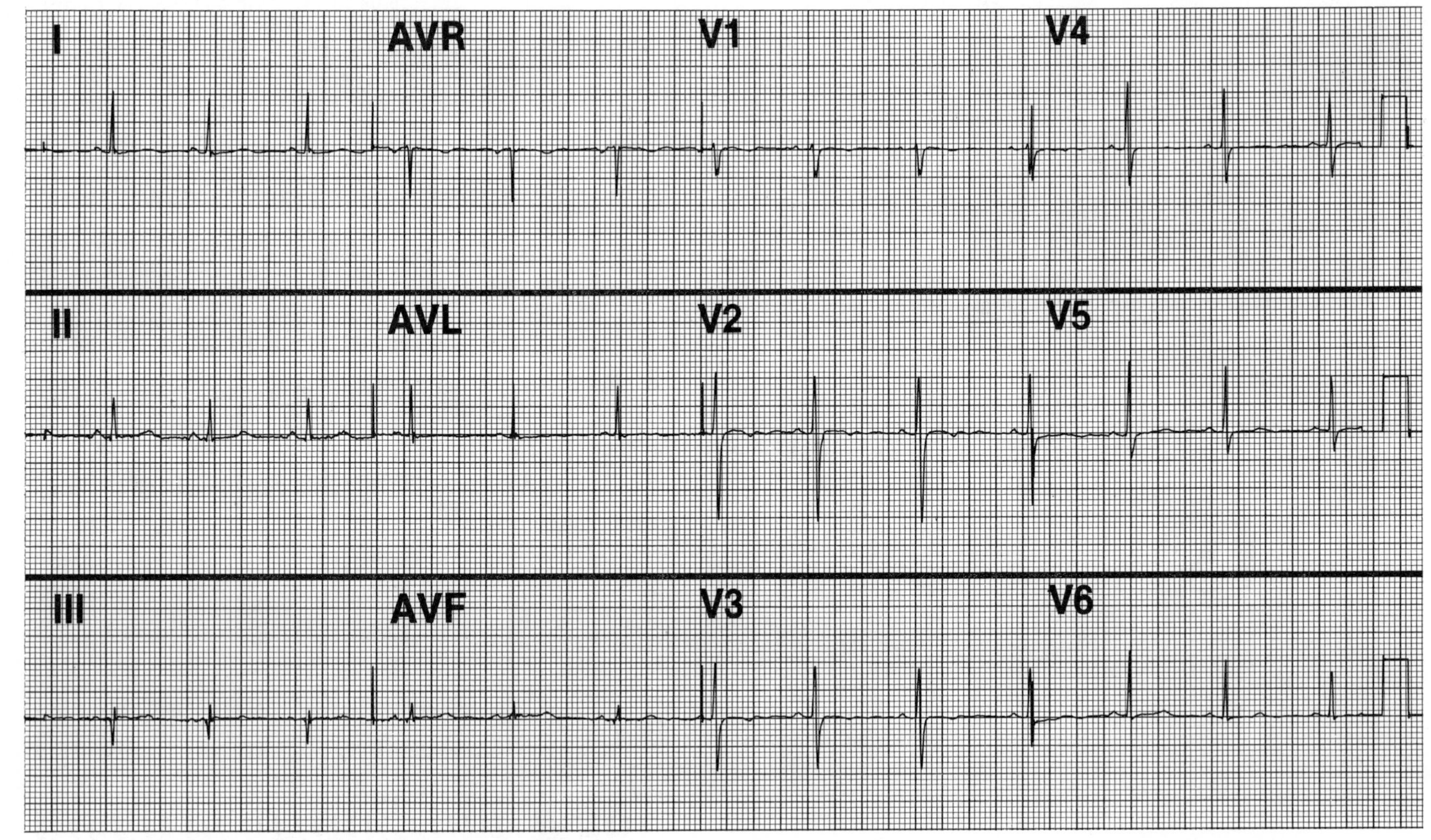
I
AVR
V1
V4
II
AVL
V2
V5
III
AVF
V3
V6

Electrocardiogram #57

Atrial Rate	83	**Beats/Minute**
Ventricular Rate	83	**Beats/Minute**
PR Interval	0.13	**Second**
QRS Duration	0.09	**Second**
QT-QTc	0.38–0.44	**Second**
QRS Complex Axis	10	**Degrees**

Rate: The atrial and ventricular rates are 83 beats per minute.

Rhythm: The PR interval is 0.13 second and constant. The rhythm is normal sinus rhythm.

Conduction Abnormalities: No criteria present in this electrocardiogram.

QRS Complex Axis: The mean QRS complex axis is 10°.

Chamber Enlargement: No criteria present in this electrocardiogram.

Infarction: No criteria present in this electrocardiogram.

ST Segment and T Wave Abnormalities: There are nonspecific T wave abnormalities seen throughout this electrocardiogram.

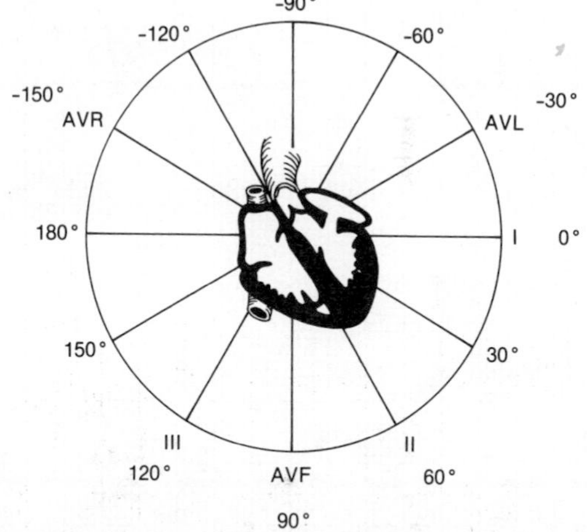

Summary

Normal sinus rhythm

Nonspecific ST segment and T wave abnormalities

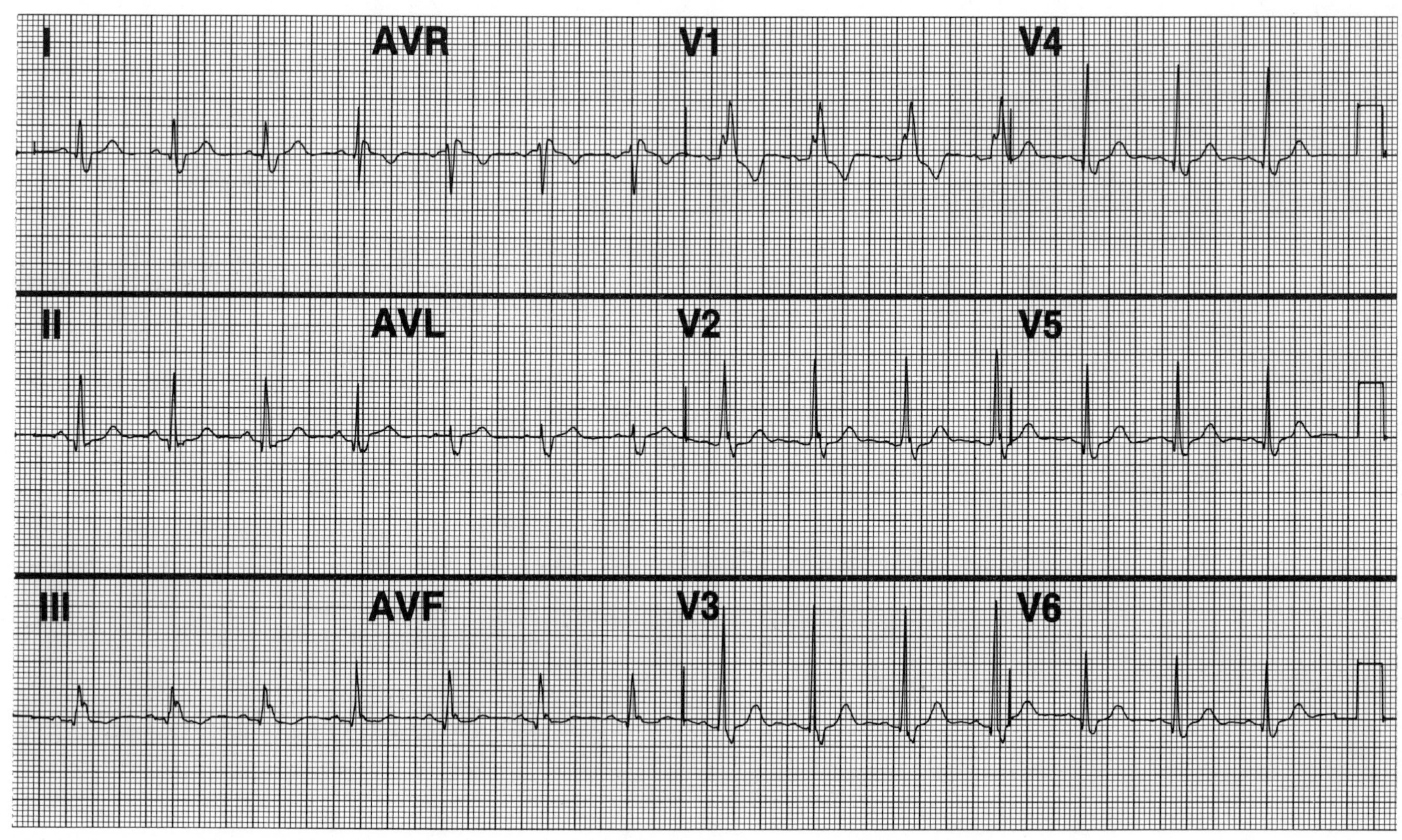
I
AVR
V1
V4
II
AVL
V2
V5
III
AVF
V3
V6

Electrocardiogram #58

Atrial Rate	**86**	**Beats/Minute**
Ventricular Rate	**86**	**Beats/Minute**
PR Interval	**0.15**	**Second**
QRS Duration	**0.14**	**Second**
QT-QTc	**0.39–0.47**	**Second**
QRS Complex Axis	**70**	**Degrees**

Rate: The atrial and ventricular rates are 86 beats per minute.

Rhythm: The PR interval is 0.15 second and constant. The rhythm is normal sinus rhythm.

Conduction Abnormalities: The QRS complex measures 0.14 second. A notched R wave is seen in lead V1. There are associated slurred S waves in leads V1, V5 and V6; therefore, the diagnosis of a right bundle branch block should be made.

QRS Complex Axis: The mean QRS complex axis is 70°.

Chamber Enlargement: No criteria present in this electrocardiogram.

Infarction: No criteria present in this electrocardiogram.

ST Segment and T Wave Abnormalities: The ST segment and T wave abnormalities seen in lead V1 are associated with the conduction abnormality.

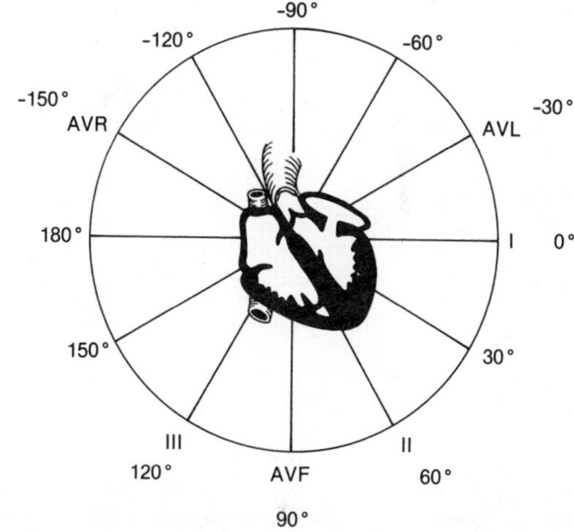

Summary

Normal sinus rhythm

Right bundle branch block

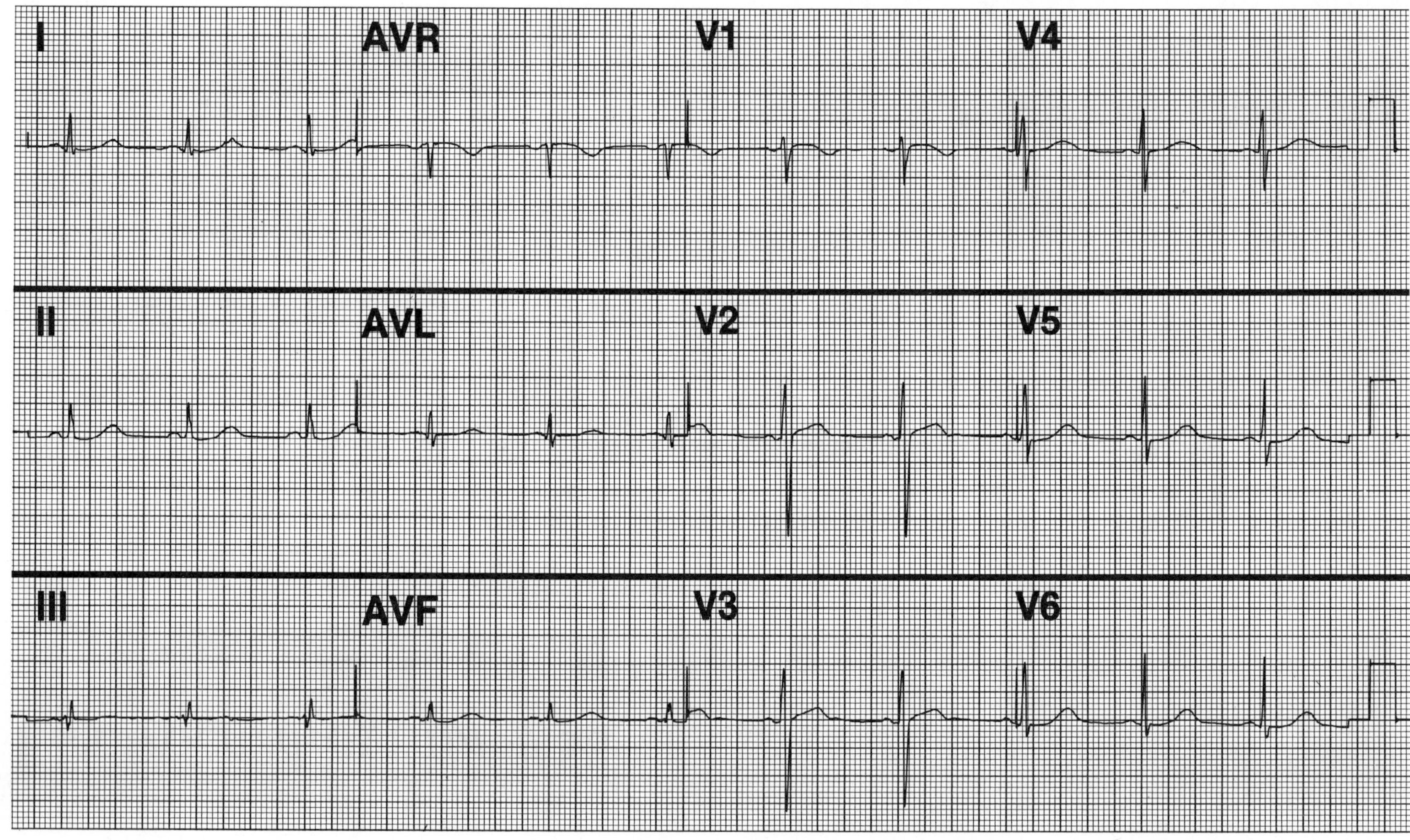
I
AVR
V1
V4
II
AVL
V2
V5
III
AVF
V3
V6

Electrocardiogram #59

Atrial Rate	70	Beats/Minute
Ventricular Rate	70	Beats/Minute
PR Interval	0.13	Second
QRS Duration	0.09	Second
QT-QTc	0.46–0.50	Second
QRS Complex Axis	40	Degrees

Rate: The atrial and ventricular rates are 70 beats per minute.

Rhythm: The PR interval is 0.13 second and constant. The rhythm is normal sinus rhythm.

Conduction Abnormalities: No criteria present in this electrocardiogram.

QRS Complex Axis: The mean QRS complex axis is 40°.

Chamber Enlargement: No criteria present in this electrocardiogram.

Infarction: No criteria present in this electrocardiogram.

ST Segment and T Wave Abnormalities: No criteria present in this electrocardiogram.

Other Findings: The only abnormality seen in this electrocardiogram is a prolonged QTc interval. The QT interval measures 0.48 second; the QTc is 0.50 second, which is prolonged. In this electrocardiogram, one should consider primary myocardial disease, electrolyte imbalance or drug effects such as those induced by the local anesthetic type antiarrhythmics, lidocaine, procainamide and quinidine.

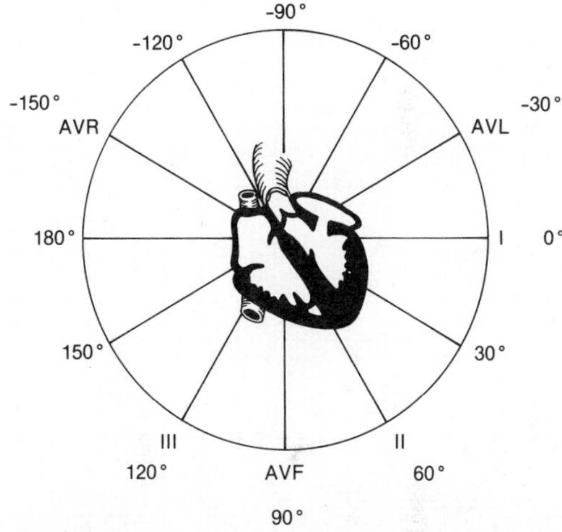

Summary

Normal sinus rhythm

Prolonged QTc interval

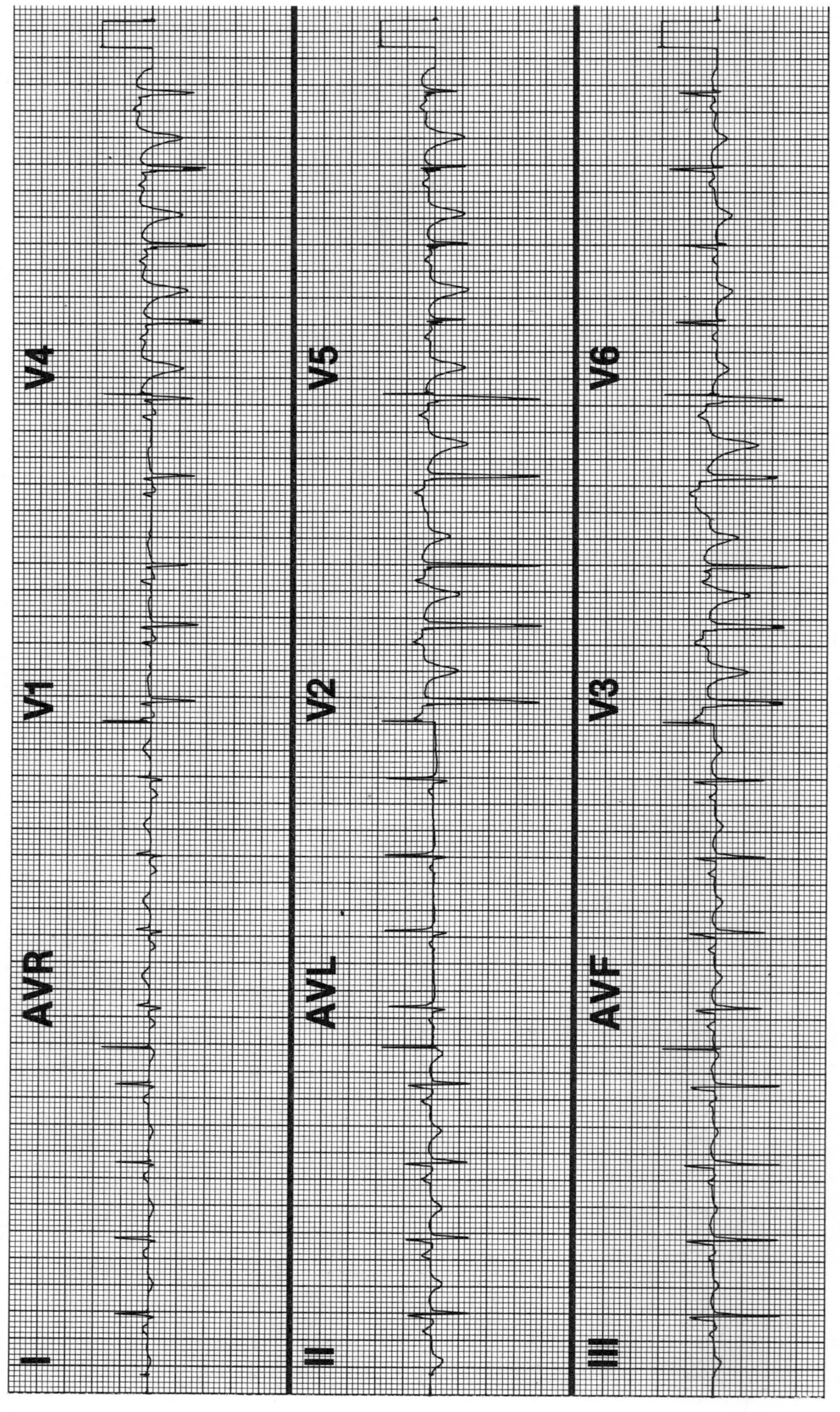
I
AVR
V1
V4
II
AVL
V2
V5
III
AVF
V3
V6

Electrocardiogram #60

Atrial Rate	**100**	**Beats/Minute**
Ventricular Rate	**100**	**Beats/Minute**
PR Interval	**0.13**	**Second**
QRS Duration	**0.08**	**Second**
QT-QTc	**0.36–0.47**	**Second**
QRS Complex Axis	**−45**	**Degrees**

Rate: The atrial and ventricular rates are 100 beats per minute.

Rhythm: The PR interval is 0.13 second and constant. The rhythm is sinus tachycardia. When one evaluates the third beat in leads V1 to V3, one will note that this beat is slightly premature. Also, the P wave preceding this beat, seen best in lead V1, is slightly wider and larger than its preceding and later beats; therefore, this is a premature supraventricular contraction. Notice that the QRS complex is identical to the normal sinus beats.

Conduction Abnormalities: A left anterior hemiblock is present in this electrocardiogram. Notice the qR complex in lead I together with the rS complex in leads II, III and AVF, which produces the mean QRS complex axis of −45°.

QRS Complex Axis: The mean QRS complex axis is −45°.

Chamber Enlargement: No criteria present in this electrocardiogram.

Infarction: The absence of R waves in leads V4 and V5 is suggestive of an anterolateral myocardial infarction, age undetermined. The QS complex seen in leads V2 and V3 is suggestive of an anteroseptal myocardial infarction, but these changes may be related to the left anterior hemiblock. Therefore, an anteroseptal myocardial infarction should not be diagnosed. The left anterior hemiblock may also mimic an anterolateral myocardial infarction, but this is less likely in this tracing.

ST Segment and T Wave Abnormalities: The ST segment and T wave abnormalities seen in the inferior leads II, III and AVF are suggestive of inferior ischemia.

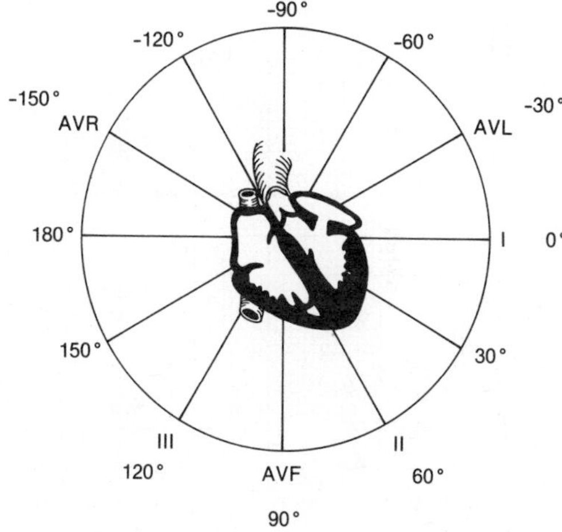

Summary

Sinus tachycardia with occasional premature supraventricular contractions

Left anterior hemiblock

Cannot rule out an anterolateral myocardial infarction, age undetermined

Inferior wall ischemia

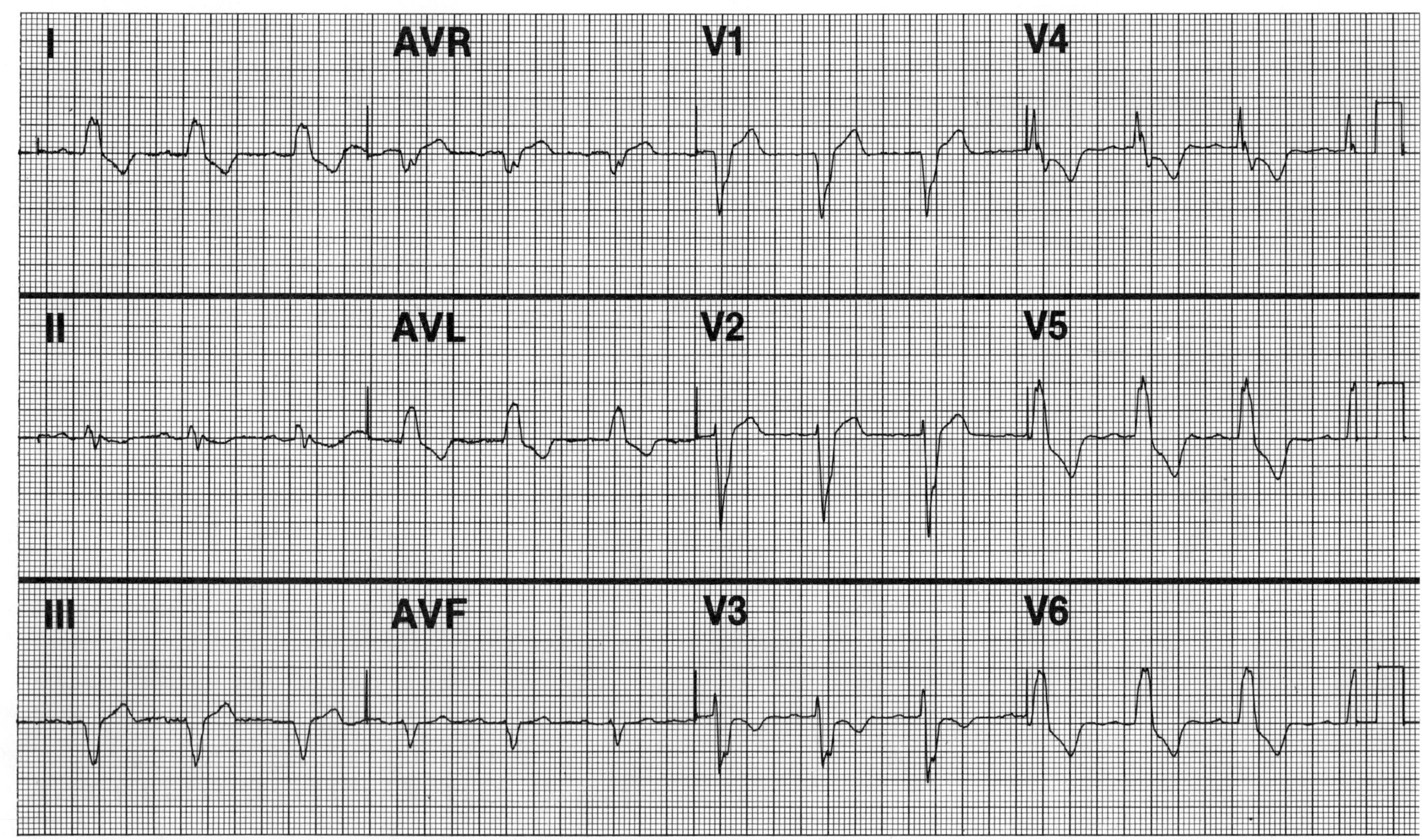
I
AVR
V1
V4
II
AVL
V2
V5
III
AVF
V3
V6

Electrocardiogram #61

Atrial Rate	79	Beats/Minute
Ventricular Rate	79	Beats/Minute
PR Interval	0.20	Second
QRS Duration	0.15	Second
QT-QTc	0.42–0.47	Second
QRS Complex Axis	−25	Degrees

Rate: The atrial and ventricular rates are 79 beats per minute.

Rhythm: The PR interval is 0.20 second and constant. The rhythm is normal sinus rhythm, borderline first degree atrioventricular block.

Conduction Abnormalities: A wide QRS complex measuring 0.15 second is present. The complex has a notching of the R wave in leads V1 and V5 and V6, with an absence of the normal septal Q waves seen in these leads. Therefore, the diagnosis of left bundle branch block should be made. The major findings in left bundle branch block include a widened QRS complex, absence of septal forces in leads I and V6, repolarization changes and a delay in the left precordial intrinsicoid deflection.

QRS Complex Axis: The mean QRS complex axis is −25°.

Chamber Enlargement: No criteria present in this electrocardiogram.

Infarction: No criteria present in this electrocardiogram.

ST Segment and T Wave Abnormalities: The ST segment and T wave abnormalities seen in these leads are secondary changes and related to the conduction abnormality.

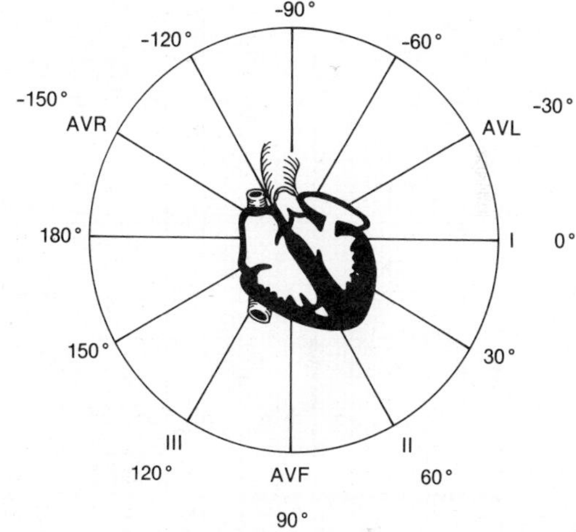

Summary

Normal sinus rhythm

Left bundle branch block

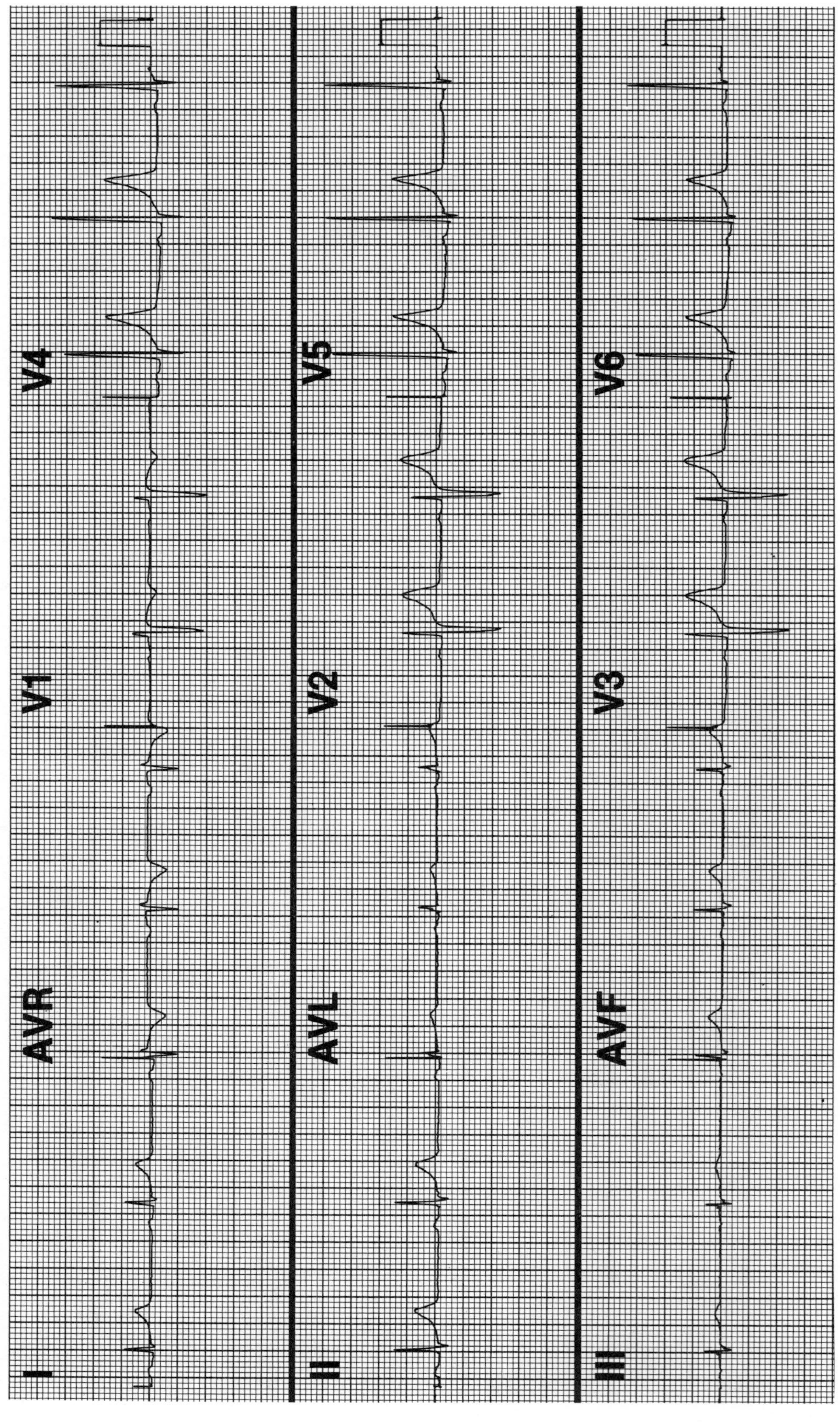
I
AVR
V1
V4
II
AVL
V2
V5
III
AVF
V3
V6

Electrocardiogram #62

Atrial Rate	**60**	**Beats/Minute**
Ventricular Rate	**60**	**Beats/Minute**
PR Interval	**0.18**	**Second**
QRS Duration	**0.08**	**Second**
QT-QTc	**0.42–0.40**	**Second**
QRS Complex Axis	**35**	**Degrees**

Rate: The atrial and ventricular rates are 60 beats per minute.

Rhythm: The PR interval is 0.18 second and constant. The rhythm is normal sinus rhythm.

Conduction Abnormalities: No criteria present in this electrocardiogram.

QRS Complex Axis: The mean QRS complex axis is 35°.

Chamber Enlargement: No criteria present in this electrocardiogram.

Infarction: No criteria present in this electrocardiogram.

ST Segment and T Wave Abnormalities: This electrocardiogram shows 1 mm ST segment elevation, seen throughout the precordial leads. Because of the ST segment takeoff, the term J point elevation is applied. This is most likely a repolarization variant, which is normal and frequently seen in young black men. However, if this patient were suffering from chest pains suggestive of pericarditis, this electrocardiogram could also be consistent with that diagnosis as well. One should therefore correlate the clinical situation with the electrocardiogram.

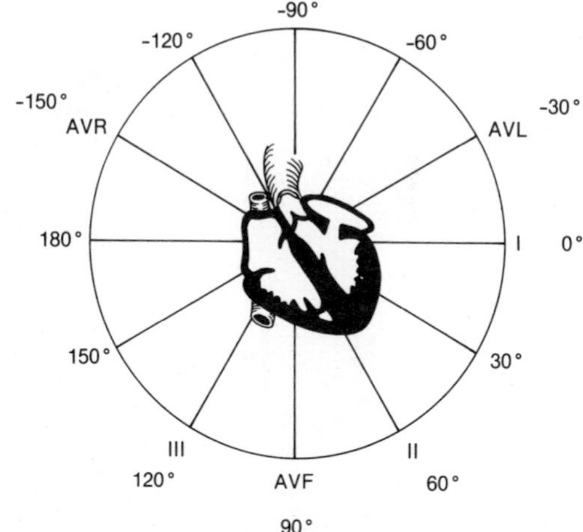

Summary

Sinus bradycardia

Repolarization variant

Otherwise normal electrocardiogram

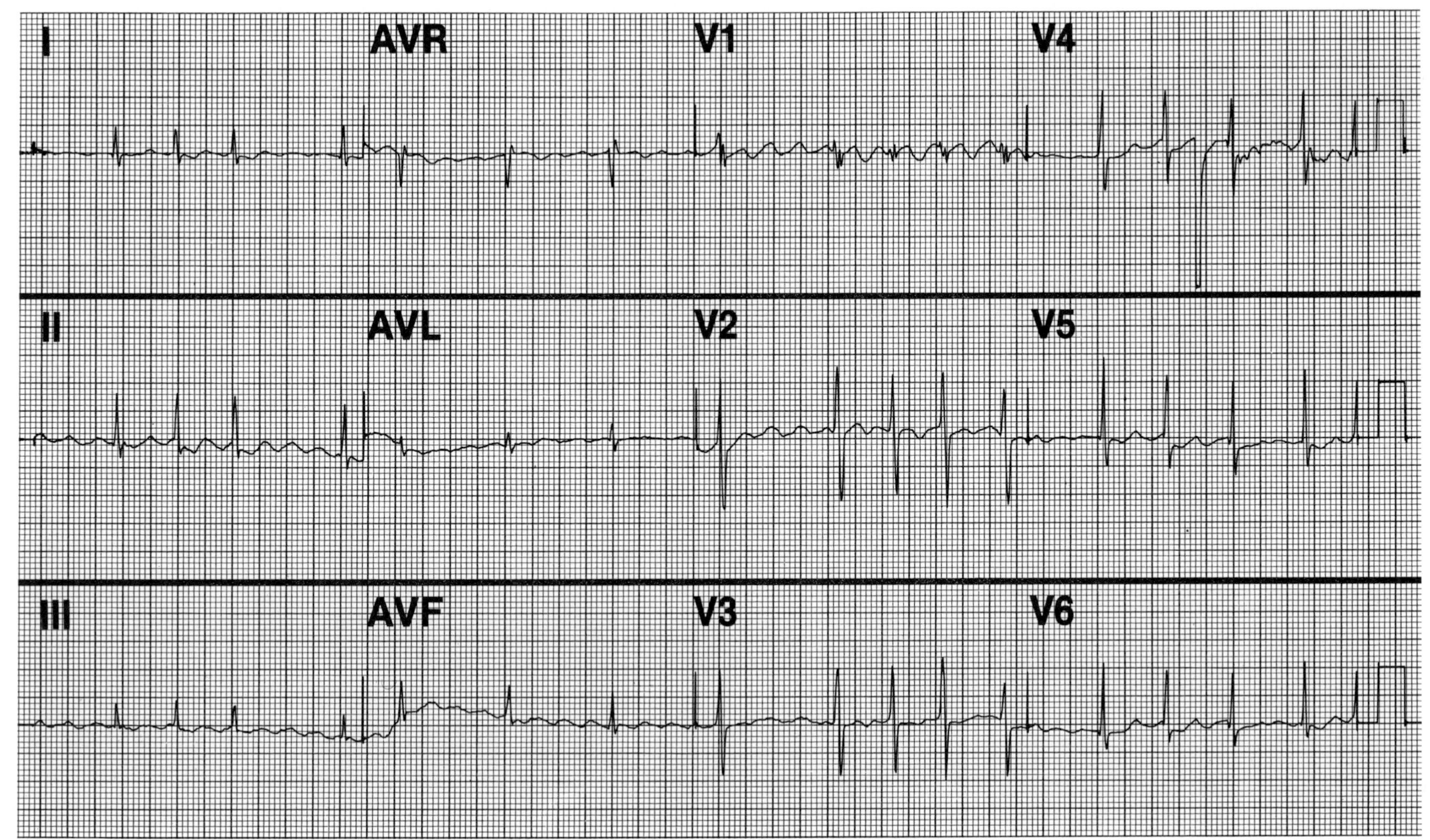
I
AVR
V1
V4
II
AVL
V2
V5
III
AVF
V3
V6

Electrocardiogram #63

Atrial Rate	300	Beats/Minute
Ventricular Rate	100	Beats/Minute
PR Interval	0.18	Second
QRS Duration	0.08	Second
QT-QTc	0.34–0.44	Second
QRS Complex Axis	60	Degrees

Rate: The ventricular rate is 100 beats per minute.

Rhythm: No P waves are seen, but a constant atrial complex is seen at approximately 300 beats per minute. The atrial and ventricular rates are variable. If one looks at the first three beats in leads I, II and III, one sees that the ventricular rate is 150 beats per minute. However, when one examines leads V1, V2 and V3, it is apparent that there are 4 atrial complexes prior to the second beat in these leads. However, 3 additional beats follow at 150 beats per minute. Therefore, this is atrial flutter with variable atrioventricular block.

Conduction Abnormalities: The variable atrioventricular block is a normal physiological effect. It is not abnormal.

QRS Complex Axis: The mean QRS complex axis is 60°.

Chamber Enlargement: No criteria present in this electrocardiogram.

Infarction: No criteria present in this electrocardiogram.

ST Segment and T Wave Abnormalities: There are nonspecific ST segment and T wave abnormalities that may be related to the atrial flutter.

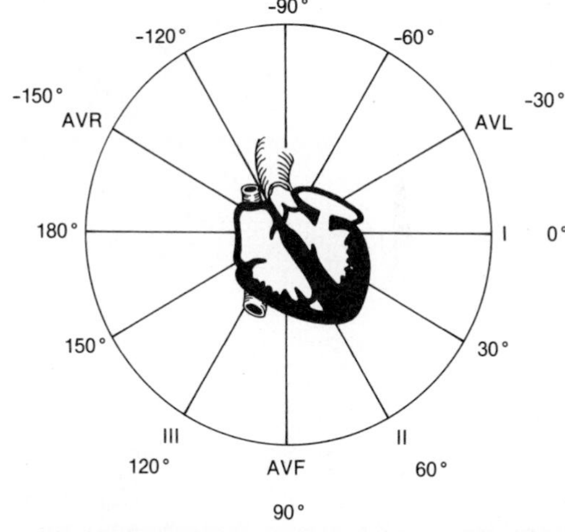

Summary

Atrial flutter with variable atrioventricular block

Nonspecific ST segment and T wave abnormalities

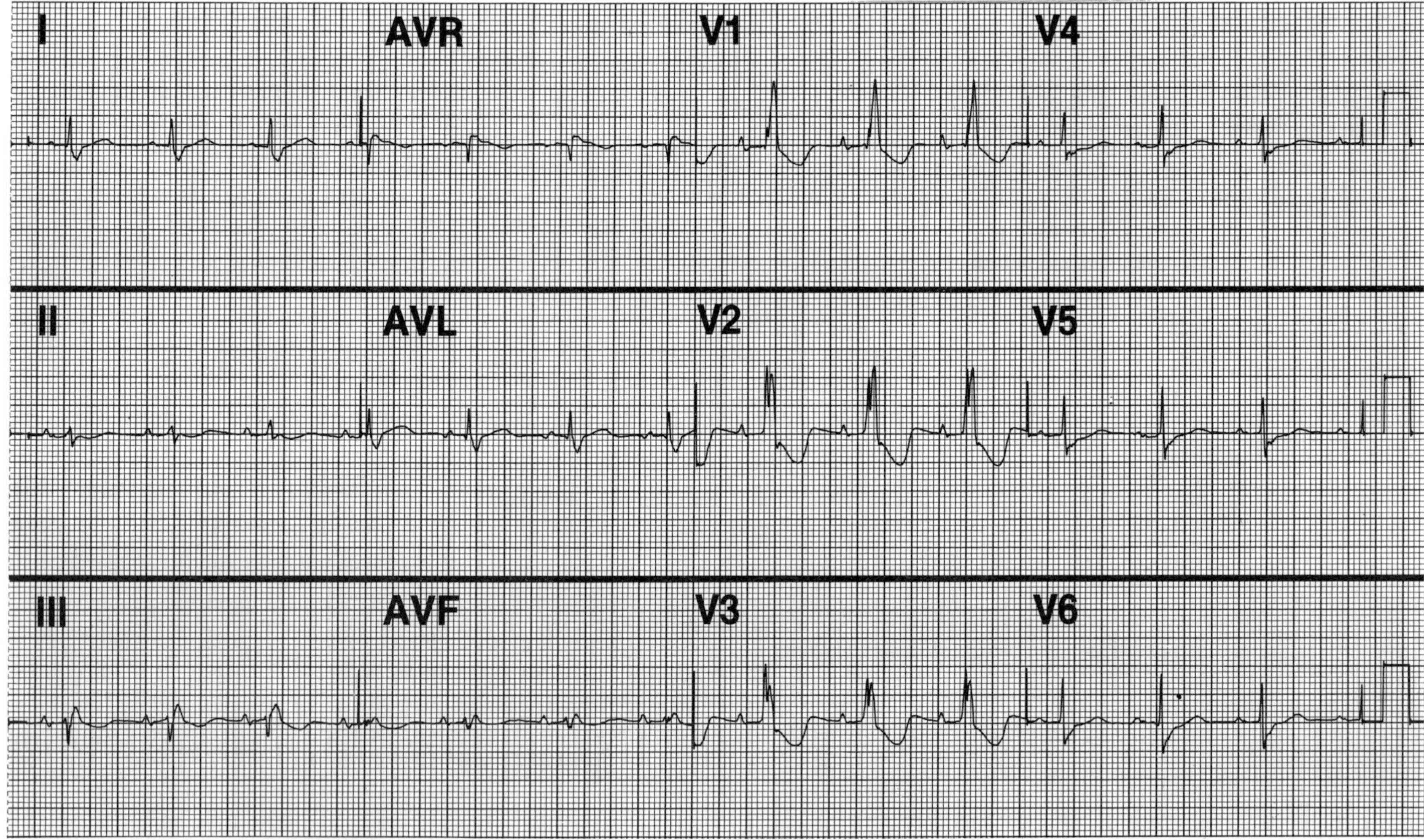
I
AVR
V1
V4
II
AVL
V2
V5
III
AVF
V3
V6

Electrocardiogram #64

Atrial Rate	83	**Beats/Minute**
Ventricular Rate	83	**Beats/Minute**
PR Interval	0.17	**Second**
QRS Duration	0.13	**Second**
QT-QTc	0.40–0.46	**Second**
QRS Complex Axis	0	**Degrees**

Rate: The atrial and ventricular rates are 83 beats per minute.

Rhythm: The PR interval is 0.17 second and constant. The rhythm is normal sinus rhythm.

Conduction Abnormalities: A QRS complex duration of 0.13 second is present that has terminal slurring seen in leads I, V5 and V6. This is associated with a notched R wave in leads V1 to V3. Therefore, the diagnosis of right bundle branch block should be made.

QRS Complex Axis: The mean QRS complex axis is 0°.

Chamber Enlargement: No criteria present in this electrocardiogram.

Infarction: No criteria present in this electrocardiogram.

ST Segment and T Wave Abnormalities: The ST segment and T wave abnormalities seen in leads V1 to V3 are related to the conduction abnormality.

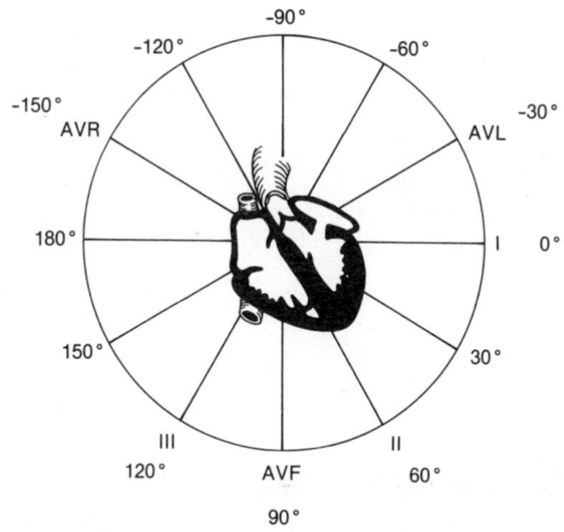

Summary

Normal sinus rhythm

Right bundle branch block

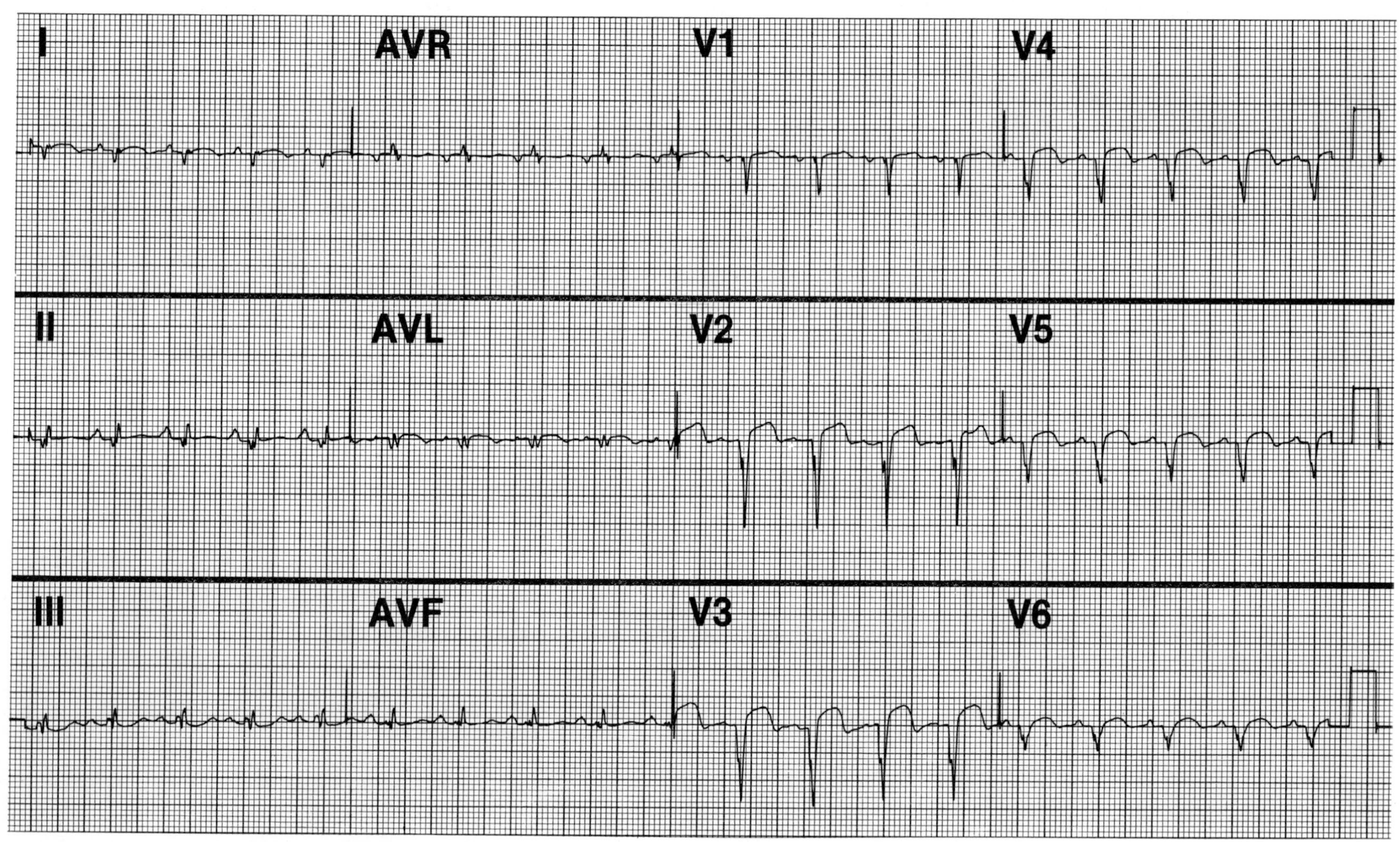
I
AVR
V1
V4
II
AVL
V2
V5
III
AVF
V3
V6

Electrocardiogram #65

Atrial Rate	**115**	**Beats/Minute**
Ventricular Rate	**115**	**Beats/Minute**
PR Interval	**0.16**	**Second**
QRS Duration	**0.10**	**Second**
QT-QTc	**0.34–0.46**	**Second**
QRS Complex Axis	**160**	**Degrees**

Rate: The atrial and ventricular rates are 115 beats per minute.

Rhythm: The PR interval is 0.16 second and constant. The rhythm is normal sinus rhythm.

Conduction Abnormalities: No criteria present in this electrocardiogram.

QRS Complex Axis: The mean QRS complex axis is 160°.

Chamber Enlargement: No criteria present in this electrocardiogram.

Infarction: The QS complex is seen throughout the precordium together with the 2 mm ST segment elevation, and T wave inversions are diagnostic of an anterior infarction, age undetermined, but possibly acute. The Qr complex seen in leads I and II are suggestive of a high lateral infarction as well. This patient suffered an anterior and high lateral infarction due to occlusion of the left main coronary artery and died 6 hours later.

ST Segment and T Wave Abnormalities: No criteria present in this electrocardiogram.

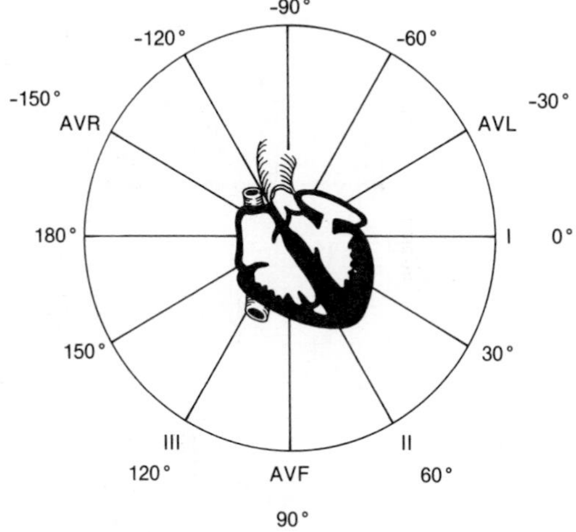

Summary

Sinus tachycardia

Anterior myocardial infarction, possibly acute

High lateral myocardial infarction, possibly acute

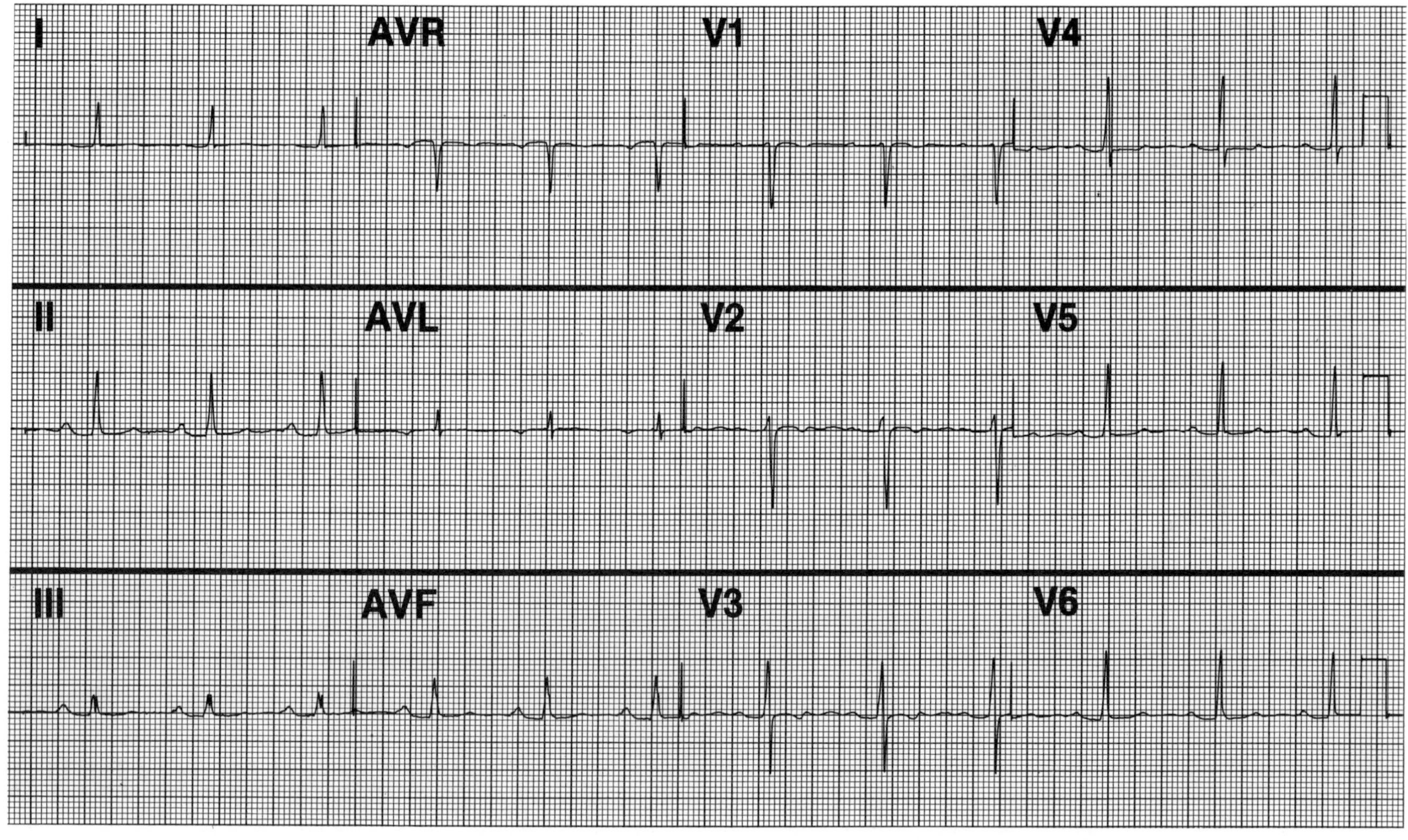
I
AVR
V1
V4
II
AVL
V2
V5
III
AVF
V3
V6

Electrocardiogram #66

Atrial Rate	71	**Beats/Minute**
Ventricular Rate	71	**Beats/Minute**
PR Interval	0.24	**Second**
QRS Duration	0.09	**Second**
QT-QTc	0.38–0.42	**Second**
QRS Complex Axis	50	**Degrees**

Rate: The atrial and ventricular rates are 71 beats per minute.

Rhythm: The diagnosis is normal sinus rhythm.

Conduction Abnormalities: The PR interval is 0.24 second and constant. First degree atrioventricular block is present.

QRS Complex Axis: The mean QRS complex axis is 50°. Leads I and AVF are both positive.

Chamber Enlargement: No criteria present in this electrocardiogram.

Infarction: No criteria present in this electrocardiogram.

ST Segment and T Wave Abnormalities: There are nonspecific T wave abnormalities seen throughout the precordial leads.

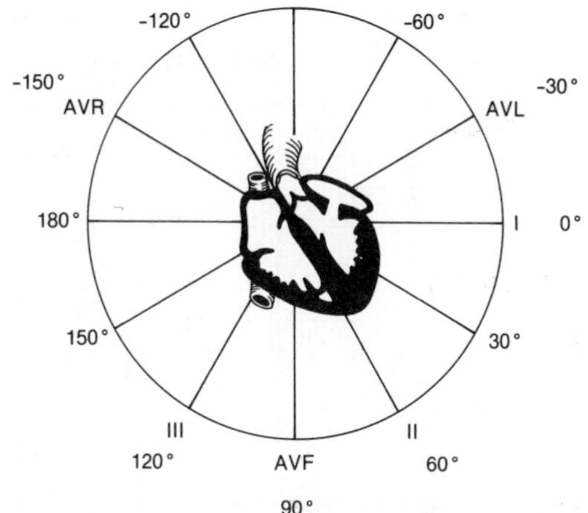

Summary

Normal sinus rhythm with first degree atrioventricular block

Nonspecific T wave abnormalities

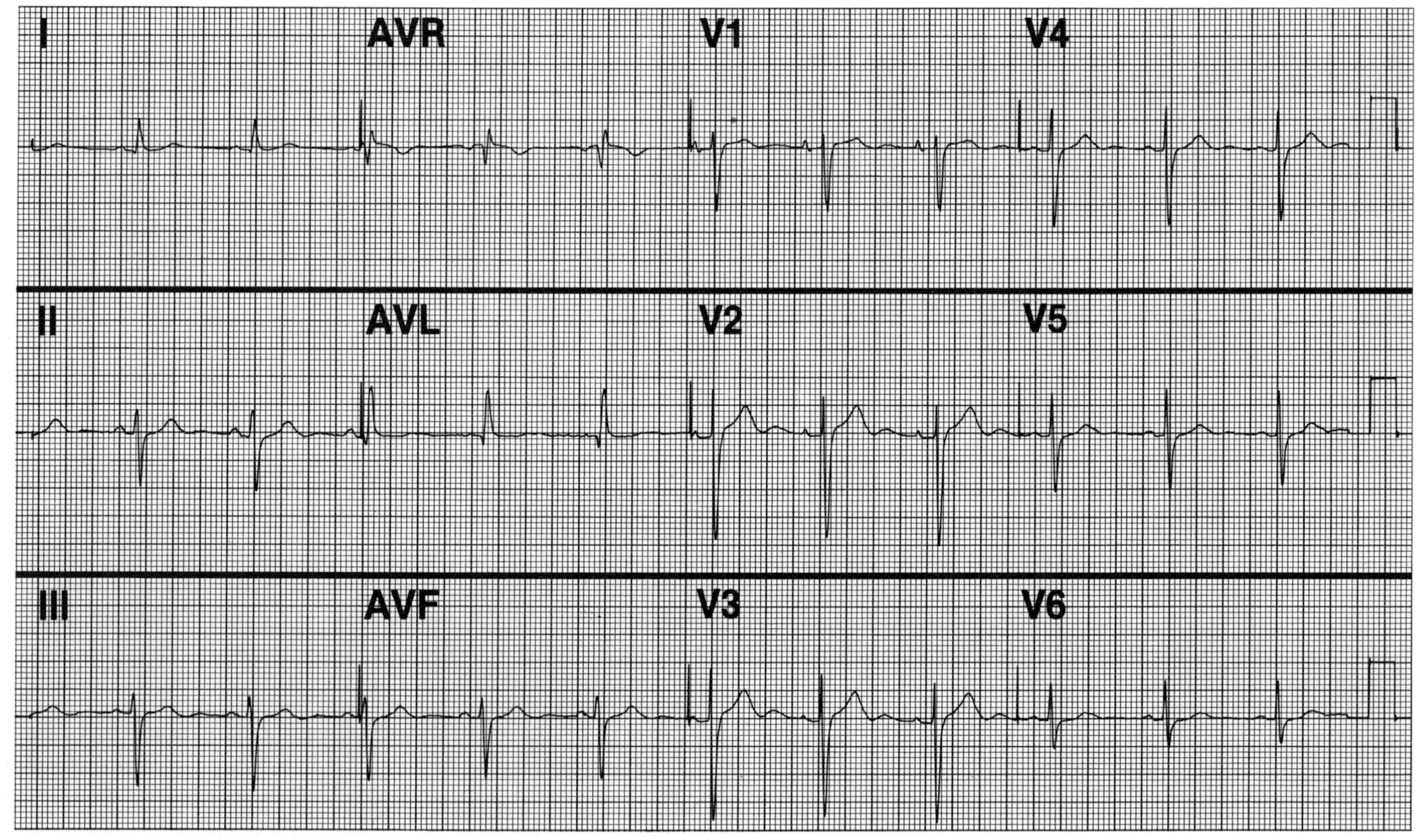
I
AVR
V1
V4
II
AVL
V2
V5
III
AVF
V3
V6

Electrocardiogram #67

Atrial Rate	**71**	**Beats/Minute**
Ventricular Rate	**71**	**Beats/Minute**
PR Interval	**0.14**	**Second**
QRS Duration	**0.11**	**Second**
QT-QTc	**0.40–0.43**	**Second**
QRS Complex Axis	**−60**	**Degrees**

Rate: The atrial and ventricular rates are 71 beats per minute.

Rhythm: The PR interval is 0.14 second and constant. The rhythm is normal sinus rhythm.

Conduction Abnormalities: The qR complex in lead I together with the rS complex in leads II, III and AVF produce the abnormal left axis deviation that is related to a left anterior hemiblock. In this type of conduction abnormality, there is a change in the direction of the electrical impulses. The initial wave of depolarization is posterior and to the right and produces a small q wave in lead I and a small r wave in lead II. The bulk of the depolarization proceeds in an upward, anterior and leftward direction. This produces the left axis deviation by inscribing a qR complex in lead I and an rS complex in lead II.

QRS Complex Axis: The mean QRS complex axis is −60° with marked left axis deviation.

Chamber Enlargement: No criteria present in this electrocardiogram.

Infarction: No criteria present in this electrocardiogram.

ST Segment and T Wave Abnormalities: No criteria present in this electrocardiogram.

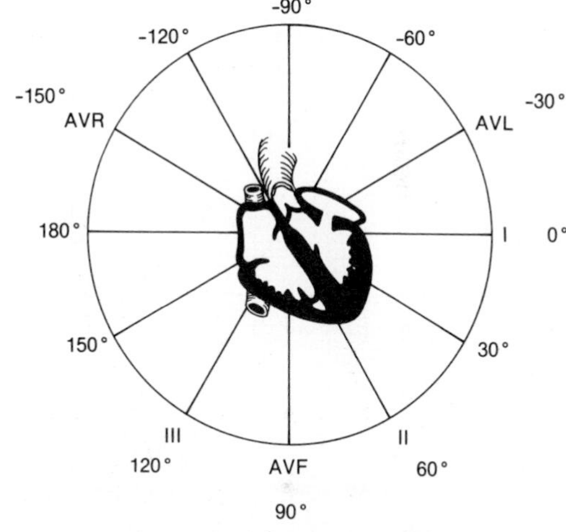

Summary

Normal sinus rhythm

Left anterior hemiblock

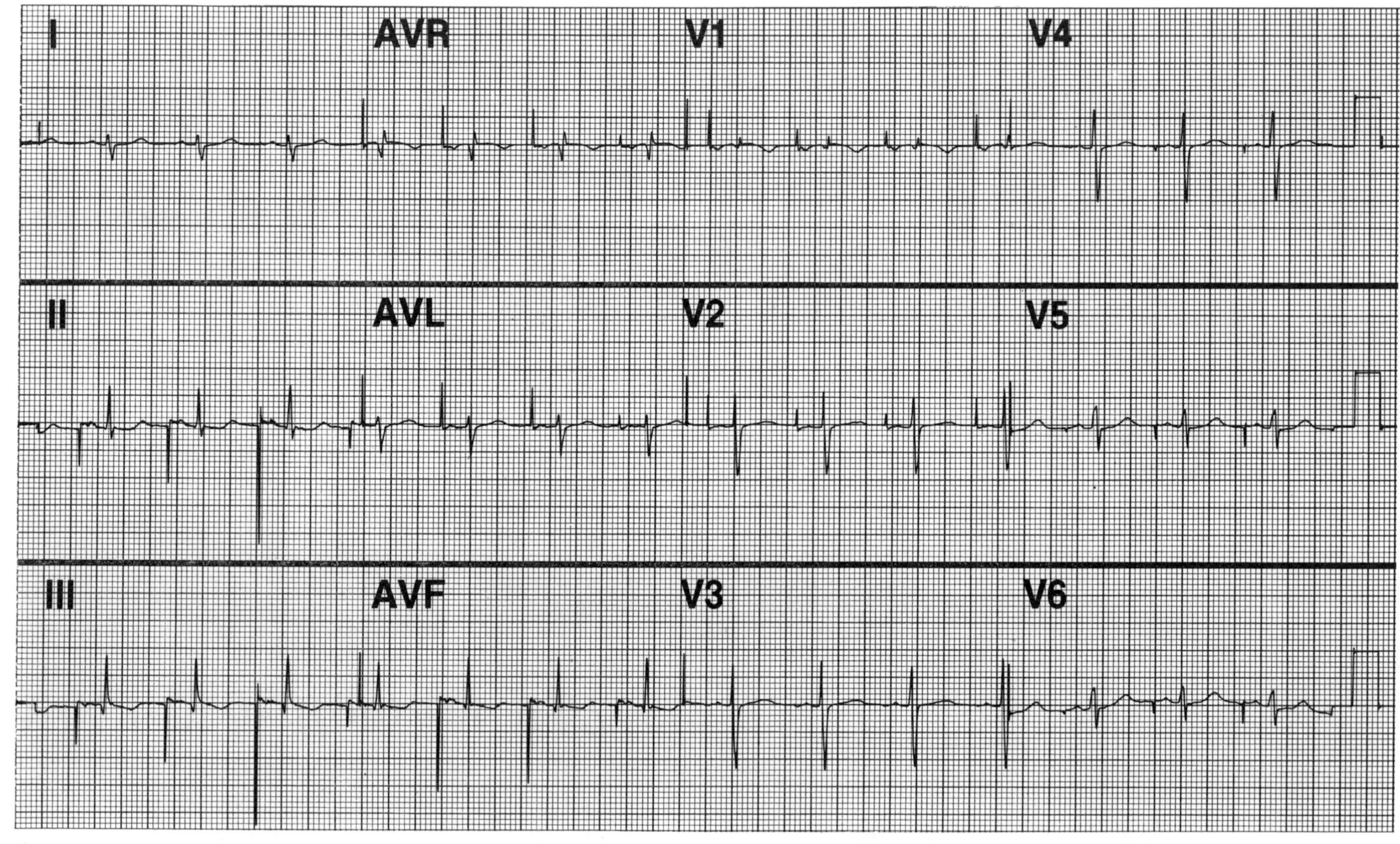
I
AVR
V1
V4
II
AVL
V2
V5
III
AVF
V3
V6

Electrocardiogram #68

Atrial Rate	**88**	**Beats/Minute**
Ventricular Rate	**88**	**Beats/Minute**
PR Interval	**0.19**	**Second**
QRS Duration	**0.08**	**Second**
QT-QTc	**0.37–0.44**	**Second**
QRS Complex Axis	**100**	**Degrees**

Rate: The atrial and ventricular rates are 88 beats per minute.

Rhythm: The PR interval is 0.19 second and constant. One should note that there is an electronic pacemaker spike seen preceding every P wave. The PR interval is therefore the "spike-R wave" interval and is set at 88 beats per minute. This patient has an atrial pacemaker. The QRS complex is normal, with no interference caused by the atrial pacemaker, which merely triggers the atrium to contract. An atrial pacemaker would be placed in a patient in whom the sinus node is either too slow or unreliable. However, atrioventricular conduction appears to be normal in this patient, since the PR interval is normal.

Conduction Abnormalities: No criteria present in this electrocardiogram.

QRS Complex Axis: The mean QRS complex axis is 100°.

Chamber Enlargement: No criteria present in this electrocardiogram.

Infarction: No criteria present in this electrocardiogram.

ST Segment and T Wave Abnormalities: There are nonspecific ST segment and T wave abnormalities.

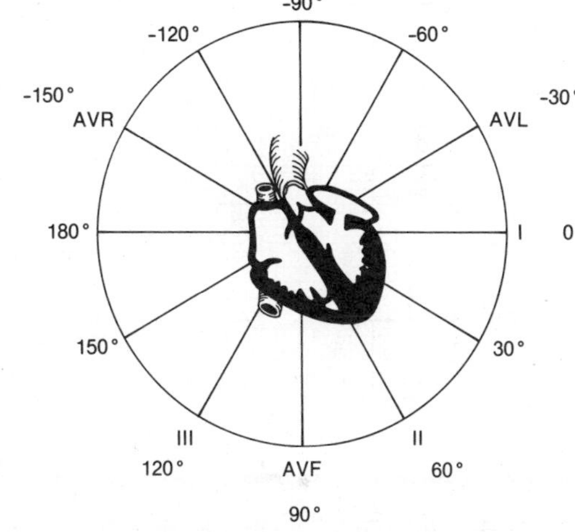

Summary

Electronic atrial pacemaker

Nonspecific ST segment and T wave abnormalities

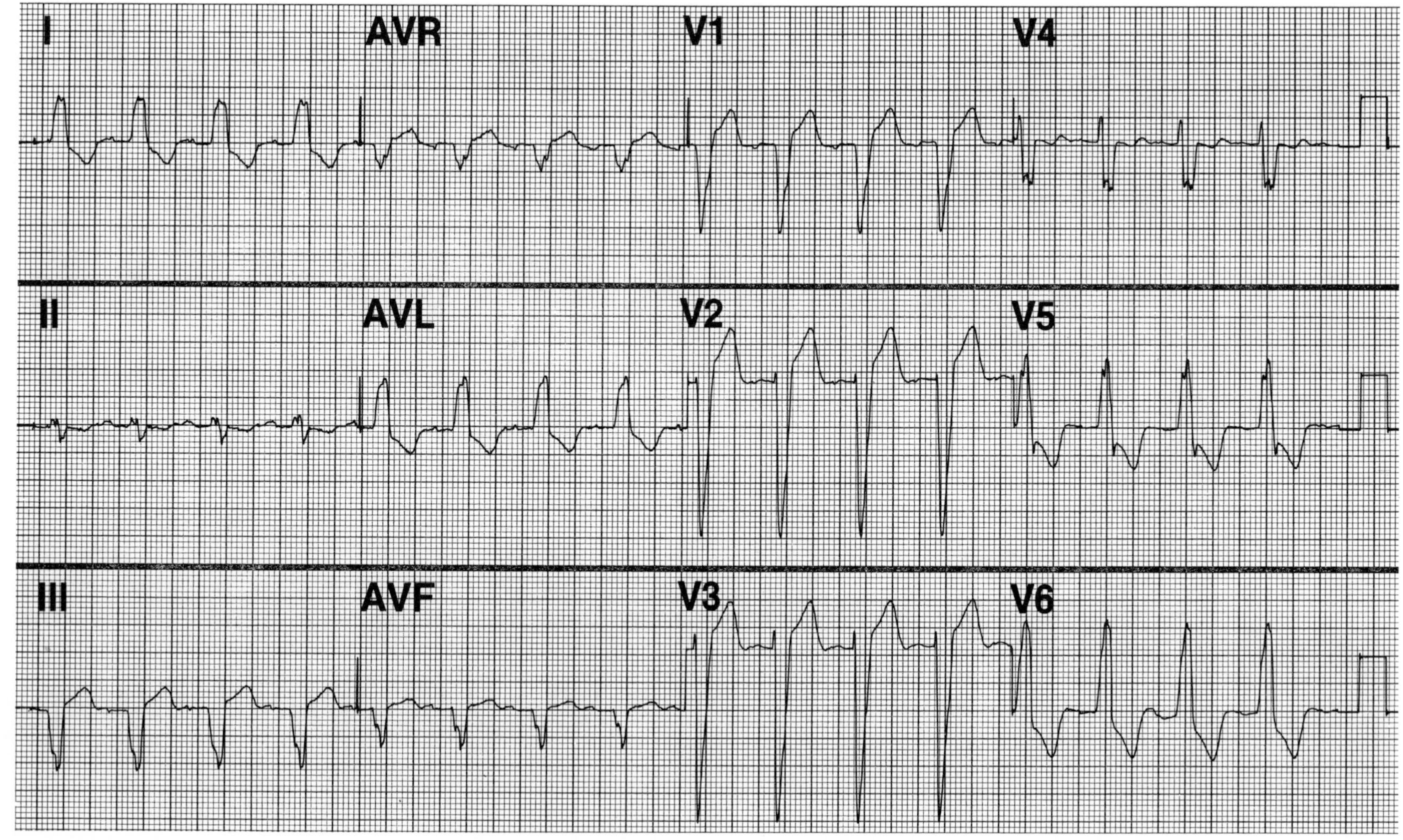
I
AVR
V1
V4
II
AVL
V2
V5
III
AVF
V3
V6

Electrocardiogram #69

Atrial Rate	100	**Beats/Minute**
Ventricular Rate	100	**Beats/Minute**
PR Interval	0.19	**Second**
QRS Duration	0.15	**Second**
QT-QTc	0.39–0.50	**Second**
QRS Complex Axis	−40	**Degrees**

Rate: The atrial and ventricular rates are 100 beats per minute.

Rhythm: The PR interval is 0.19 second and constant. The diagnosis is normal sinus rhythm.

Conduction Abnormalities: The QRS complex measures 0.15 second and is notched in leads I, AVL, V5 and V6. In addition, the normal septal depolarization from left to right is not seen in this electrocardiogram. This abnormality of septal depolarization and the resulting electrocardiographic changes are caused by a left bundle branch block. The QS complex seen in lead V1 and the small R waves and prominent S waves seen in leads V1 to V3 are related to this conduction abnormality.

QRS Complex Axis: The mean QRS complex axis is −40°, abnormal left axis deviation.

Chamber Enlargement: No criteria present in this electrocardiogram.

Infarction: No criteria present in this electrocardiogram.

ST Segment and T Wave Abnormalities: No criteria present in this electrocardiogram.

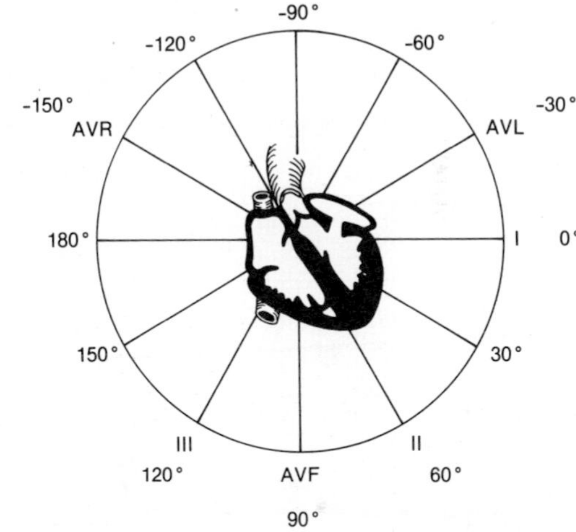

Summary

Normal sinus rhythm

Abnormal left axis deviation

Left bundle branch block

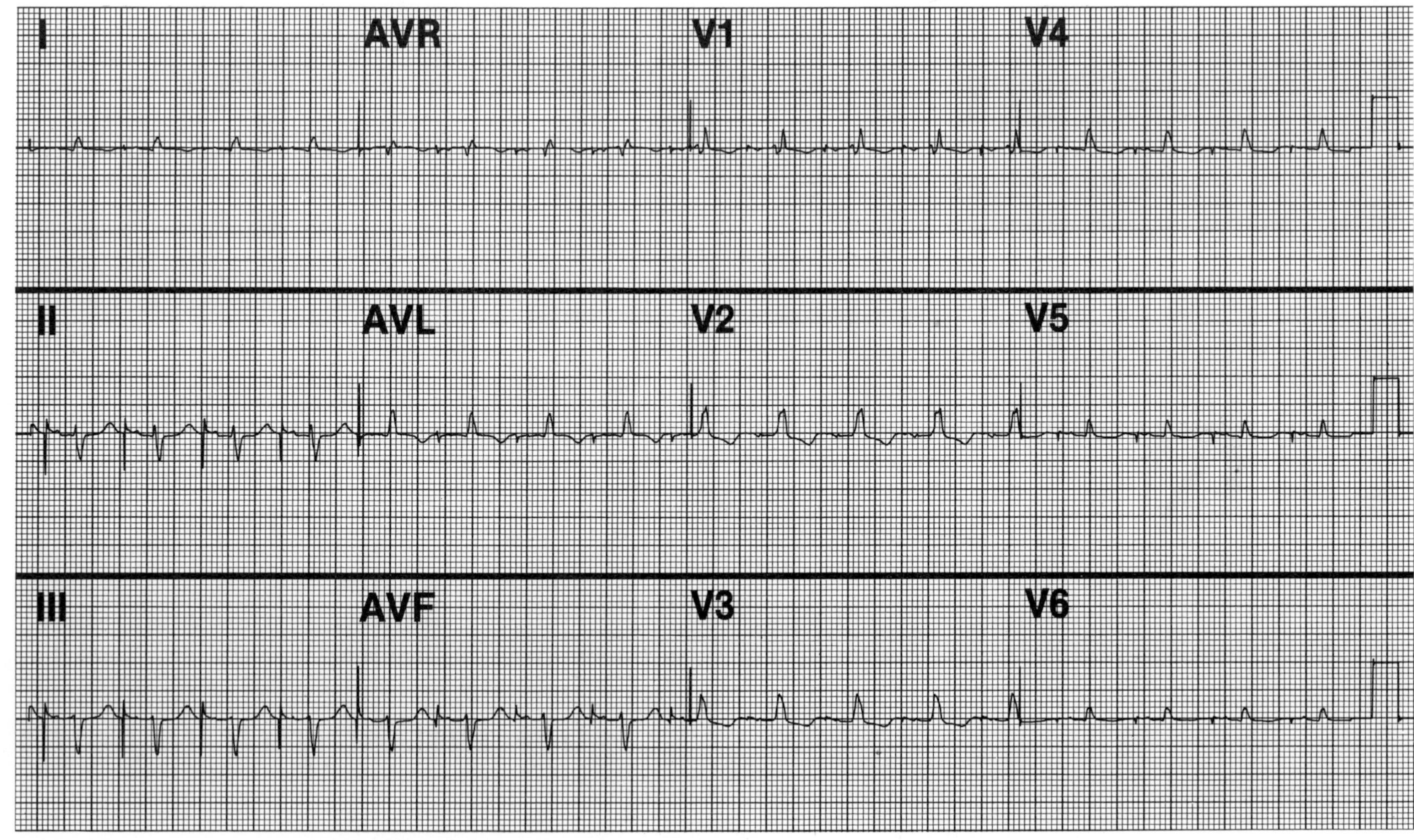
I
AVR
V1
V4
II
AVL
V2
V5
III
AVF
V3
V6

Electrocardiogram #70

Atrial Rate	**100**	**Beats/Minute**
Ventricular Rate	**100**	**Beats/Minute**
PR Interval	**0.20**	**Second**
QRS Duration	**0.09**	**Second**
QT-QTc	**0.33–0.43**	**Second**
QRS Complex Axis	**−60**	**Degrees**

Rate: The atrial and ventricular rates are 100 beats per minute.

Rhythm: The PR interval is 0.20 second. There is a prominent spike seen preceding each P wave, which is caused by an electronic atrial pacemaker. This patient has an atrial pacemaker that was implanted because of an unreliable sinus node. The patient may have had slow atrial fibrillation or atrial flutter, and the atrial pacemaker, by triggering atrial contraction, allows for the "atrial kick" that contributes approximately 10 to 15 per cent to the cardiac output. In patients with mitral stenosis, the atrial contribution may be as much as 25 to 30 per cent of the total cardiac output.

Conduction Abnormalities: This patient has a widened QRS complex of 0.09 second and a leftward axis. A left anterior hemiblock is present, which produces the qR complex in lead I and the rS complex in leads II, III and AVF.

QRS Complex Axis: The mean QRS complex axis is −60°. The left axis is related to a left anterior hemiblock.

Chamber Enlargement: No criteria present in this electrocardiogram.

Infarction: No criteria present in this electrocardiogram.

ST Segment and T Wave Abnormalities: No criteria present in this electrocardiogram.

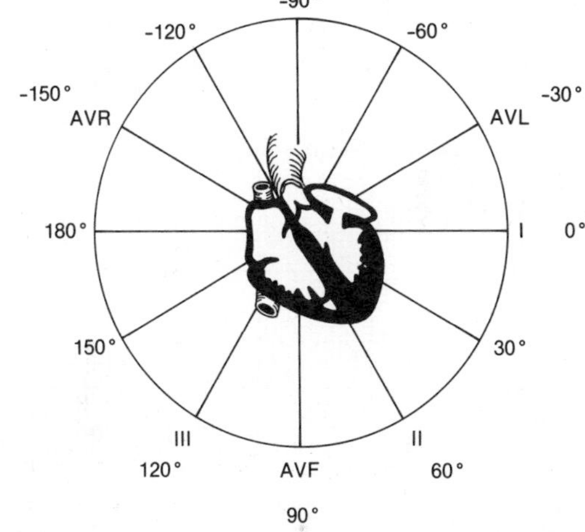

Summary

Electronic atrial pacemaker

Left anterior hemiblock

Abnormal left axis deviation

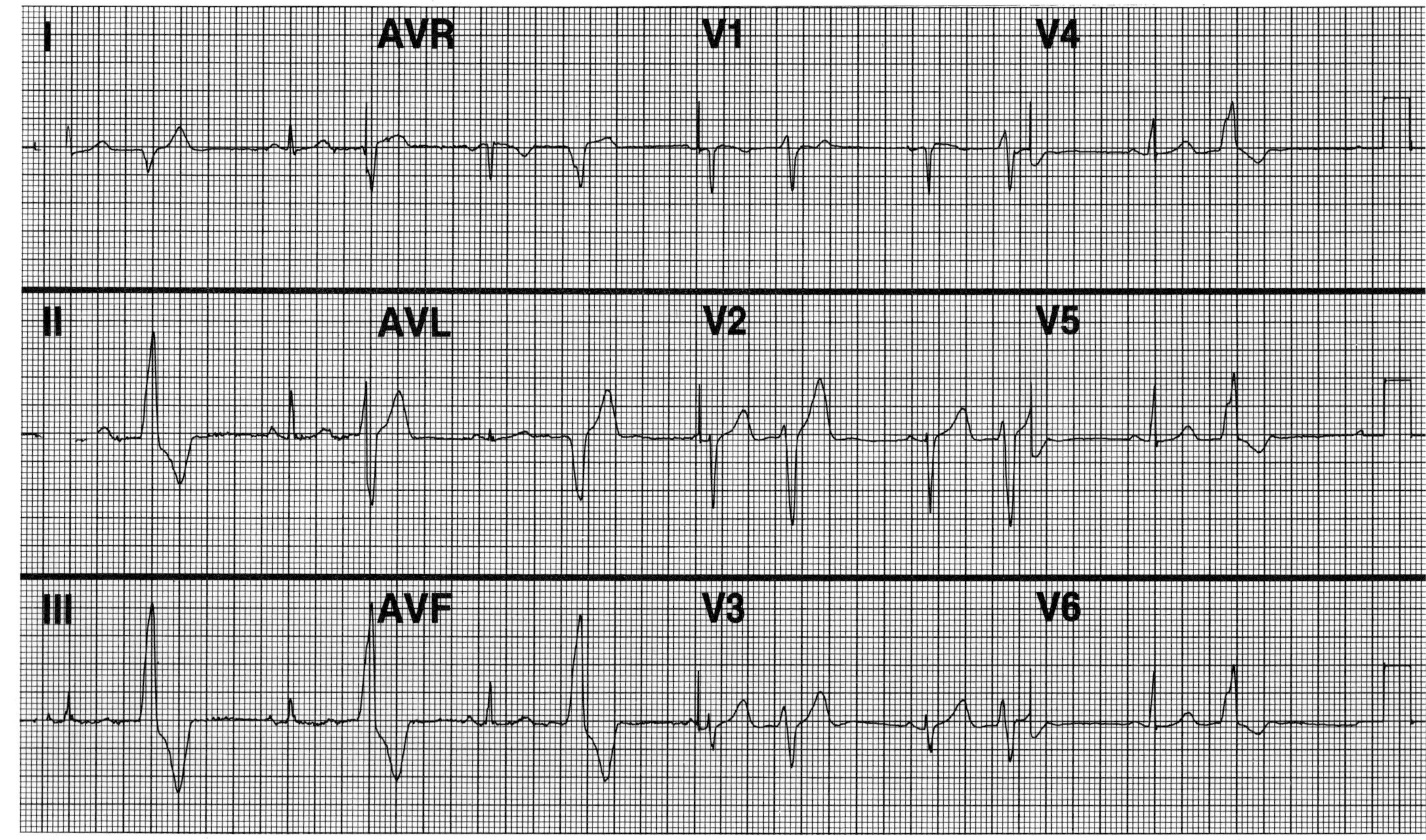
I
AVR
V1
V4
II
AVL
V2
V5
III
AVF
V3
V6

Electrocardiogram #71

Atrial Rate	75	Beats/Minute
Ventricular Rate	75	Beats/Minute
PR Interval	0.16	Second
QRS Duration	0.07	Second
QT-QTc	0.36–0.40	Second
QRS Complex Axis	60	Degrees

Rate: The atrial and ventricular rates are 75 beats per minute.

Rhythm: The PR interval is 0.16 second and constant on alternate beats. The basic rhythm is normal sinus rhythm. There is, however, a wide ventricular complex alternating with every sinus beat. These are frequent premature ventricular contractions. The alteration of normal sinus beats followed by a ventricular premature contraction is called bigeminy.

Conduction Abnormalities: No criteria present in this electrocardiogram.

QRS Complex Axis: The mean QRS complex axis is 60°. One needs to measure the QRS complex axis only in the beats that are of sinus origin.

Chamber Enlargement: No criteria present in this electrocardiogram.

Infarction: No criteria present in this electrocardiogram.

ST Segment and T Wave Abnormalities: No criteria present in this electrocardiogram.

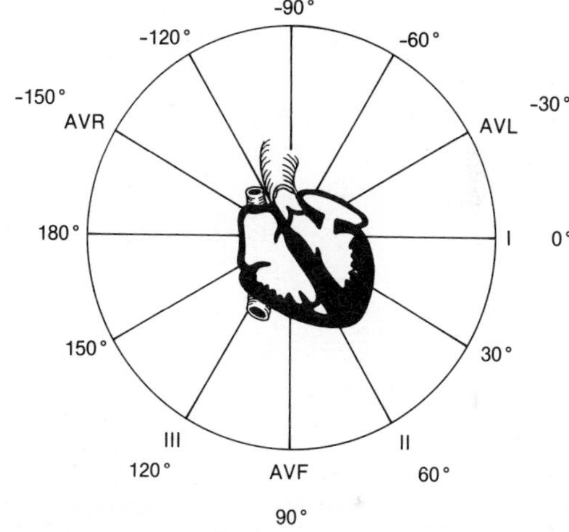

Summary

Normal sinus rhythm with frequent premature ventricular contractions forming bigeminy

Otherwise normal electrocardiogram

I AVR V1 V4

II AVL V2 V5

III AVF V3 V6

Electrocardiogram #72

Atrial Rate	**81**	**Beats/Minute**
Ventricular Rate	**81**	**Beats/Minute**
PR Interval	**0.13**	**Second**
QRS Duration	**0.08**	**Second**
QT-QTc	**0.38–0.44**	**Second**
QRS Complex Axis	**−25**	**Degrees**

Rate: The atrial and ventricular rates are 81 beats per minute.

Rhythm: The PR interval is 0.13 second and constant. The rhythm is normal sinus rhythm.

Conduction Abnormalities: No criteria present in this electrocardiogram.

QRS Complex Axis: The mean QRS complex axis is −25°.

Chamber Enlargement: No criteria present in this electrocardiogram.

Infarction: The QS complexes seen in leads V1 to V2 and the Q wave in lead V4 are diagnostic of an anteroseptal infarction. There is 2 mm elevation in leads V2 and V3, with upright T waves in these leads. The diagnosis of anteroseptal infarction, age undetermined, should be made. Anteroseptal wall myocardial infarctions are usually the result of occlusion of the left anterior descending artery of the left coronary artery.

ST Segment and T Wave Abnormalities: There are nonspecific ST segment and T wave abnormalities seen in the inferior leads II, III and AVF.

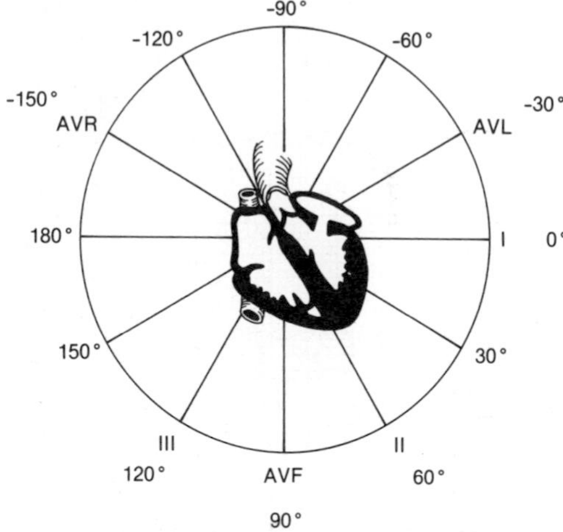

Summary

Normal sinus rhythm

Anteroseptal myocardial infarction, age undetermined

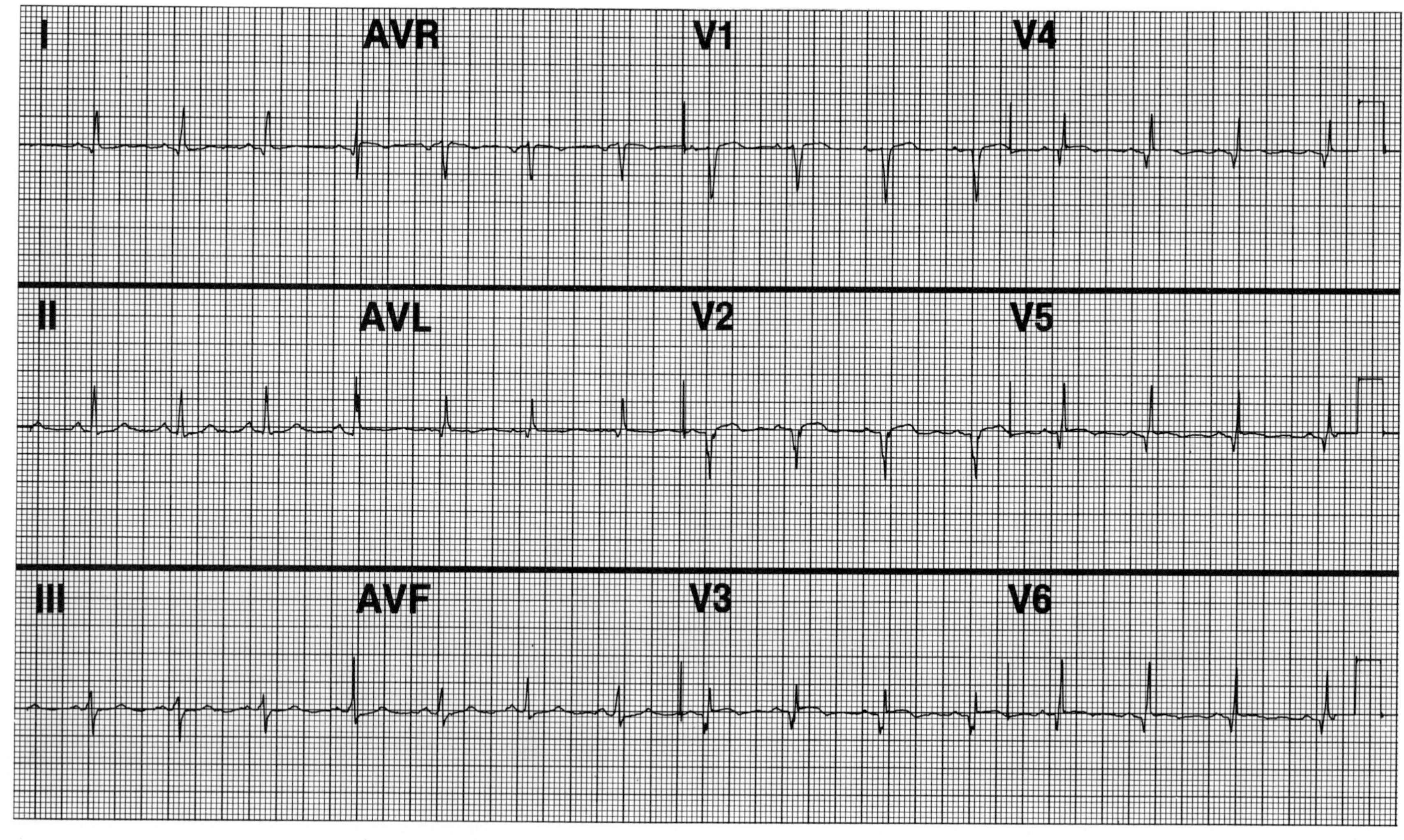
I
AVR
V1
V4
II
AVL
V2
V5
III
AVF
V3
V6

Electrocardiogram #73

Atrial Rate	88	**Beats/Minute**
Ventricular Rate	88	**Beats/Minute**
PR Interval	0.14	**Second**
QRS Duration	0.09	**Second**
QT-QTc	0.32–0.40	**Second**
QRS Complex Axis	25	**Degrees**

Rate: The atrial and ventricular rates are 88 beats per minute.

Rhythm: The PR interval is 0.14 second and constant. The rhythm is normal sinus rhythm.

Conduction Abnormalities: No criteria present in this electrocardiogram.

QRS Complex Axis: The mean QRS complex axis is 25°.

Chamber Enlargement: No criteria present in this electrocardiogram.

Infarction: QS complexes are seen in leads V1 and V2 as well as prominent Q waves in leads V3 to V4. There is ST segment elevation seen in these leads as well as T wave inversions. The diagnosis of an anterolateral infarction, age undetermined, should be made.

ST Segment and T Wave Abnormalities: See the preceding discussion under infarction.

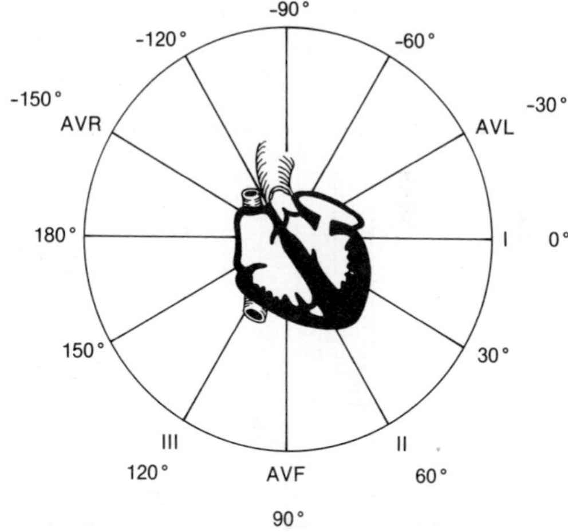

Summary

Normal sinus rhythm

Anterolateral myocardial infarction, age undetermined

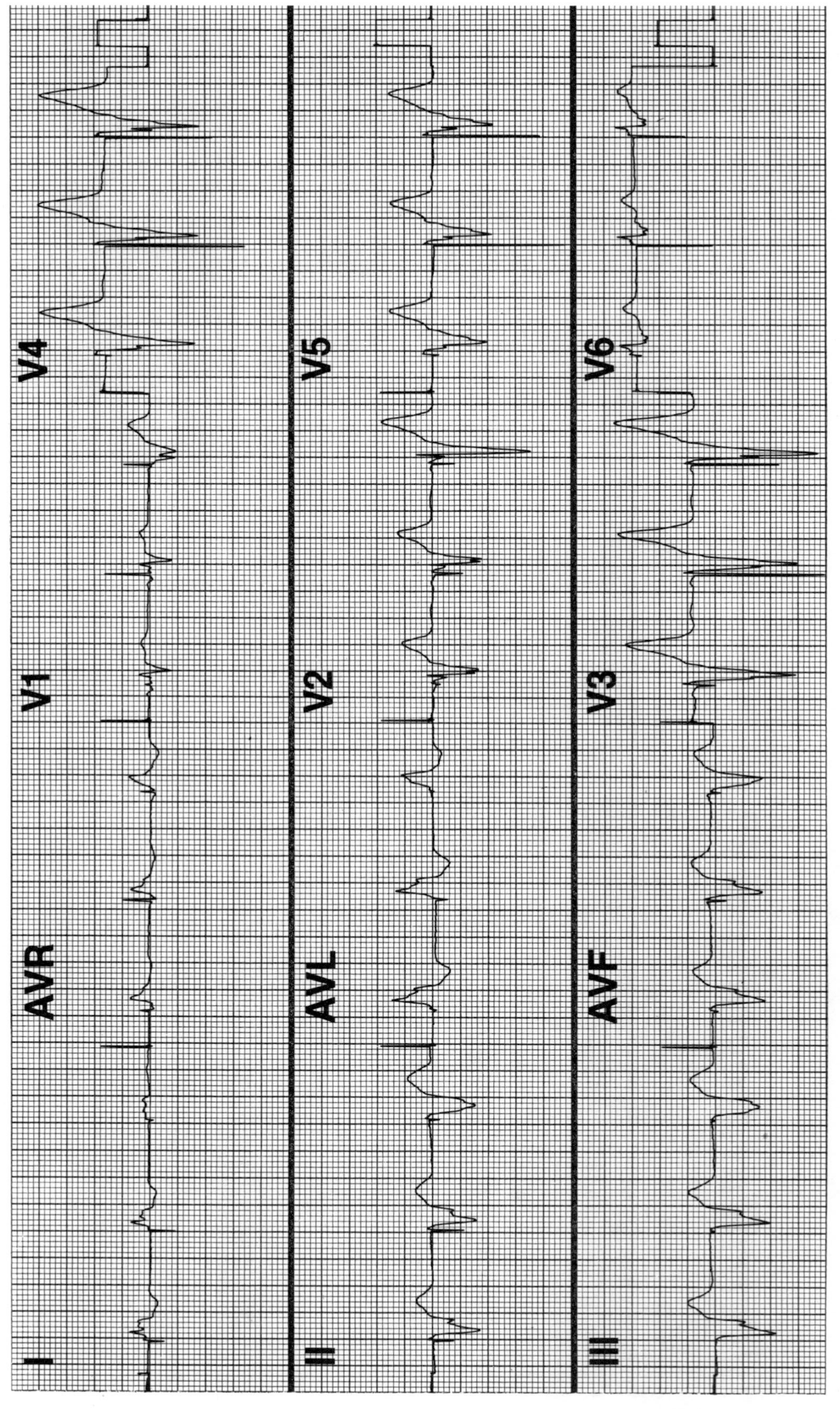
I
AVR
V1
V4
II
AVL
V2
V5
III
AVF
V3
V6

Electrocardiogram #74

Atrial Rate	—	**Beats/Minute**
Ventricular Rate	75	**Beats/Minute**
PR Interval	—	**Second**
QRS Duration	0.19	**Second**
QT-QTc	0.42–0.47	**Second**
QRS Complex Axis	−75	**Degrees**

Rate: The ventricular rate is 75 beats per minute.

Rhythm: No P waves are seen in this electrocardiogram. Each QRS complex measures 0.19 second and follows an electronic pacing spike. Therefore, a ventricular pacemaker is present in this electrocardiogram.

Conduction Abnormalities: This electrocardiogram may appear similar to those tracings showing a left bundle branch block. This is related to the conduction abnormalities seen when an electronic ventricular pacemaker is placed in the right ventricle and stimulates the right ventricle first. Therefore, conduction of the septum is right to left, as one sees in a left bundle branch block. By looking at this tracing, one can determine that a ventricular pacemaker is present and is located in the right ventricle, which is its usual position.

QRS Complex Axis: The mean QRS complex axis is −75°.

Chamber Enlargement: No criteria present in this electrocardiogram.

Infarction: No criteria present in this electrocardiogram.

ST Segment and T Wave Abnormalities: No criteria present in this electrocardiogram.

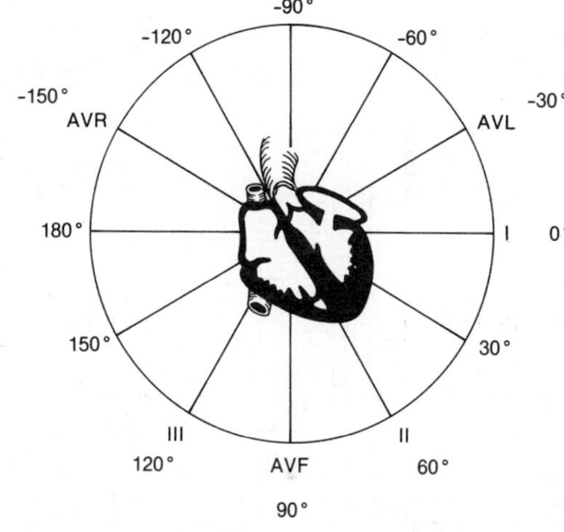

Summary

Electronic ventricular pacemaker

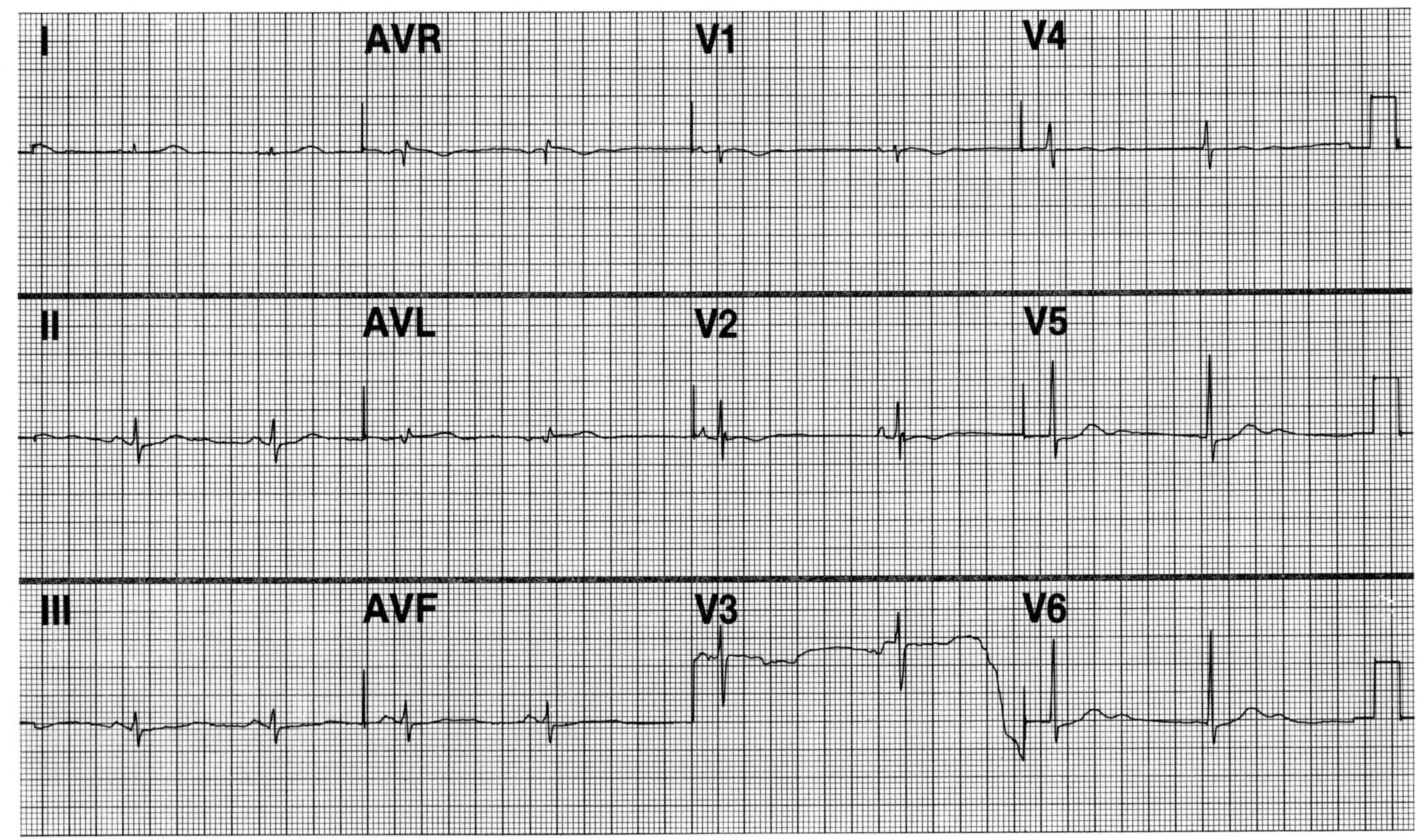
I
AVR
V1
V4
II
AVL
V2
V5
III
AVF
V3
V6

Electrocardiogram #75

Atrial Rate	50	**Beats/Minute**
Ventricular Rate	50	**Beats/Minute**
PR Interval	0.12	**Second**
QRS Duration	0.08	**Second**
QT-QTc	0.43–0.40	**Second**
QRS Complex Axis	40	**Degrees**

Rate: The atrial and ventricular rates are 50 beats per minute.

Rhythm: The PR interval is 0.12 second. The rhythm is normal sinus rhythm with sinus arrhythmia.

Conduction Abnormalities: No criteria present in this electrocardiogram.

QRS Complex Axis: The mean QRS complex axis is 40°.

Chamber Enlargement: No criteria present in this electrocardiogram.

Infarction: No criteria present in this electrocardiogram.

ST Segment and T Wave Abnormalities: There are nonspecific T wave abnormalities.

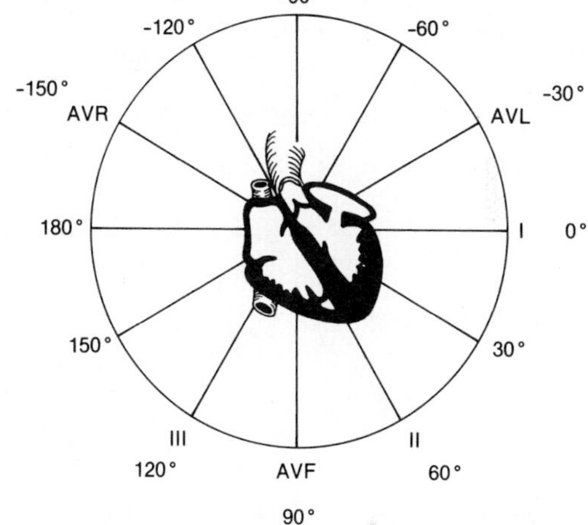

Summary

Normal sinus rhythm with short PR interval

Nonspecific T wave abnormalities

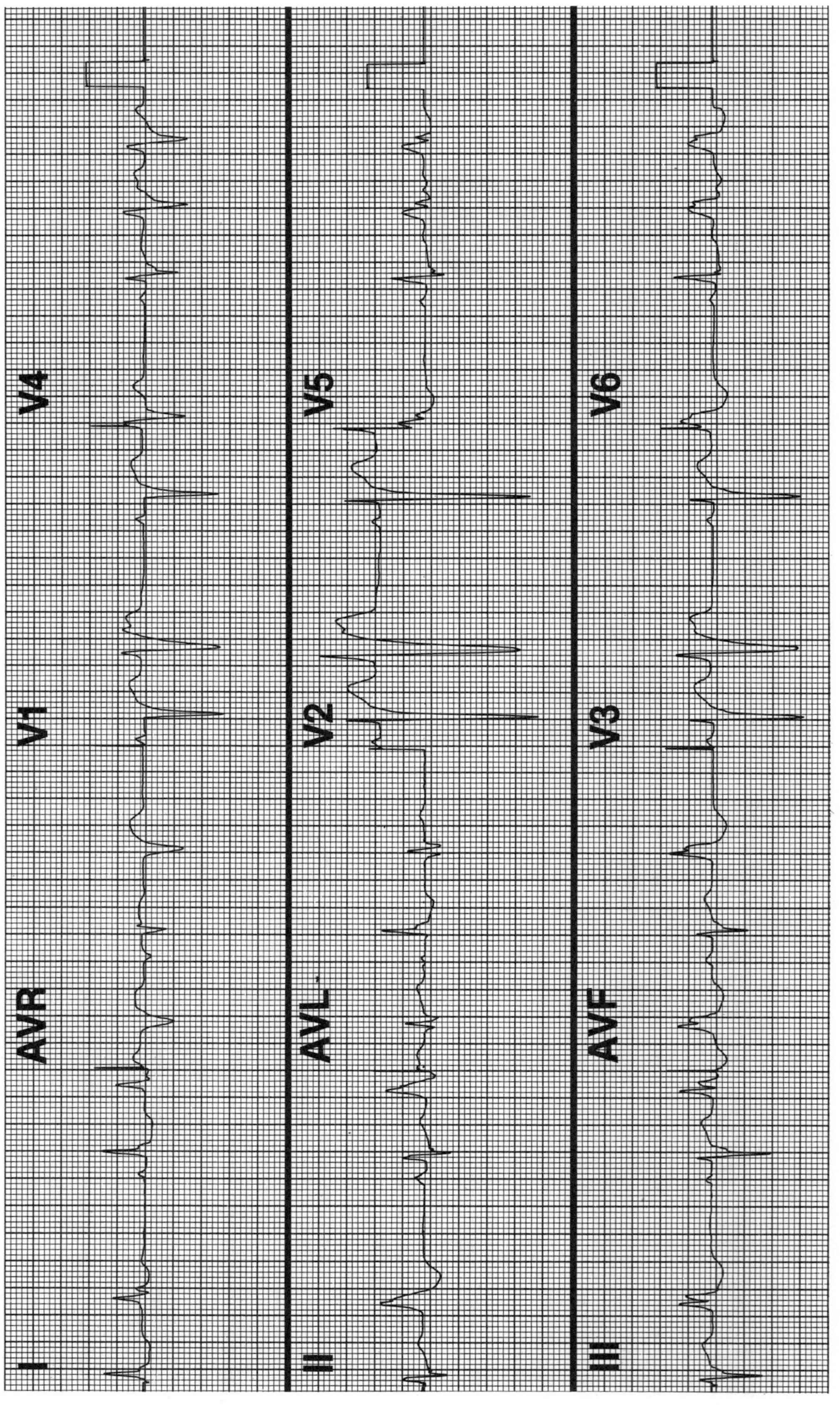
I
AVR
V1
V4
II
AVL
V2
V5
III
AVF
V3
V6

Electrocardiogram #76

Atrial Rate	**80**	**Beats/Minute**
Ventricular Rate	**80**	**Beats/Minute**
PR Interval	**0.18**	**Second**
QRS Duration	**0.10**	**Second**
QT-QTc	**0.36–0.42**	**Second**
QRS Complex Axis	**−30**	**Degrees**

Rate: The atrial and ventricular rates are 80 beats per minute.

Rhythm: The PR interval is 0.18 second and constant. The diagnosis is normal sinus rhythm. In addition, frequent wide ventricular complexes are seen. The second beat in leads I, II and III is a ventricular premature contraction, while the first and third complexes in leads AVR, AVL and AVF are ventricular premature contractions. The second beat in leads V1, V2 and V3 as well as the first, third and fourth complexes in leads V4, V5 and V6 are ventricular premature contractions. Consecutive premature ventricular contractions are termed a couplet or salvo. When three premature ventricular contractions are consecutive, the term ventricular tachycardia is used.

Conduction Abnormalities: Besides the abnormal conduction of the ventricular complexes, there are no criteria present in this electrocardiogram.

QRS Complex Axis: The mean QRS complex axis is −30°, left axis deviation. Other criteria for left anterior hemiblock are not present.

Chamber Enlargement: No criteria present in this electrocardiogram.

Infarction: No criteria present in this electrocardiogram.

ST Segment and T Wave Abnormalities: There are nonspecific T wave abnormalities.

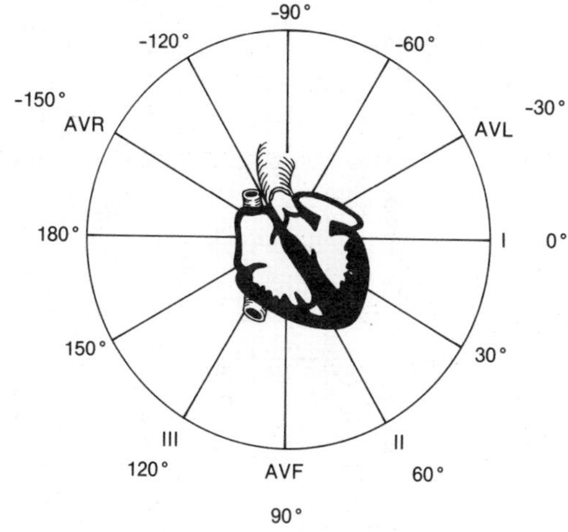

Summary

Normal sinus rhythm with frequent premature ventricular contractions occasionally forming couplets

Abnormal left axis deviation

Nonspecific T wave abnormalities

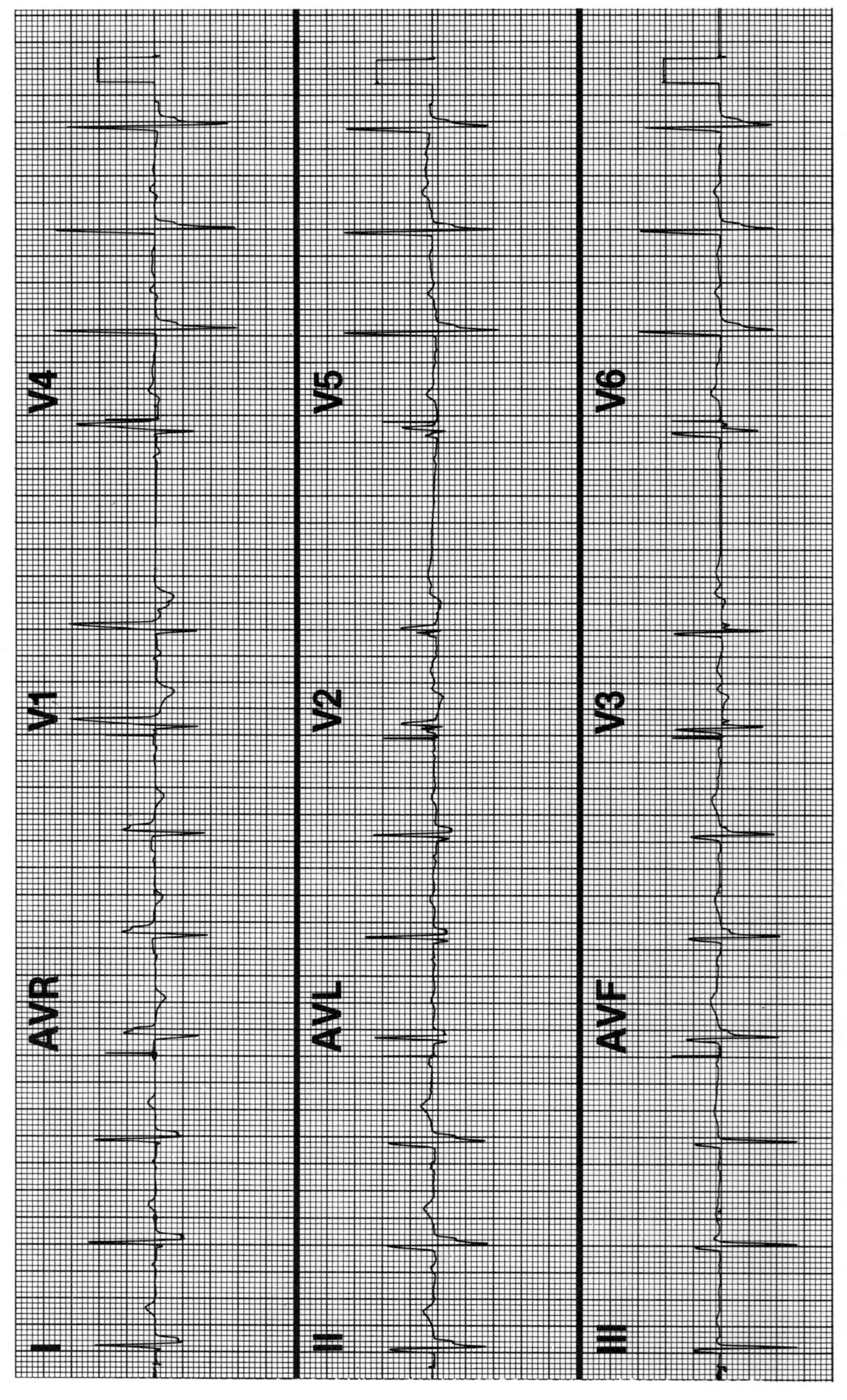
I
AVR
V1
V4
II
AVL
V2
V5
III
AVF
V3
V6

Electrocardiogram #77

Atrial Rate	**83**	**Beats/Minute**
Ventricular Rate	**83**	**Beats/Minute**
PR Interval	**0.20**	**Second**
QRS Duration	**0.13**	**Second**
QT-QTc	**0.40–0.42**	**Second**
QRS Complex Axis	**−40**	**Degrees**

Rate: The atrial and ventricular rates are 83 beats per minute.

Rhythm: The PR interval is 0.20 second and constant. The rhythm is normal sinus rhythm. Although this rhythm is perfectly regular with a constant PR interval, after the second beat in leads V1, V2 and V3, a pause will be seen. Notice the decending limb of the T wave of this beat—there is a deformation of this slope resulting from an early P wave that has found the atrioventricular node refractory. Therefore, this pause is related to a blocked atrial premature contraction.

Conduction Abnormalities: The QRS complex measures 0.13 second. An rsR′ complex is seen in lead V2 together with terminal slurring of the S wave in leads I, V5 and V6, which is diagnostic of a right bundle branch block. In addition, there is an abnormal left axis deviation, and a diagnosis of a left anterior hemiblock should be made. There is a qRS complex in lead I and an rS complex in leads II, III and AVF that produce this abnormal axis deviation.

QRS Complex Axis: The mean QRS complex axis is −40,° abnormal left axis deviation. This is caused by the left anterior hemiblock.

Chamber Enlargement: The R wave in lead AVL is 12 mm. Therefore, the voltage criteria for left ventricular hypertrophy is present.

Infarction: No criteria present in this electrocardiogram.

ST Segment and T Wave Abnormalities: There is flattening of the T wave in lead AVL and in the leads of the left precordium. This is related to the left ventricular hypertrophy.

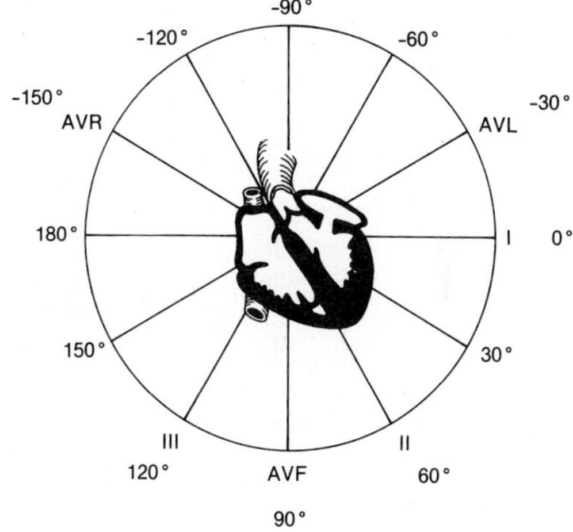

Summary

Normal sinus rhythm with a blocked atrial premature contraction

Abnormal left axis deviation

Right bundle branch block

Left ventricular hypertrophy

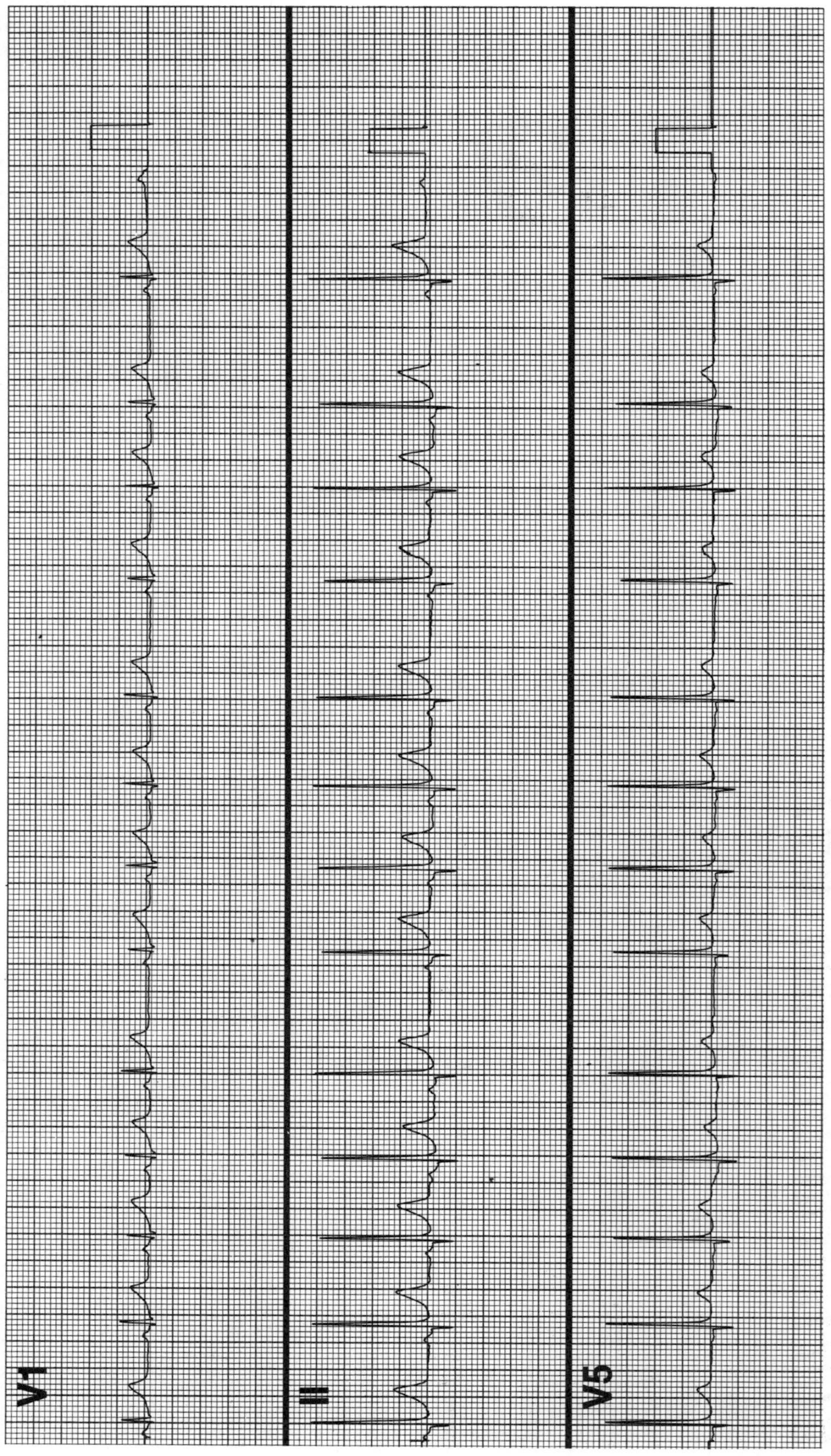
V1
II
V5

Electrocardiogram #78

Atrial Rate	80	**Beats/Minute**
Ventricular Rate	80	**Beats/Minute**
PR Interval	0.13	**Second**
QRS Duration	0.08	**Second**
QT-QTc	0.37–0.43	**Second**
QRS Complex Axis	—	**Degrees**

Rate: The atrial and ventricular rates are 80 beats per minute.

Rhythm: The PR interval is 0.13 second and constant. Therefore, it is normal sinus rhythm. However, in the rhythm strip seen here, there is a marked irregularity despite the fact that each QRS complex is preceded by a P wave, and the PR interval is constant. The rhythm is, therefore, a marked sinus arrhythmia. Sinus arrhythmia can be seen in young healthy individuals or in individuals with severe lung disease.

Conduction Abnormalities: No criteria present in this electrocardiogram.

QRS Complex Axis: The mean QRS complex axis cannot be determined from the tracings provided.

Chamber Enlargement: No criteria present in this electrocardiogram.

Infarction: No criteria present in this electrocardiogram.

ST Segment and T Wave Abnormalities: No criteria present in this electrocardiogram.

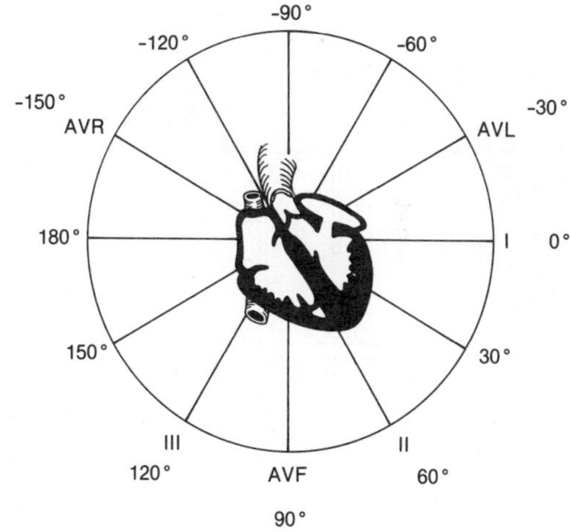

Summary

Normal sinus rhythm with marked sinus arrhythmia

Otherwise normal electrocardiogram

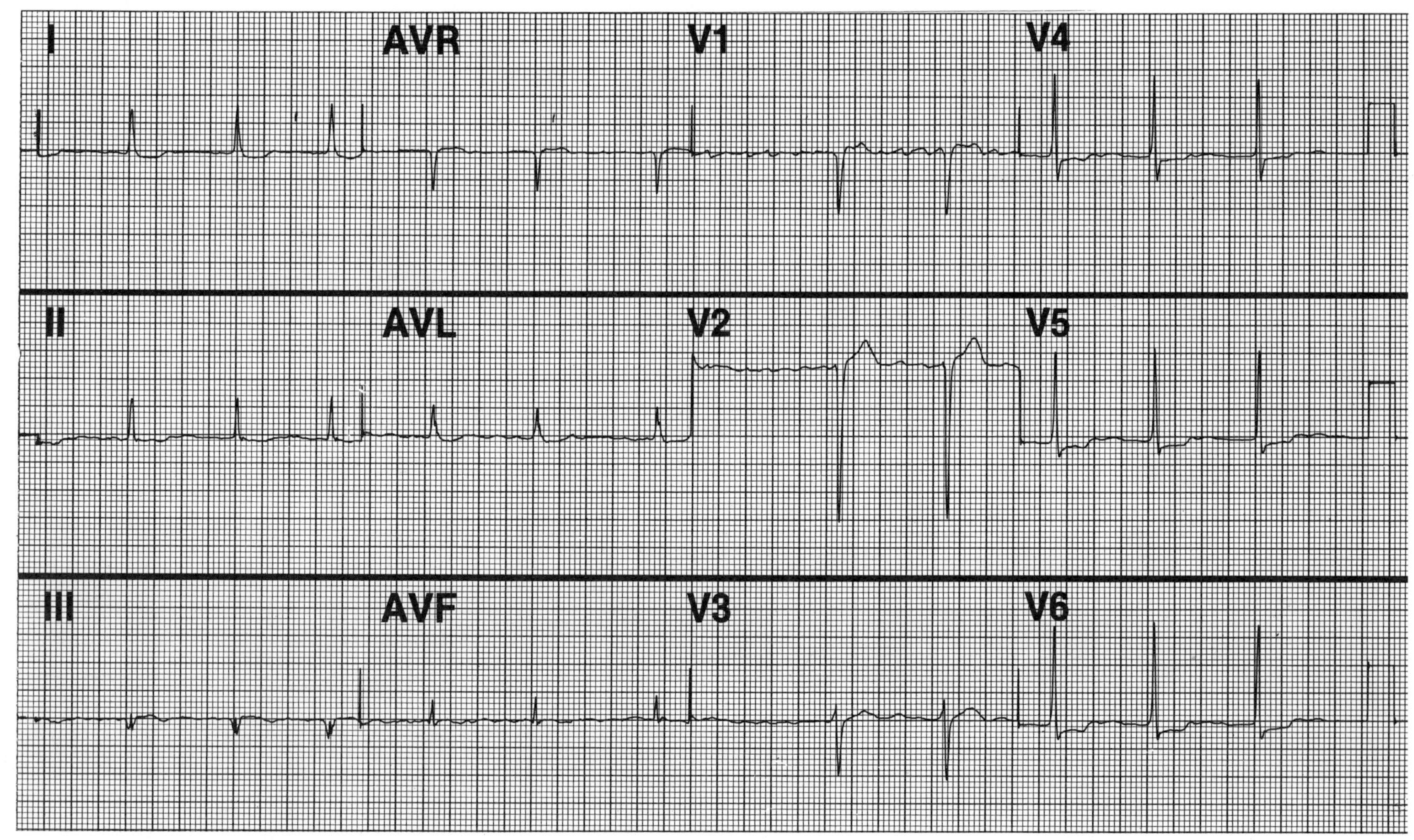
I
AVR
V1
V4
II
AVL
V2
V5
III
AVF
V3
V6

Electrocardiogram #79

Atrial Rate	—	Beats/Minute
Ventricular Rate	70	Beats/Minute
PR Interval	—	Second
QRS Duration	0.10	Second
QT-QTc	0.36–0.40	Second
QRS Complex Axis	15	Degrees

Rate: The average ventricular rate is 70 beats per minute.

Rhythm: No P waves are seen in this electrocardiogram. The baseline is undulating, and the QRS complexes are irregularly irregular. The rhythm is, therefore, atrial fibrillation.

Conduction Abnormalities: No criteria present in this electrocardiogram.

QRS Complex Axis: The mean QRS complex axis is 15°.

Chamber Enlargement: No criteria present in this electrocardiogram.

Infarction: Despite the fact that there is a QS complex in lead V1, a small micro R wave is seen in lead V2 that develops normally through the precordial leads. The diagnosis of an anteroseptal infarction should not be made.

ST Segment and T Wave Abnormalities: There are nonspecific ST segment and T wave abnormalities.

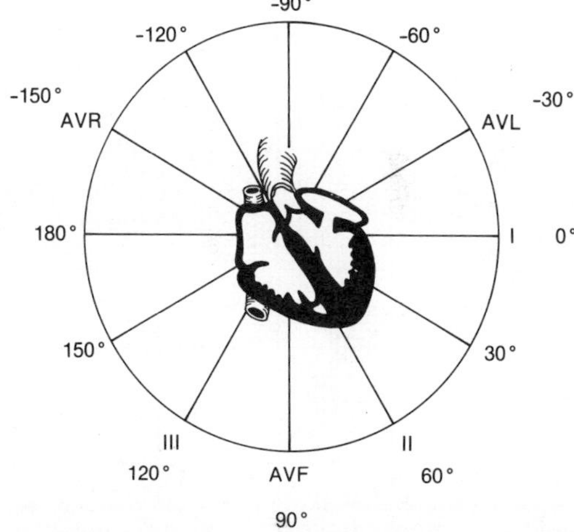

Summary

Coarse atrial fibrillation

Nonspecific ST segment and T wave abnormalities

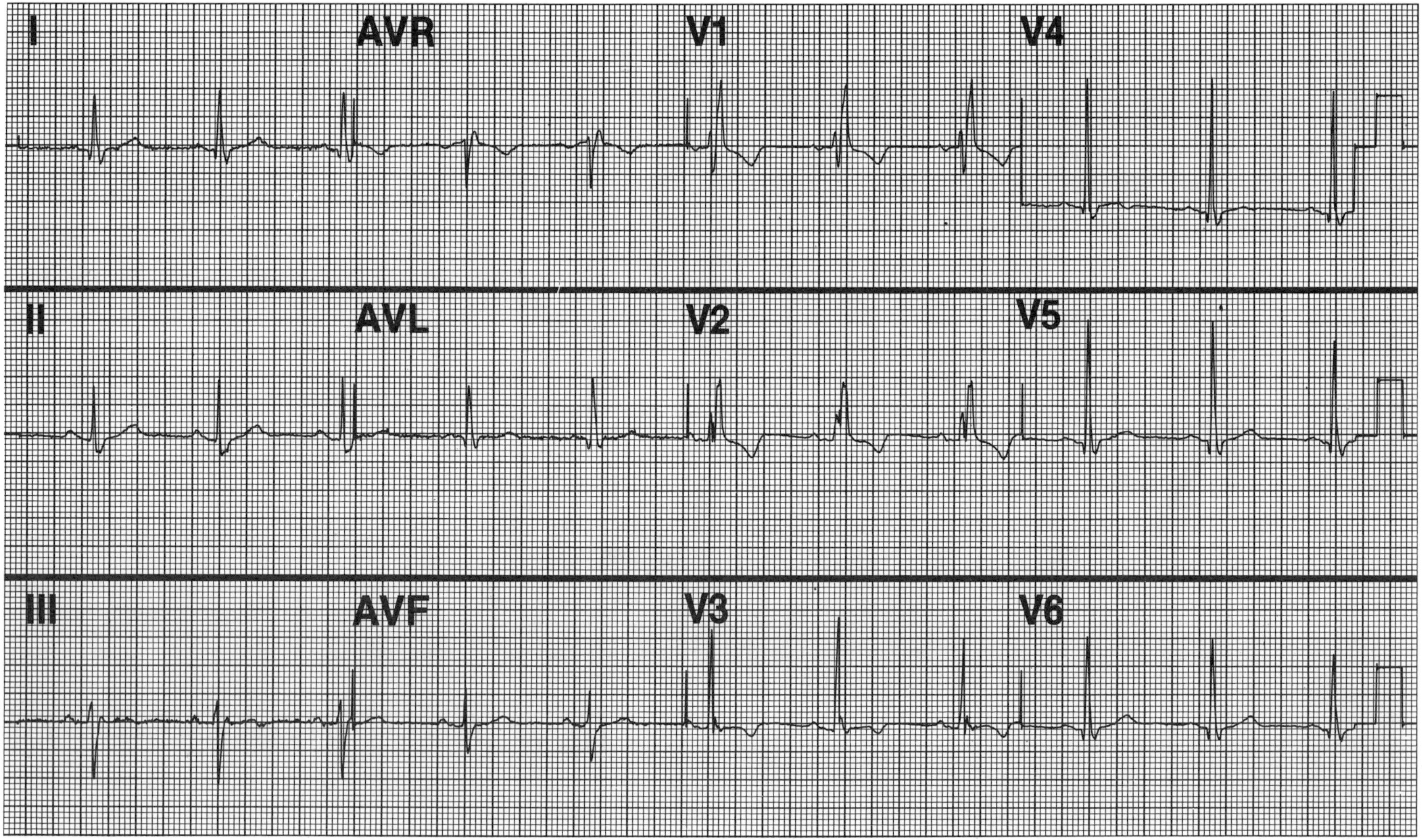
I
AVR
V1
V4
II
AVL
V2
V5
III
AVF
V3
V6

Electrocardiogram #80

Atrial Rate	65	Beats/Minute
Ventricular Rate	65	Beats/Minute
PR Interval	0.17	Second
QRS Duration	0.13	Second
QT-QTc	0.41–0.43	Second
QRS Complex Axis	5	Degrees

Rate: The atrial and ventricular rates are 65 beats per minute.

Rhythm: The PR interval is 0.17 second and constant. The rhythm is normal sinus rhythm.

Conduction Abnormalities: The QRS complex is wide and measures 0.13 second. An rSR′ complex is seen in lead V1, and the terminal delay in leads I, V5 and V6 makes the diagnosis of a right bundle branch block.

QRS Complex Axis: The mean QRS complex axis is 5°.

Chamber Enlargement: No criteria present in this electrocardiogram.

Infarction: No criteria present in this electrocardiogram.

ST Segment and T Wave Abnormalities: The ST segment and T wave abnormalities are secondary to the conduction abnormalities.

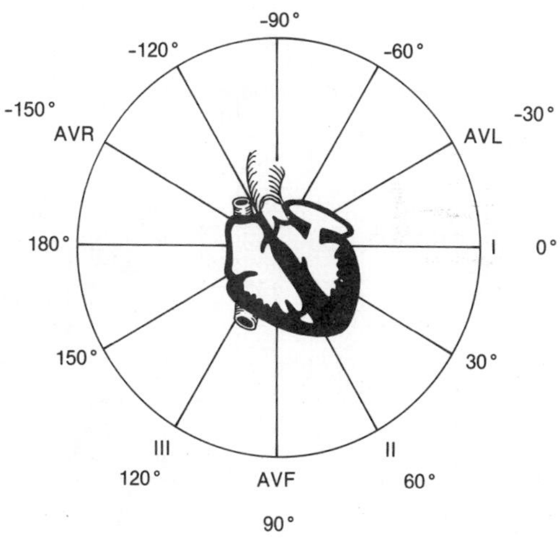

Summary

Normal sinus rhythm

Right bundle branch block

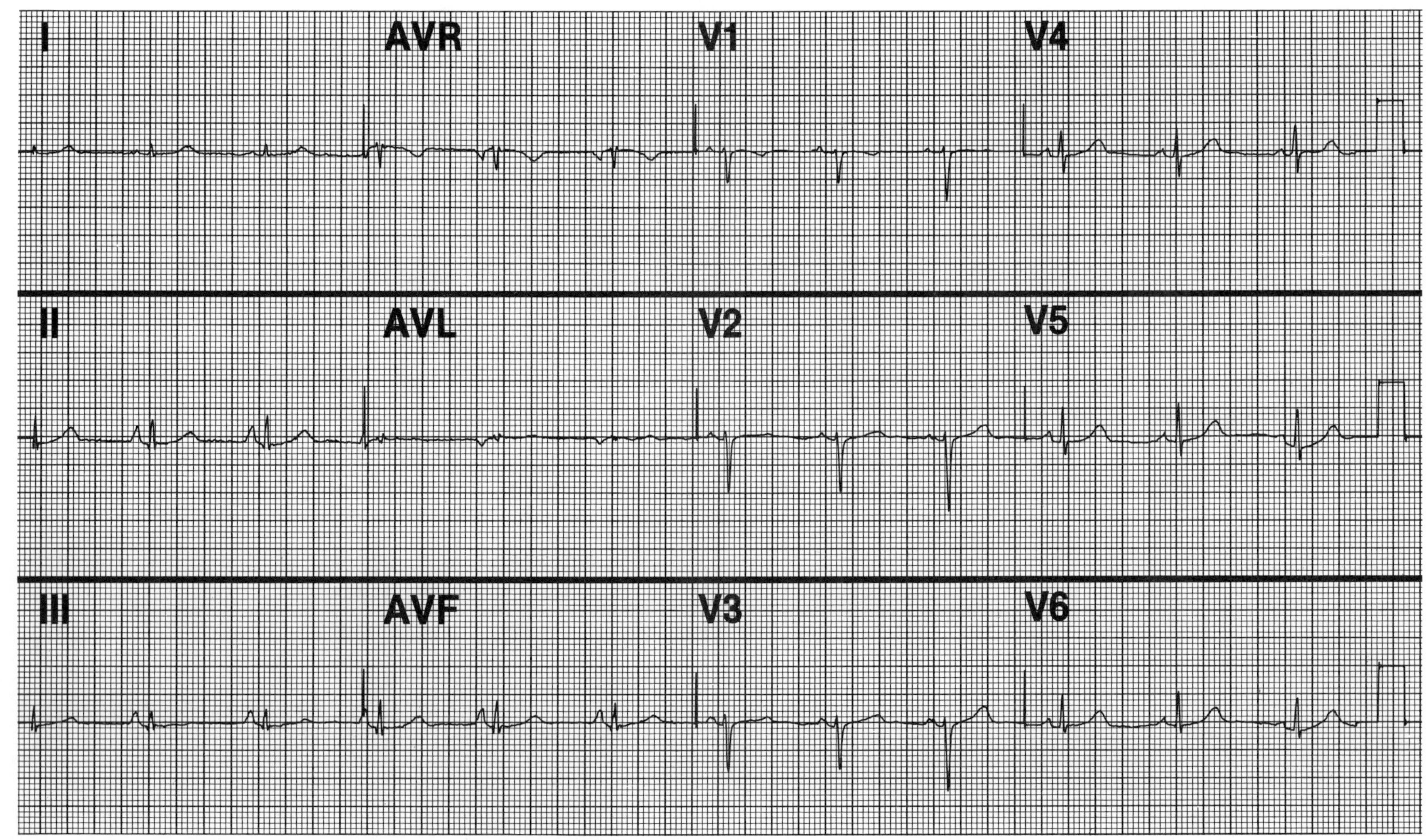
I
AVR
V1
V4
II
AVL
V2
V5
III
AVF
V3
V6

Electrocardiogram #81

Atrial Rate	**73**	**Beats/Minute**
Ventricular Rate	**73**	**Beats/Minute**
PR Interval	**0.13**	**Second**
QRS Duration	**0.08**	**Second**
QT-QTc	**0.40–0.43**	**Second**
QRS Complex Axis	**60**	**Degrees**

Rate: The atrial and ventricular rates are 73 beats per minute.

Rhythm: The PR interval is 0.13 second and constant. The rhythm is normal sinus rhythm.

Conduction Abnormalities: No criteria present in this electrocardiogram.

QRS Complex Axis: The mean QRS complex axis is 60°.

Chamber Enlargement: The prominent P waves seen in the inferior leads II, III and AVF are indicative of right atrial enlargement. The P waves measure 3 mm in lead II.

Infarction: No criteria present in this electrocardiogram.

ST Segment and T Wave Abnormalities: No criteria present in this electrocardiogram.

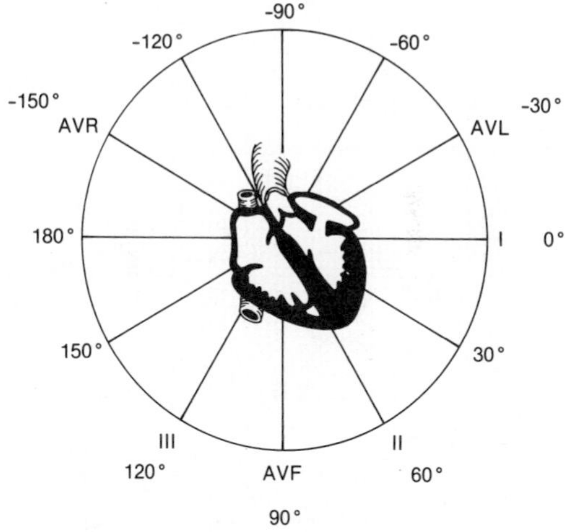

Summary

Normal sinus rhythm

Right atrial enlargement

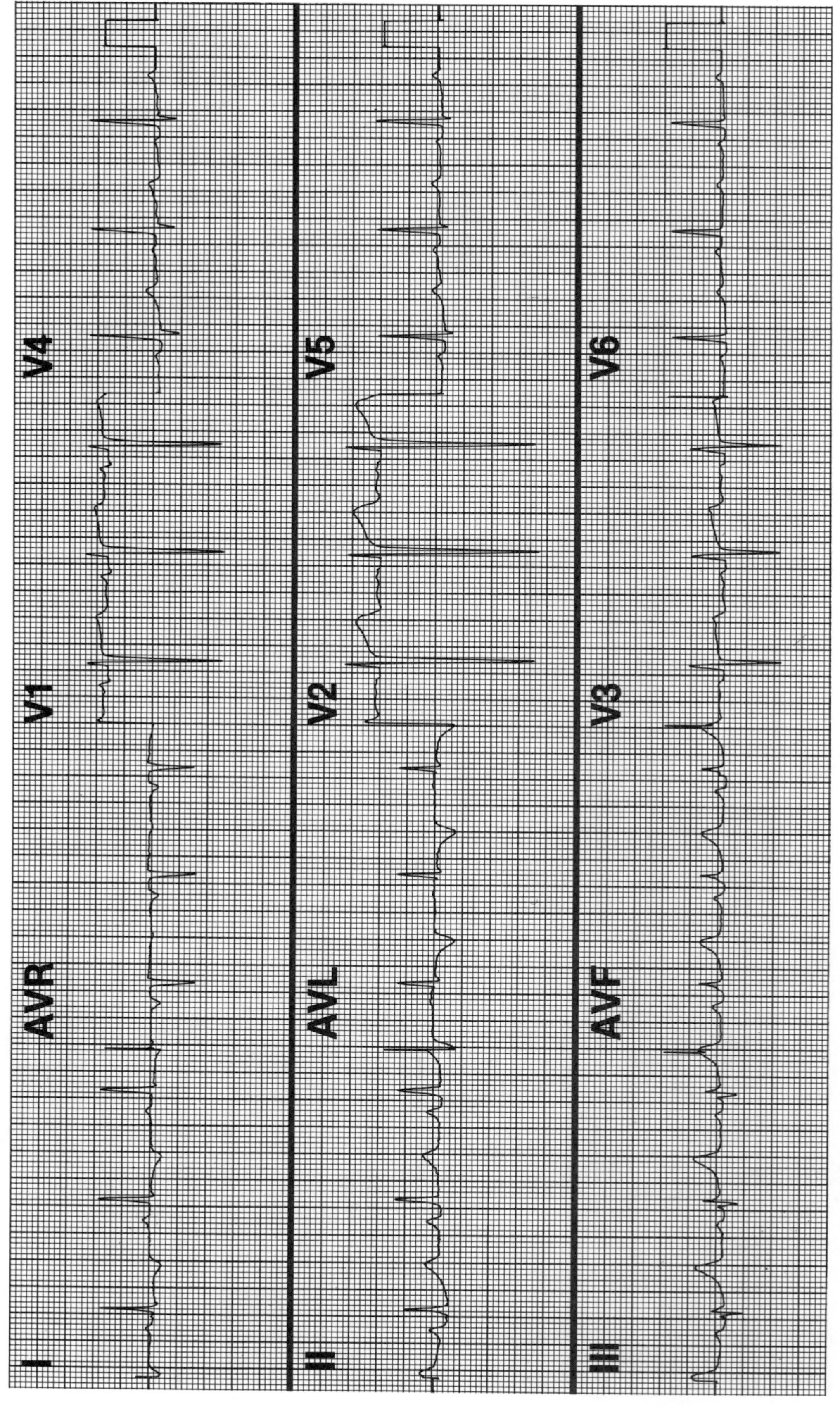
I
AVR
V1
V4
II
AVL
V2
V5
III
AVF
V3
V6

Electrocardiogram #82

Atrial Rate	73	Beats/Minute
Ventricular Rate	73	Beats/Minute
PR Interval	0.18	Second
QRS Duration	0.09	Second
QT-QTc	0.45–0.50	Second
QRS Complex Axis	30	Degrees

Rate: The atrial and ventricular rates are 73 beats per minute.

Rhythm: The PR interval is 0.18 second and constant. The rhythm is normal sinus rhythm.

Conduction Abnormalities: No criteria present in this electrocardiogram.

QRS Complex Axis: The mean QRS complex axis is 30°.

Chamber Enlargement: No criteria present in this electrocardiogram.

Infarction: No criteria present in this electrocardiogram.

ST Segment and T Wave Abnormalities: The ST segment and T wave abnormalities seen in leads I and AVL are suggestive of lateral ischemia.

Other Findings: The QTc interval measures 0.50 second and is prolonged. An important cause of prolongation of the QT interval is hypocalcemia. A prolonged QT interval predisposes to the R on T phenomenon, which can result in ventricular tachycardia (see Ventricular Tachycardia, page 52 and Chapter 4, Review of Complexes).

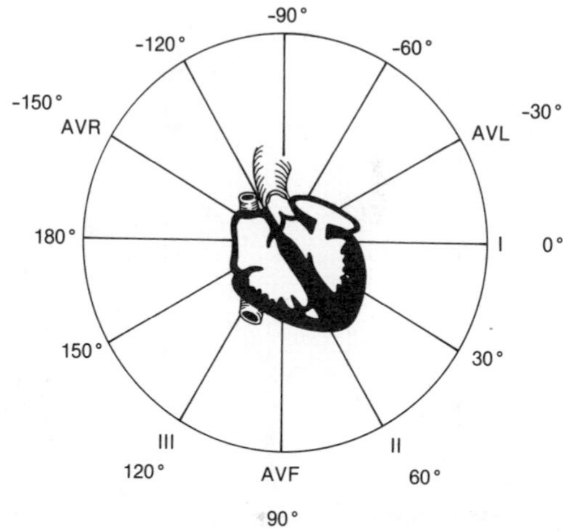

Summary

Normal sinus rhythm

Lateral wall ischemia

Prolonged QTc interval

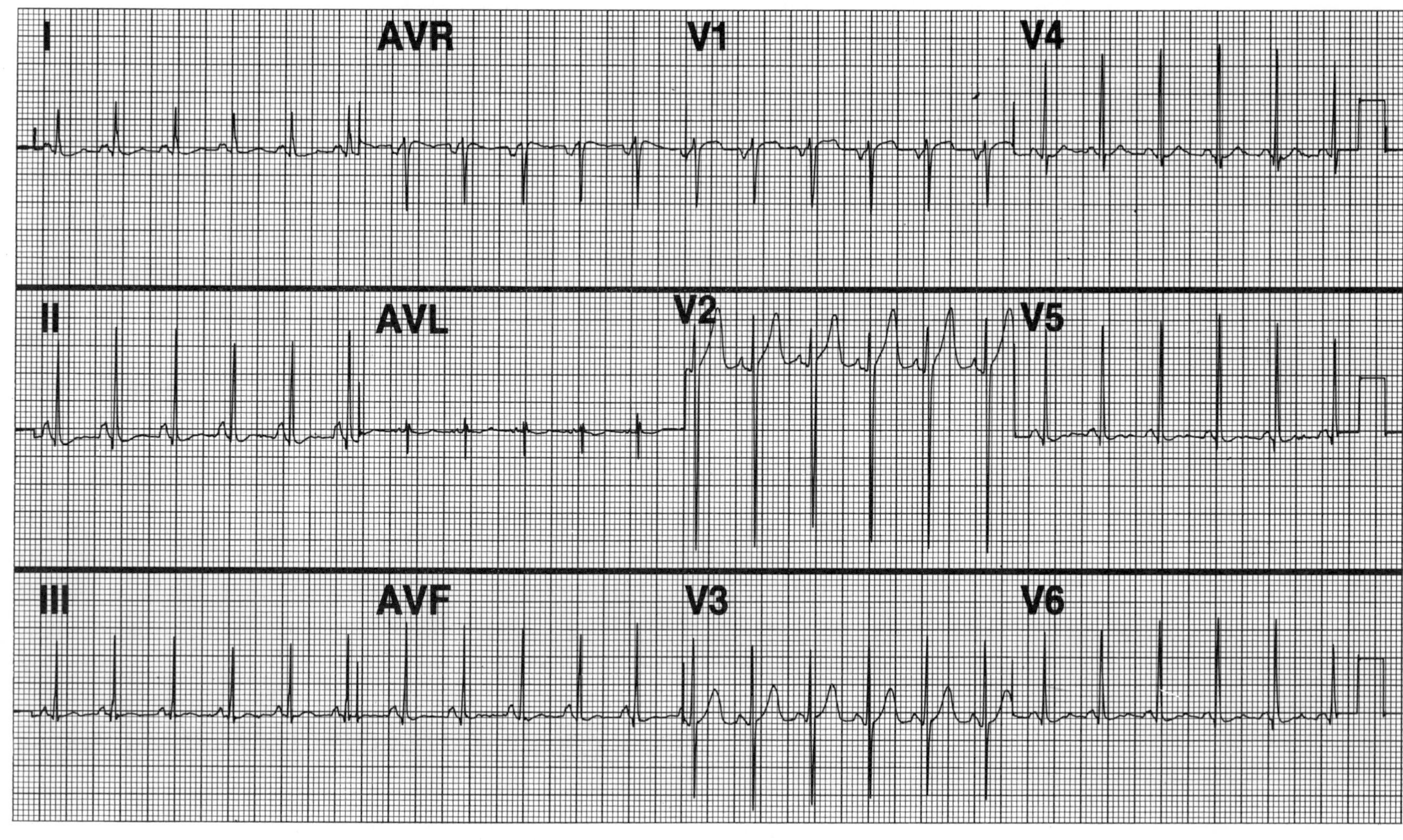
I
AVR
V1
V4
II
AVL
V2
V5
III
AVF
V3
V6

Electrocardiogram #83

Atrial Rate	**136**	**Beats/Minute**
Ventricular Rate	**136**	**Beats/Minute**
PR Interval	**0.09**	**Second**
QRS Duration	**0.06**	**Second**
QT-QTc	**0.28–0.43**	**Second**
QRS Complex Axis	**60**	**Degrees**

Rate: The atrial and ventricular rates are 136 beats per minute.

Rhythm: The PR interval is 0.09 second and constant. The diagnosis is sinus tachycardia with a short PR interval.

Conduction Abnormalities: No criteria present in this electrocardiogram.

QRS Complex Axis: The mean QRS complex axis is 60°.

Chamber Enlargement: Biatrial enlargement is seen in this electrocardiogram. Notice the peaking of the P waves in leads II and AVF. The P waves measure 2.5 mm in lead II. The marked negative component of the P wave in lead V1 suggests left atrial enlargement. These findings are indicative of right and left atrial enlargement, respectively. The notching of the P wave in lead I is indicative of left atrial enlargement as well. In addition, the S wave voltage in lead V2 and the R wave voltage in lead V6 equal 49 mm. One should suspect that left ventricular hypertrophy is present.

Infarction: No criteria present in this electrocardiogram.

ST Segment and T Wave Abnormalities: There are ST segment and T wave abnormalities seen in the lateral leads that are secondary changes to the left ventricular hypertrophy.

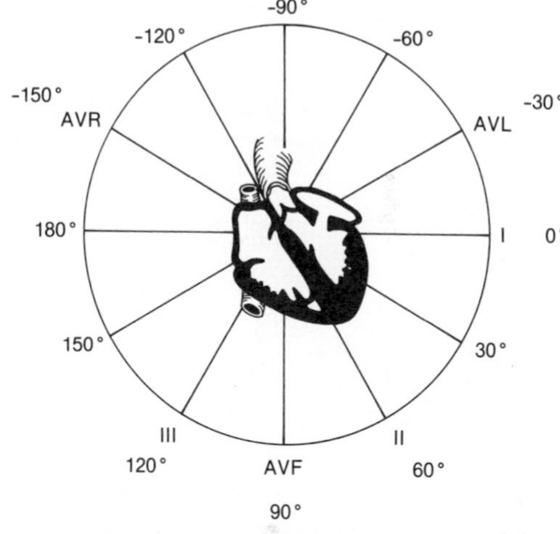

Summary

Sinus tachycardia with short PR interval

Biatrial enlargement

Left ventricular hypertrophy

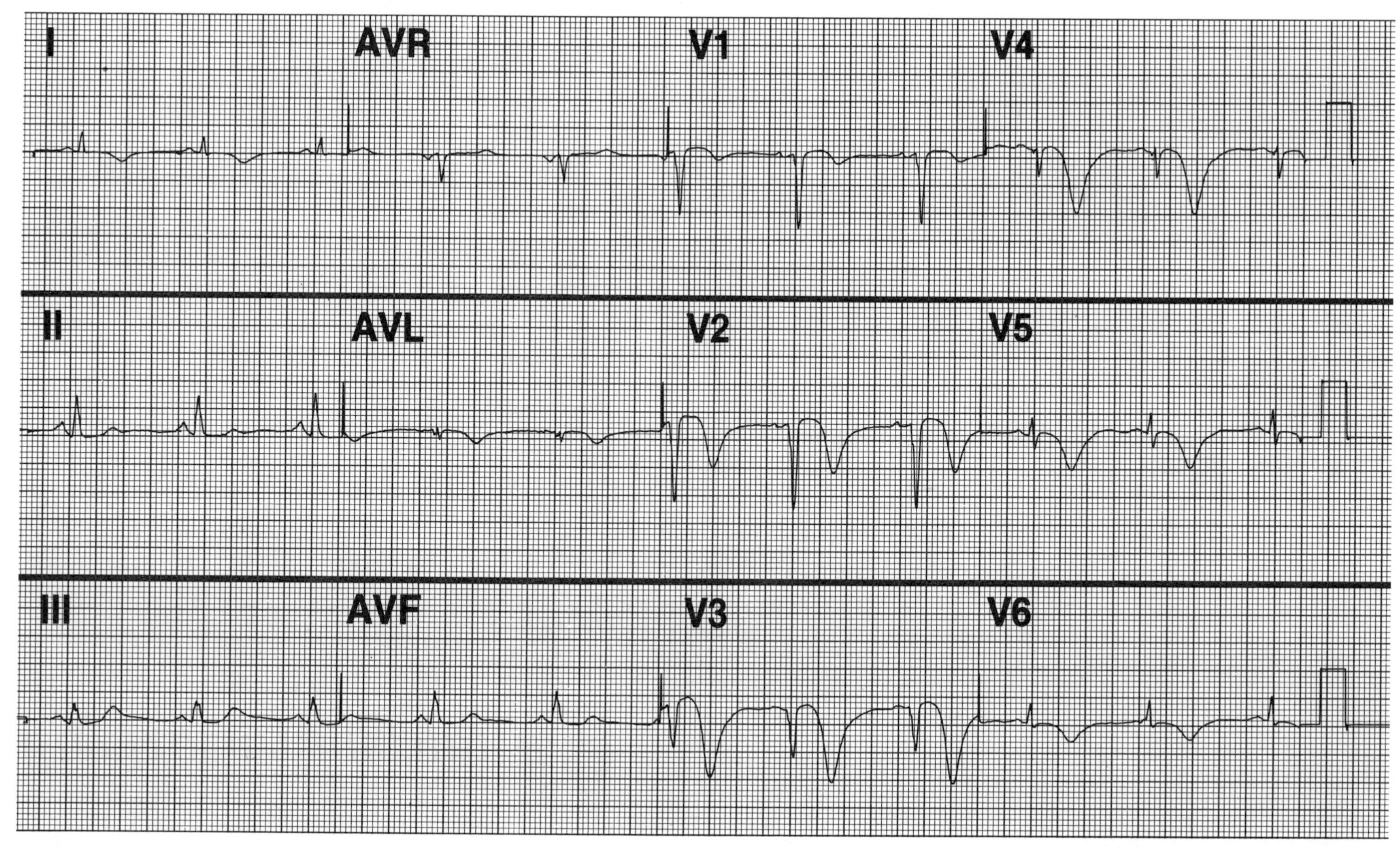
I
AVR
V1
V4
II
AVL
V2
V5
III
AVF
V3
V6

Electrocardiogram #84

Atrial Rate	65	Beats/Minute
Ventricular Rate	65	Beats/Minute
PR Interval	0.14	Second
QRS Duration	0.09	Second
QT-QTc	0.52–0.54	Second
QRS Complex Axis	70	Degrees

Rate: The atrial and ventricular rates are 65 beats per minute.

Rhythm: The PR interval is 0.14 second and constant. The diagnosis is normal sinus rhythm.

Conduction Abnormalities: No criteria present in this electrocardiogram.

QRS Complex Axis: The mean QRS complex axis is 70°.

Chamber Enlargement: No criteria present in this electrocardiogram.

Infarction: The marked abnormality in this tracing is related to the anteroseptal myocardial infarction, possibly acute. The QS complex seen in leads V1 to V3 together with the 2 mm ST segment elevation and marked symmetric T inversion seen in leads V1 to V6 supports this diagnosis.

ST Segment and T Wave Abnormalities: There are symmetric T wave inversions in leads V4 to V6 indicative of ischemia.

Other Findings: The QRS is prolonged secondary to the ischemia and infarction.

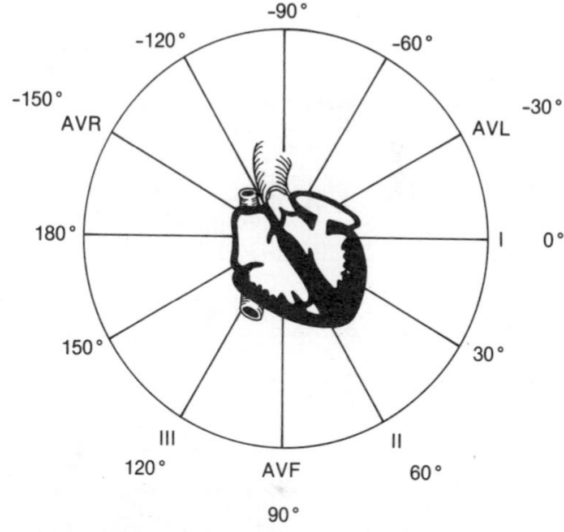

Summary

Normal sinus rhythm

Anteroseptal myocardial infarction, possibly acute

Lateral wall ischemia

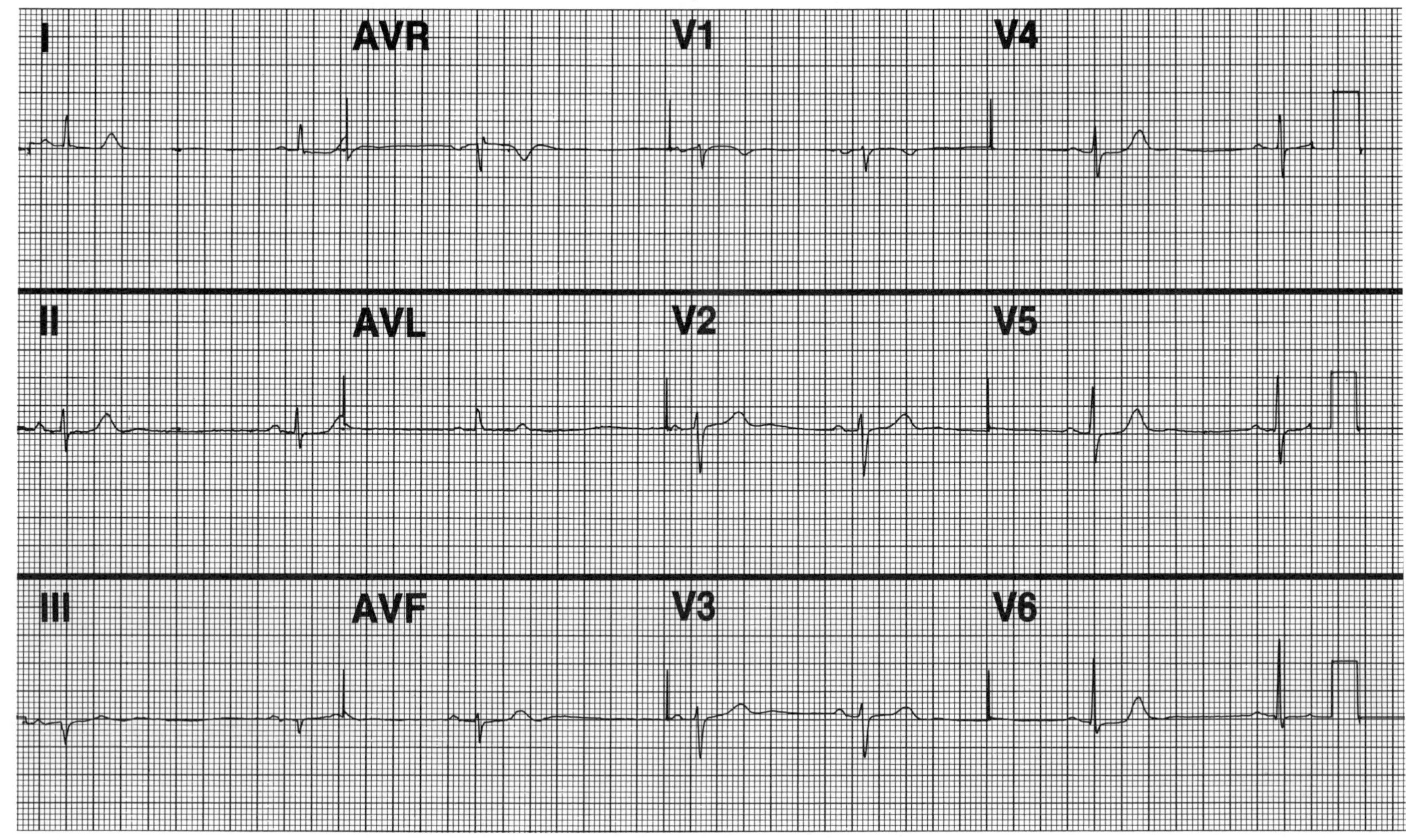

I
AVR
V1
V4
II
AVL
V2
V5
III
AVF
V3
V6

Electrocardiogram #85

Atrial Rate	**38**	**Beats/Minute**
Ventricular Rate	**38**	**Beats/Minute**
PR Interval	**0.18**	**Second**
QRS Duration	**0.08**	**Second**
QT-QTc	**0.50–0.40**	**Second**
QRS Complex Axis	**−15**	**Degrees**

Rate: The atrial and ventricular rates are 38 beats per minute.

Rhythm: The PR interval is 0.18 second and constant. The diagnosis is marked sinus bradycardia with sinus arrhythmia. Patients with this degree of bradycardia should be carefully evaluated for evidence of sick sinus syndrome or the bradycardia-tachycardia syndrome. These patients may have periods of syncope related to decreased cardiac output and decreased cerebral profusion. These individuals frequently will require an electronic pacemaker.

Conduction Abnormalities: No criteria present in this electrocardiogram.

QRS Complex Axis: The mean QRS complex axis is −15°.

Chamber Enlargement: No criteria present in this electrocardiogram.

Infarction: No criteria present in this electrocardiogram.

ST Segment and T Wave Abnormalities: No criteria present in this electrocardiogram.

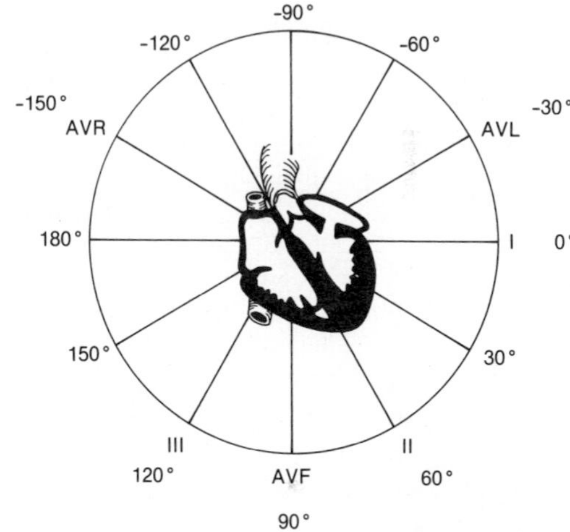

Summary

Marked sinus bradycardia with sinus arrhythmia

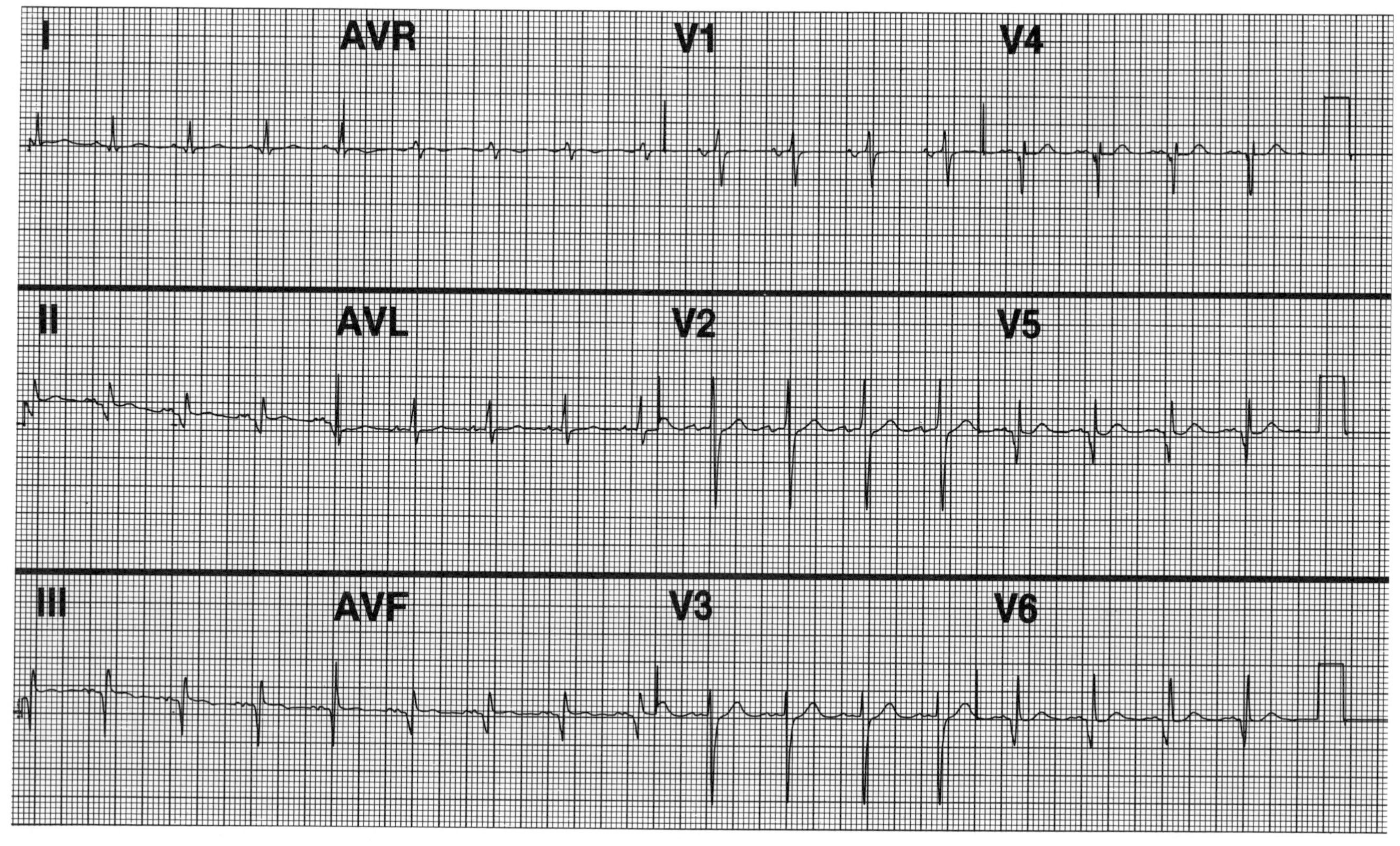
I
AVR
V1
V4
II
AVL
V2
V5
III
AVF
V3
V6

Electrocardiogram #86

Atrial Rate	**107**	**Beats/Minute**
Ventricular Rate	**107**	**Beats/Minute**
PR Interval	**0.14**	**Second**
QRS Duration	**0.09**	**Second**
QT-QTc	**0.31–0.40**	**Second**
QRS Complex Axis	**−5**	**Degrees**

Rate: The atrial and ventricular rates are 107 beats per minute.

Rhythm: The PR interval is 0.14 second and constant. The rhythm is sinus tachycardia.

Conduction Abnormalities: No criteria present in this electrocardiogram.

QRS Complex Axis: The mean QRS complex axis is −5°.

Chamber Enlargement: No criteria present in this electrocardiogram.

Infarction: The prominent Q wave seen in the inferior leads II, III and AVF together with the ½ mm ST segment elevation and T wave abnormalities seen in the same leads is diagnostic of an inferior infarction, age undetermined. In addition, there are prominent Q waves seen in leads V4 to V6 that are indicative of an anterolateral infarction. These electrocardiographic patterns are diagnostic of an inferolateral infarction, which may be related to an occlusion of the right coronary artery or left circumflex artery.

ST Segment and T Wave Abnormalities: No criteria present in this electrocardiogram.

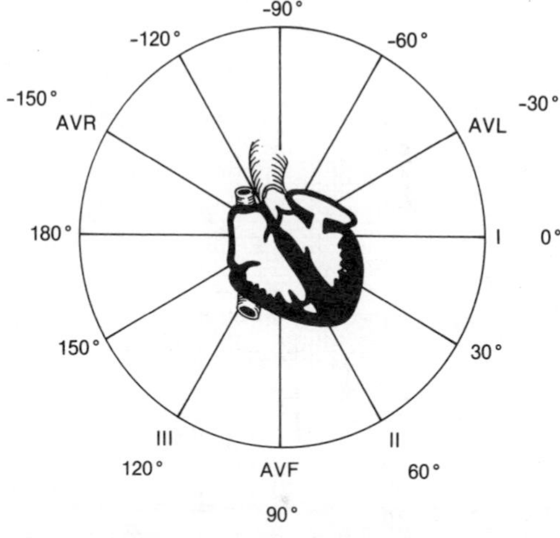

Summary

Sinus tachycardia

Inferolateral myocardial infarction, age undetermined

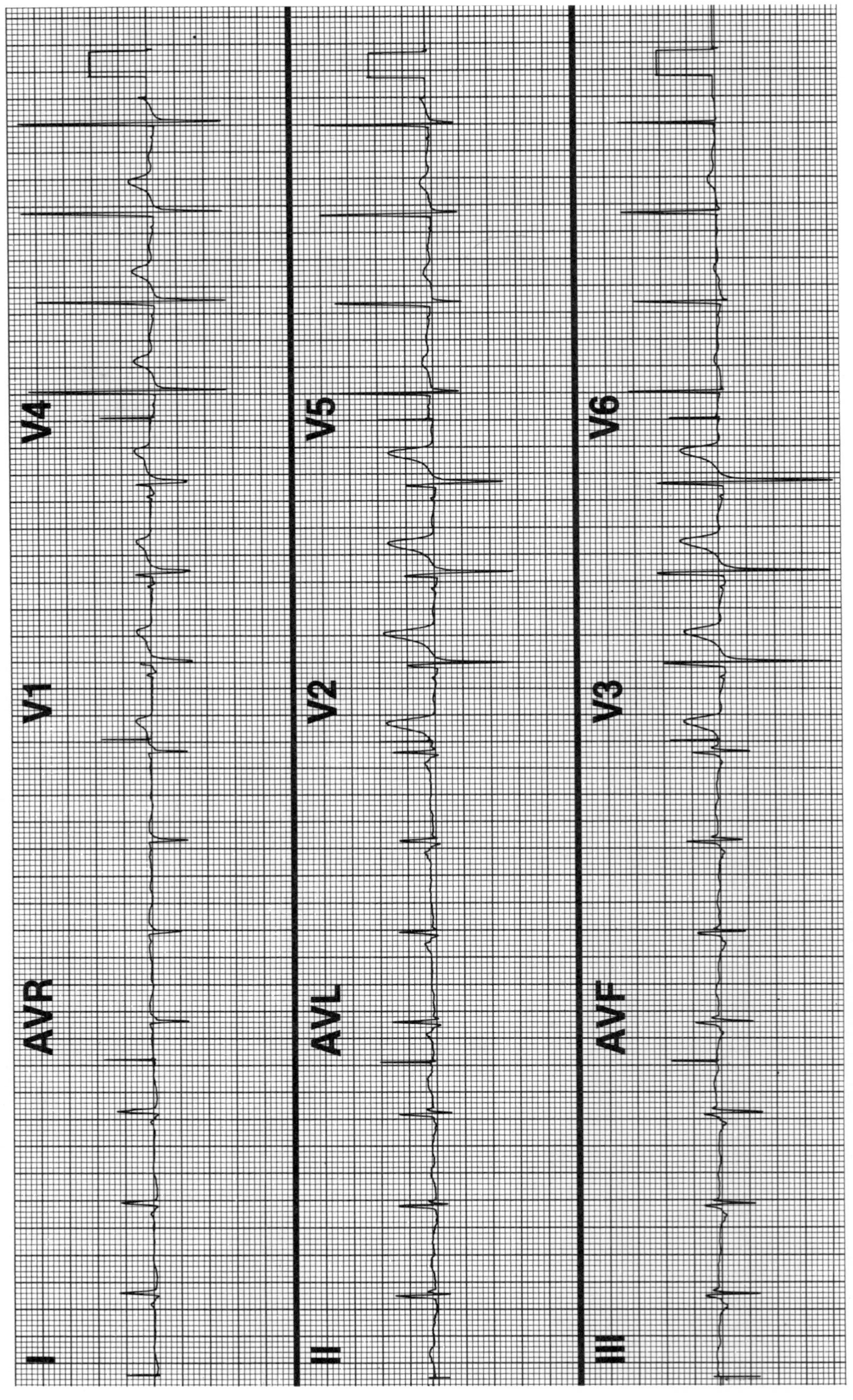
I
AVR
V1
V4
II
AVL
V2
V5
III
AVF
V3
V6

Electrocardiogram #87

Atrial Rate	91	Beats/Minute
Ventricular Rate	91	Beats/Minute
PR Interval	0.12	Second
QRS Duration	0.08	Second
QT-QTc	0.35–0.41	Second
QRS Complex Axis	0	Degrees

Rate: The atrial and ventricular rates are 91 beats per minute.

Rhythm: The PR interval is 0.12 second and constant. In addition, the P wave is inverted in leads II, III and AVF. This unusual P wave axis is caused by an ectopic atrial rhythm. The term low atrial or coronary sinus rhythm has been applied to the presence of a short PR interval and inverted P waves in leads II, III and AVF.

Conduction Abnormalities: No criteria present in this electrocardiogram.

QRS Complex Axis: The mean QRS complex axis is 0°.

Chamber Enlargement: No criteria present in this electrocardiogram.

Infarction: No criteria present in this electrocardiogram.

ST Segment and T Wave Abnormalities: There are nonspecific T wave abnormalities.

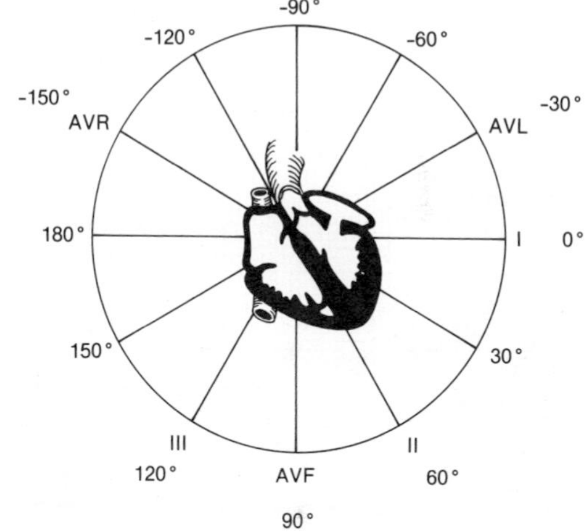

Summary

Ectopic atrial rhythm

Nonspecific T wave abnormalities

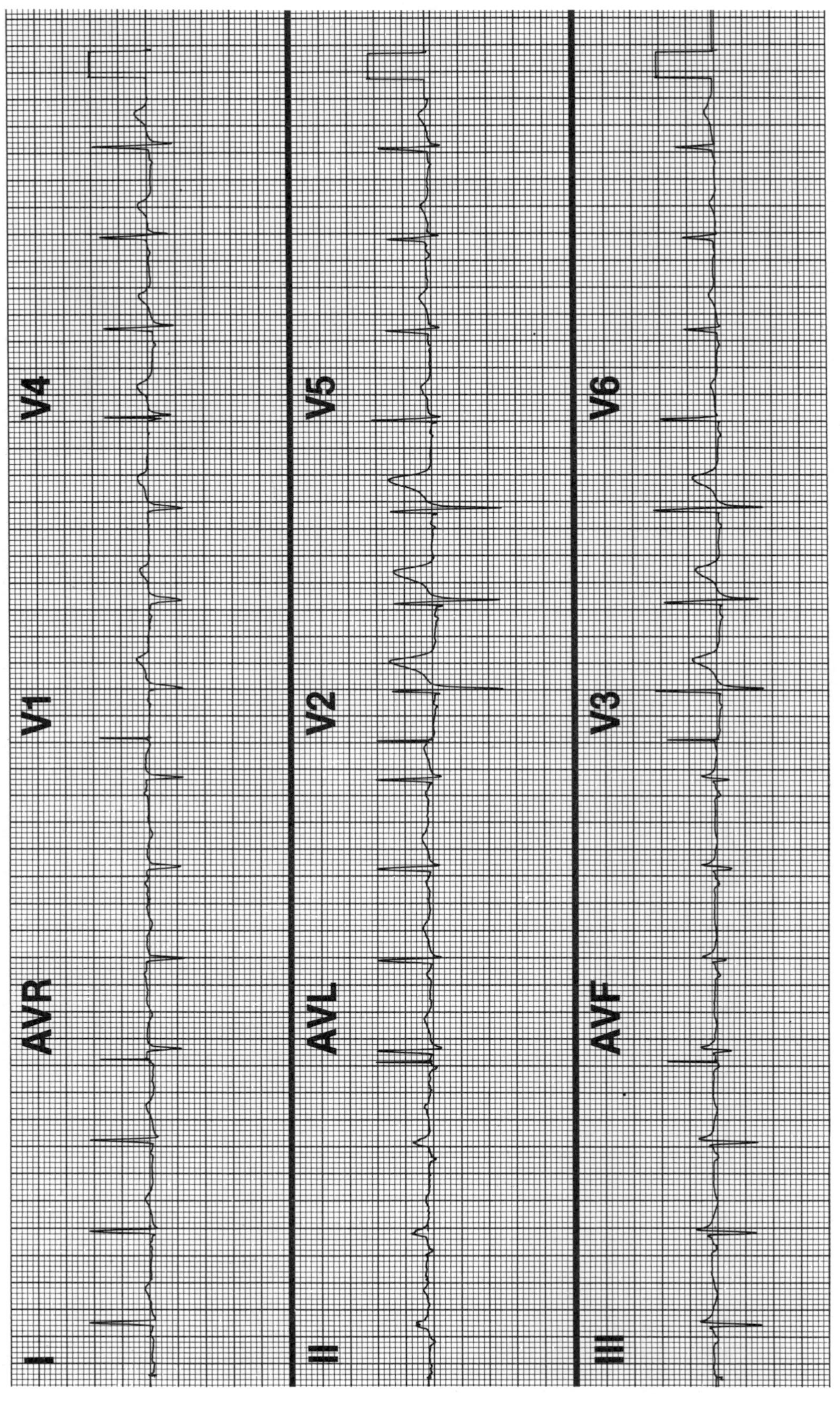
I
AVR
V1
V4
II
AVL
V2
V5
III
AVF
V3
V6

Electrocardiogram #88

Atrial Rate	**88**	**Beats/Minute**
Ventricular Rate	**88**	**Beats/Minute**
PR Interval	**0.13**	**Second**
QRS Duration	**0.09**	**Second**
QT-QTc	**0.36–0.43**	**Second**
QRS Complex Axis	**−10**	**Degrees**

Rate: The atrial and ventricular rates are 88 beats per minute.

Rhythm: The PR interval is 0.13 second. The P wave is inverted in leads II, III and AVF. This short PR interval is suggestive of a junctional rhythm or a coronary sinus rhythm. Coronary sinus rhythm is a low atrial or borderline junctional rhythm.

Conduction Abnormalities: No criteria present in this electrocardiogram.

QRS Complex Axis: The mean QRS complex axis is −10°.

Chamber Enlargement: No criteria present in this electrocardiogram.

Infarction: There is a QS complex in lead V1 and small Q wave in leads V2 and V3 that are diagnostic of an anteroseptal infarction, age undetermined.

ST Segment and T Wave Abnormalities: No criteria present in this electrocardiogram.

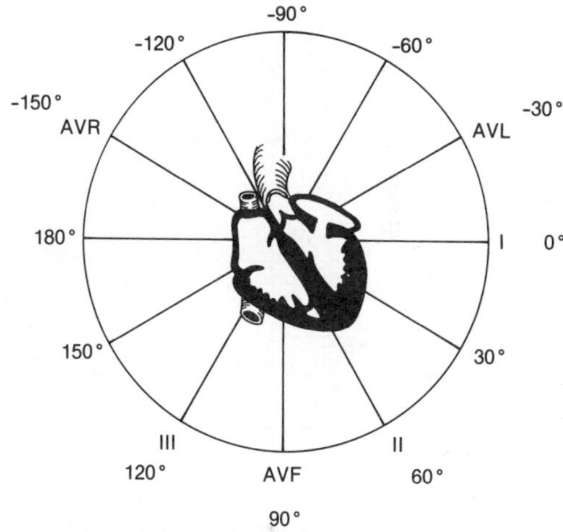

Summary

Ectopic atrial rhythm

Anteroseptal myocardial infarction, age undetermined

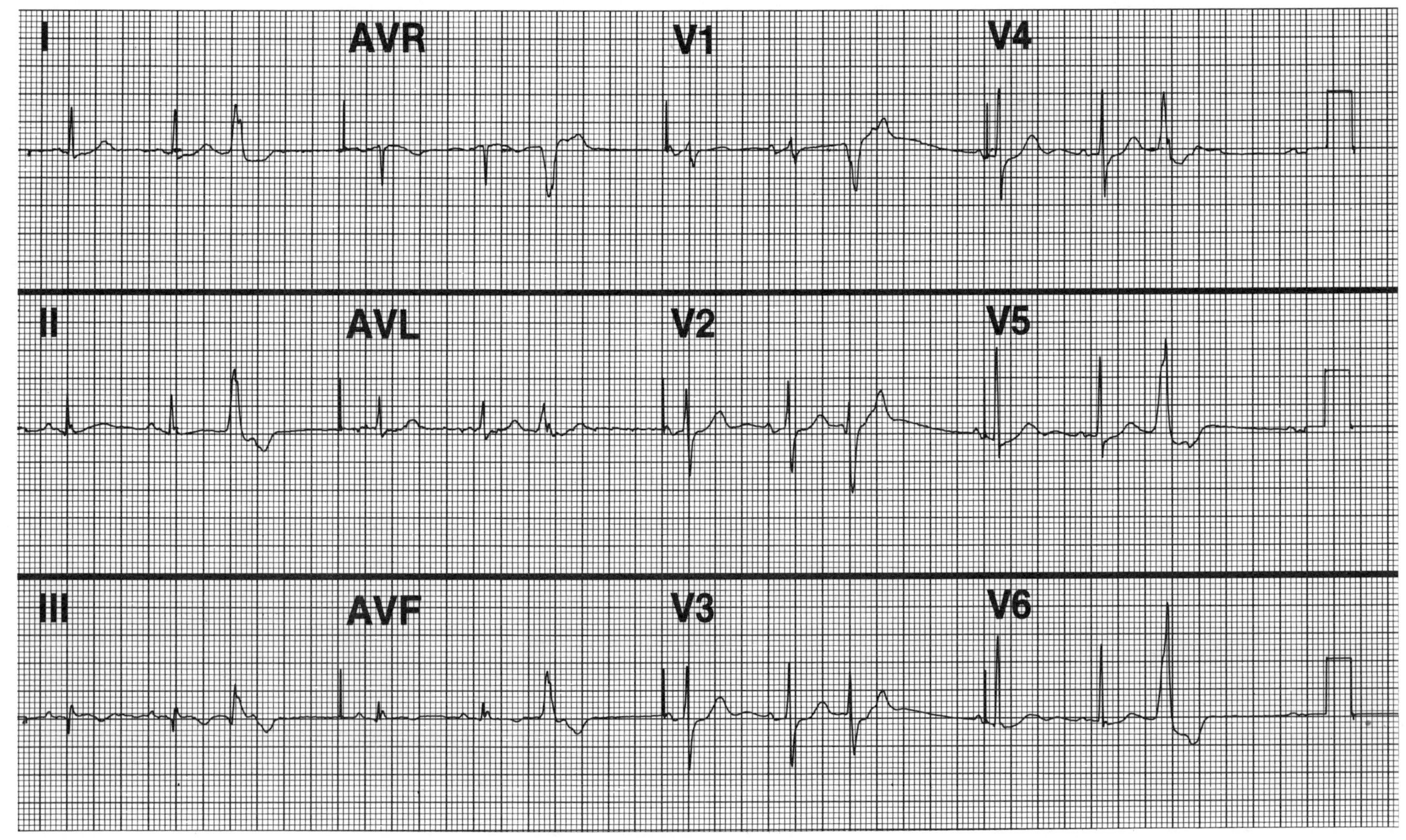
I
AVR
V1
V4
II
AVL
V2
V5
III
AVF
V3
V6

Electrocardiogram #89

Atrial Rate	79	**Beats/Minute**
Ventricular Rate	79	**Beats/Minute**
PR Interval	0.16	**Second**
QRS Duration	0.10	**Second**
QT-QTc	0.38–0.42	**Second**
QRS Complex Axis	20	**Degrees**

Rate: The atrial and ventricular rates are 79 beats per minute.

Rhythm: The PR interval is 0.16 second and constant. The rhythm is normal sinus rhythm. In addition, however, there are frequent premature ventricular contractions. These are seen as the third beat in each of the lead groups. Notice that the interval between the sinus QRS complex and the beginning of the premature ventricular contraction is 0.40 second. This is called the coupling interval. Although this interval can vary, with unifocal premature ventricular contractions it is usually fixed.

Conduction Abnormalities: No criteria present in this electrocardiogram.

QRS Complex Axis: The mean QRS complex axis is 20°.

Chamber Enlargement: No criteria present in this electrocardiogram.

Infarction: No criteria present in this electrocardiogram.

ST Segment and T Wave Abnormalities: No criteria present in this electrocardiogram.

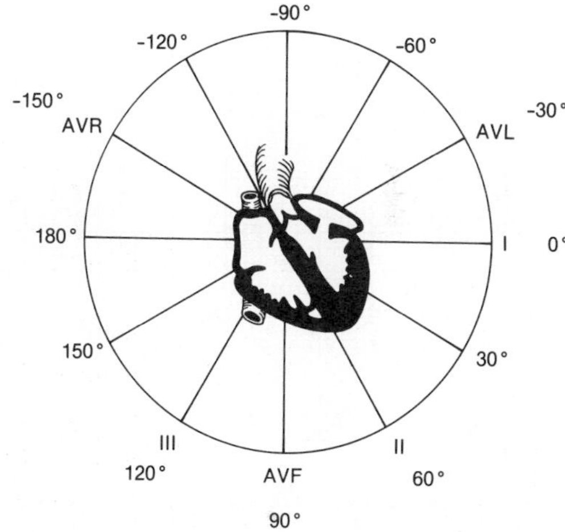

Summary

Normal sinus rhythm with frequent premature ventricular contractions

Otherwise normal electrocardiogram

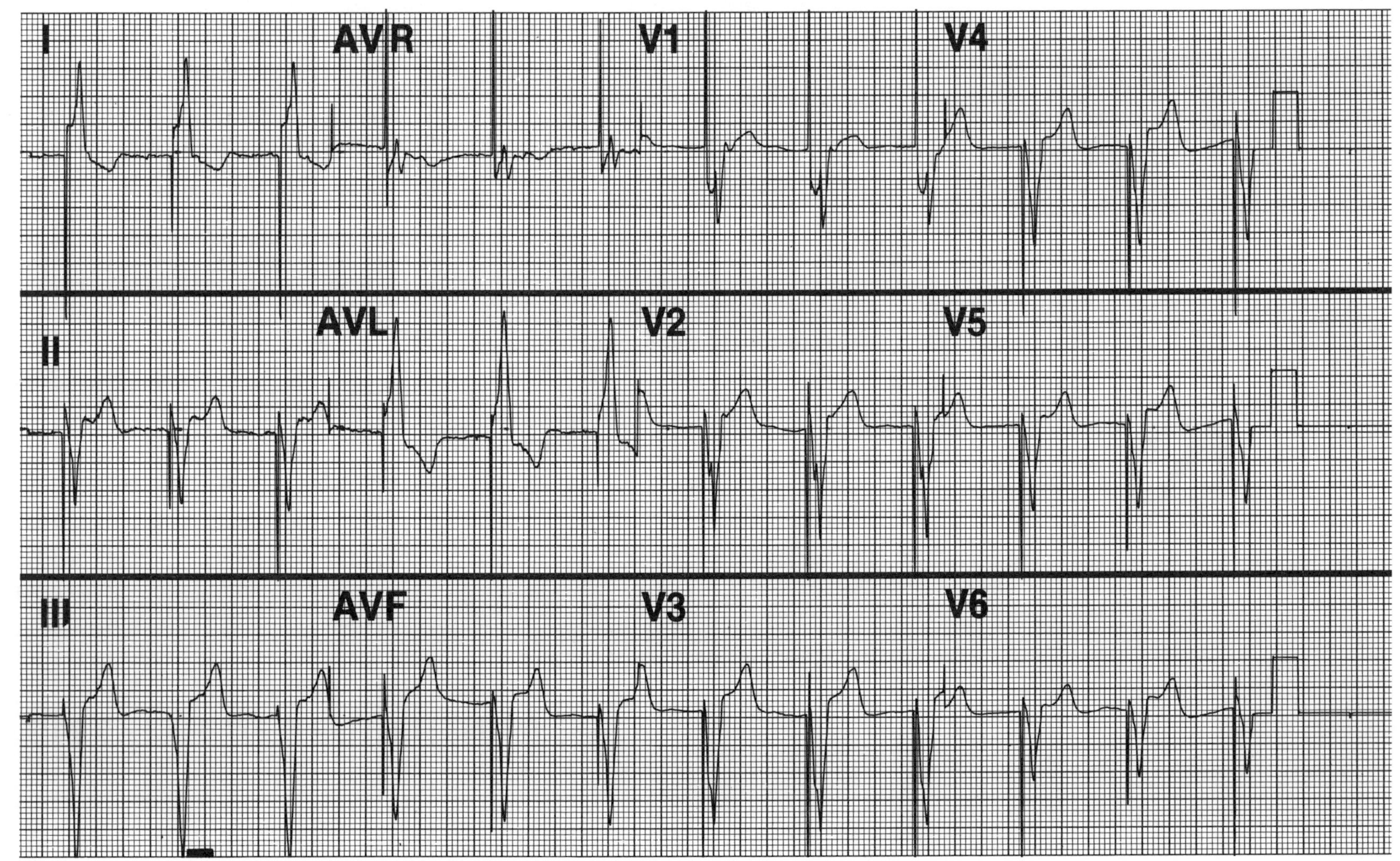
I
AVR
V1
V4
II
AVL
V2
V5
III
AVF
V3
V6

Electrocardiogram #90

Atrial Rate	—	**Beats/Minute**
Ventricular Rate	75	**Beats/Minute**
PR Interval	—	**Second**
QRS Duration	0.18	**Second**
QT-QTc	0.44–0.49	**Second**
QRS Complex Axis	−45	**Degrees**

Rate: The ventricular rate is 75 beats per minute.

Rhythm: No P waves are seen in this electrocardiogram. A prominent electronic pacemaker spike is seen preceding each QRS complex at a rate of 72 beats per minute.

Conduction Abnormalities: An electronic pacemaker spike is seen preceding each QRS complex. A left bundle branch block pattern is seen in leads I and AVL indicative of septal depolarization from the right to the left. One therefore recognizes that the pacemaker is present in the right ventricular cavity. When one has diagnosed the presence of an electronic ventricular pacemaker, it is very difficult to determine whether any further abnormality exists.

QRS Complex Axis: The mean QRS complex axis is −45°.

Chamber Enlargement: No criteria present in this electrocardiogram.

Infarction: No criteria present in this electrocardiogram.

ST Segment and T Wave Abnormalities: The marked repolarization abnormalities seen are secondary to the pacemaker.

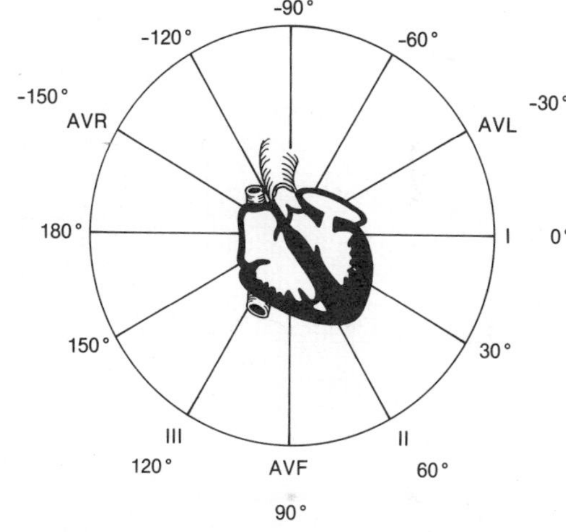

> *Summary*
>
> Electronic ventricular pacemaker

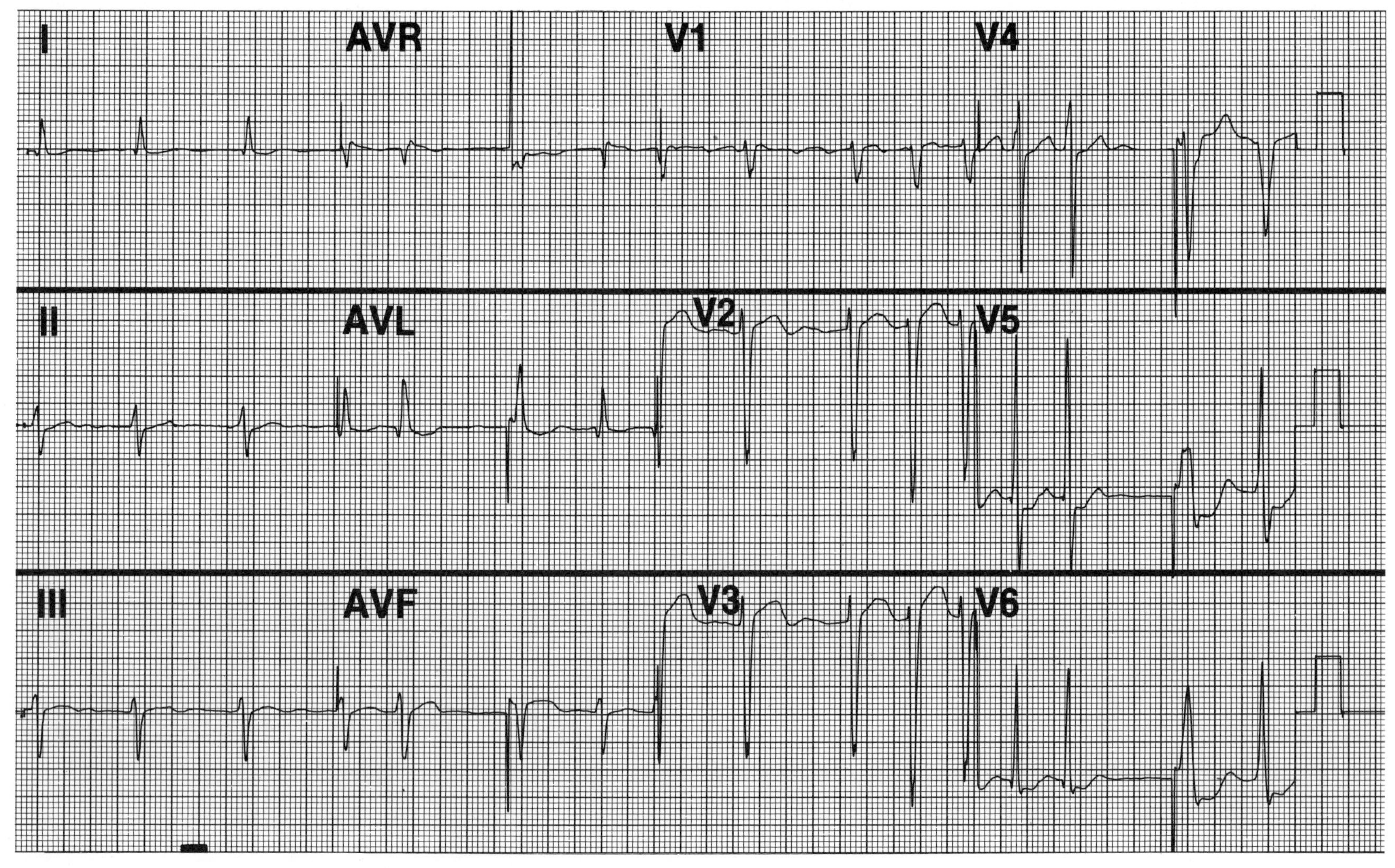
I
AVR
V1
V4
II
AVL
V2
V5
III
AVF
V3
V6

Electrocardiogram #91

Atrial Rate	—	**Beats/Minute**
Ventricular Rate	90	**Beats/Minute**
PR Interval	—	**Second**
QRS Duration	0.10	**Second**
QT-QTc	0.34–0.42	**Second**
QRS Complex Axis	−45	**Degrees**

Rate: The ventricular rate is 90 beats per minute.

Rhythm: No P waves are seen in this electrocardiogram. The basic rhythm is atrial fibrillation; however, a pacing spike may be seen preceding the third complex in leads AVR, AVL and AVF and in the third complex in leads V1, V2 and V3. This pacemaker spike is not seen preceding any of the other beats. Therefore, the pacemaker is on demand and is called a demand electronic pacemaker.

Conduction Abnormalities: A left anterior hemiblock is present. Notice the qR complex in lead I and the rS complex in leads II, III and AVF. The initial wave of depolarization is posterior and to the right and produces a small q wave in lead I and a small r wave in lead II. The bulk of depolarization proceeds in an upward, anterior and leftward direction. This produces the left axis deviation by inscribing a qR complex in lead I and an rS complex in lead II.

QRS Complex Axis: The mean QRS complex axis is −45°, abnormal left axis deviation.

Chamber Enlargement: Voltage criteria for left ventricular hypertrophy is present. The voltage of the S wave in lead V2 and the voltage of the R wave in lead V6 equals 40 mm. This is most likely the result of left ventricular hypertrophy. However, a left anterior hemiblock may mimic left ventricular hypertrophy.

Infarction: No criteria present in this electrocardiogram.

ST Segment and T Wave Abnormalities: The ST segment and T wave abnormalities seen are most likely related to the left ventricular hypertrophy and/or the left anterior hemiblock.

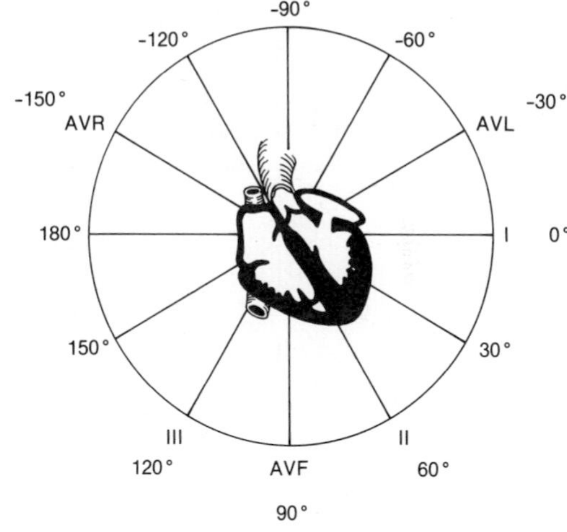

Summary

Atrial fibrillation

Demand electronic pacemaker

Left anterior hemiblock

Left ventricular hypertrophy

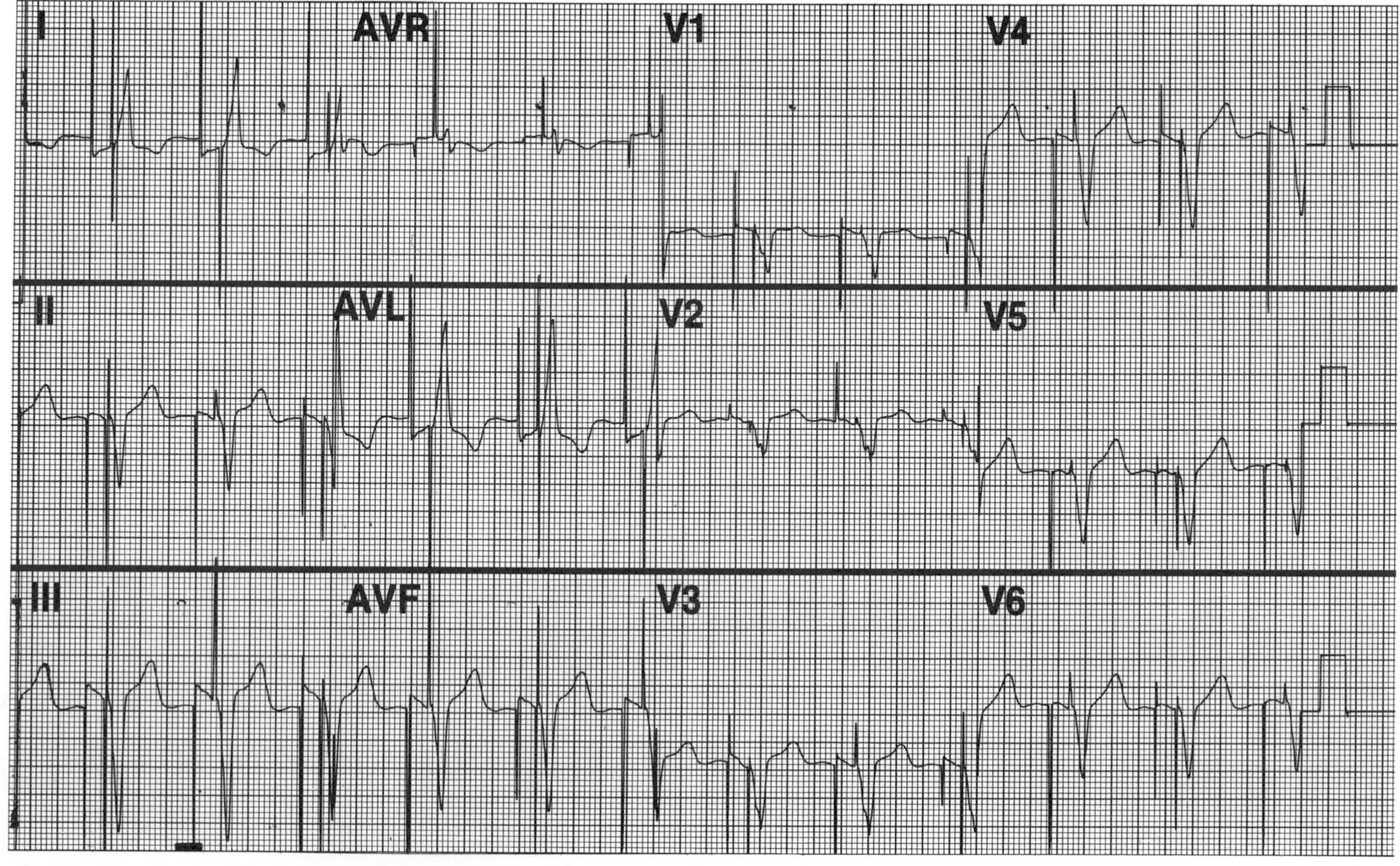
I
AVR
V1
V4
II
AVL
V2
V5
III
AVF
V3
V6

Electrocardiogram #92

Atrial Rate	**75**	**Beats/Minute**
Ventricular Rate	**75**	**Beats/Minute**
PR Interval	**0.15**	**Second**
QRS Duration	**0.18**	**Second**
QT-QTc	**0.44–0.49**	**Second**
QRS Complex Axis	**−60**	**Degrees**

Rate: The atrial and ventricular rates are 75 beats per minute.

Rhythm: The PR interval is 0.15 second. The rhythm is electrically paced.

Conduction Abnormalities: This electrocardiogram may at first be rather confusing. There are three complexes seen for each cardiac cycle. There is first an atrial spike, followed by a 0.15 second delay. This in turn is followed by another pacing spike, which is followed by the QRS complex. This patient has an atrioventricular sequential or dual-chamber electronic pacemaker. In this type of pacemaker, an atrial impulse is provided, which after a constant period, a ventricular impulse stimulates the ventricles.

QRS Complex Axis: The mean QRS complex axis is −60°. The axis deviation is probably the result of the electronic pacemaker.

Chamber Enlargement: No criteria present in this electrocardiogram.

Infarction: No criteria present in this electrocardiogram.

ST Segment and T Wave Abnormalities: No criteria present in this electrocardiogram.

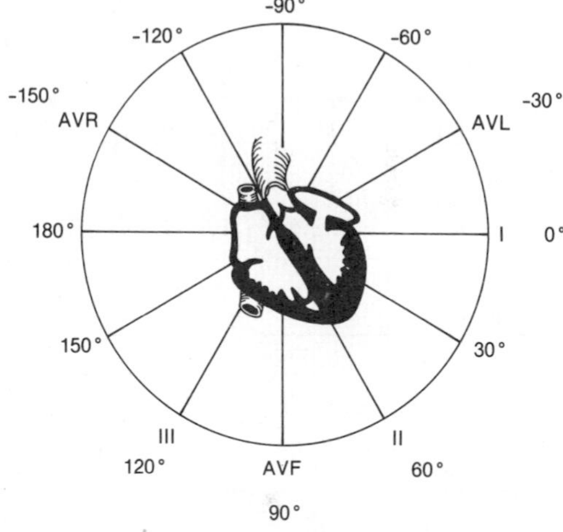

Summary

Atrioventricular sequential or dual chamber pacemaker.

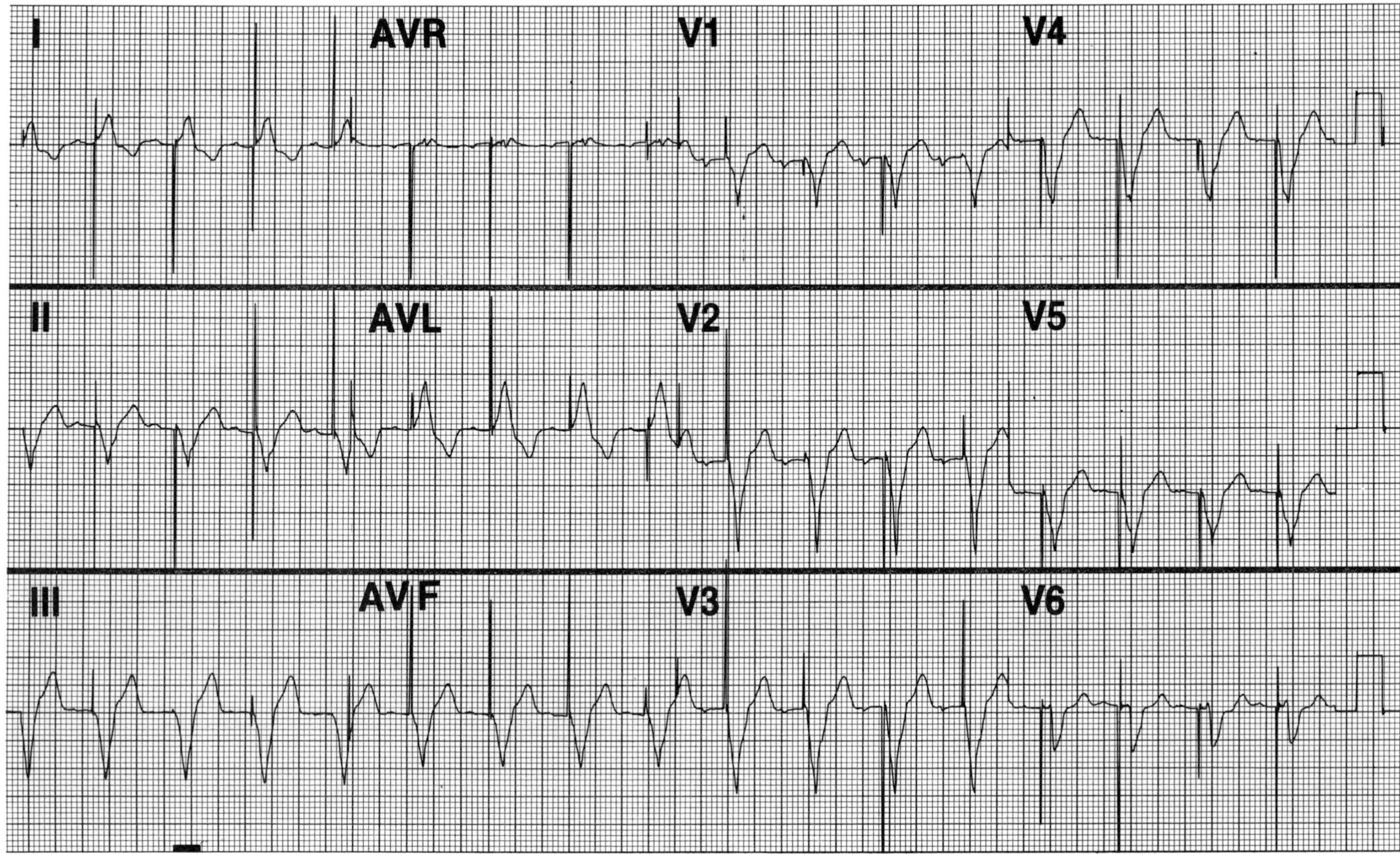
I
AVR
V1
V4
II
AVL
V2
V5
III
AVF
V3
V6

Electrocardiogram #93

Atrial Rate	**100**	**Beats/Minute**
Ventricular Rate	**100**	**Beats/Minute**
PR Interval	**0.18**	**Second**
QRS Duration	**0.19**	**Second**
QT-QTc	**0.39–0.50**	**Second**
QRS Complex Axis	**−60**	**Degrees**

Rate: The atrial and ventricular rates are 100 beats per minute.

Rhythm: The rhythm is electrically paced.

Conduction Abnormalities: An electronic pacing spike may be seen preceding each QRS complex. The QRS complex has the configuration of a left bundle branch block pattern. This is caused by the abnormal septal depolarization from right to left. This type of left bundle branch block pattern is seen when the pacing wires are present in the right ventricle.

QRS Complex Axis: The mean QRS complex axis is −60°.

Chamber Enlargement: No criteria present in this electrocardiogram.

Infarction: No criteria present in this electrocardiogram.

ST Segment and T Wave Abnormalities: No criteria present in this electrocardiogram.

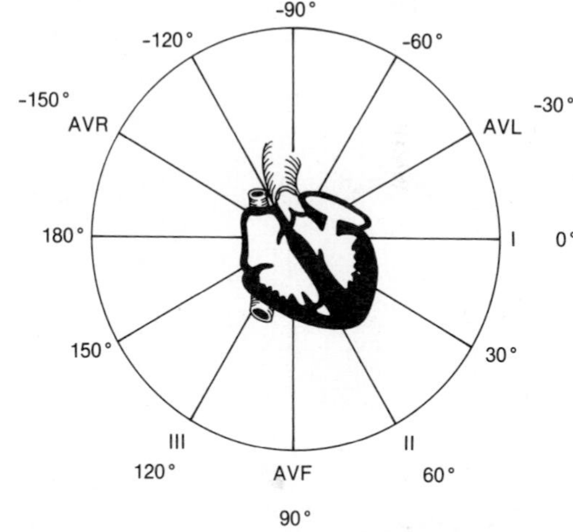

Summary

Electronic ventricular pacemaker

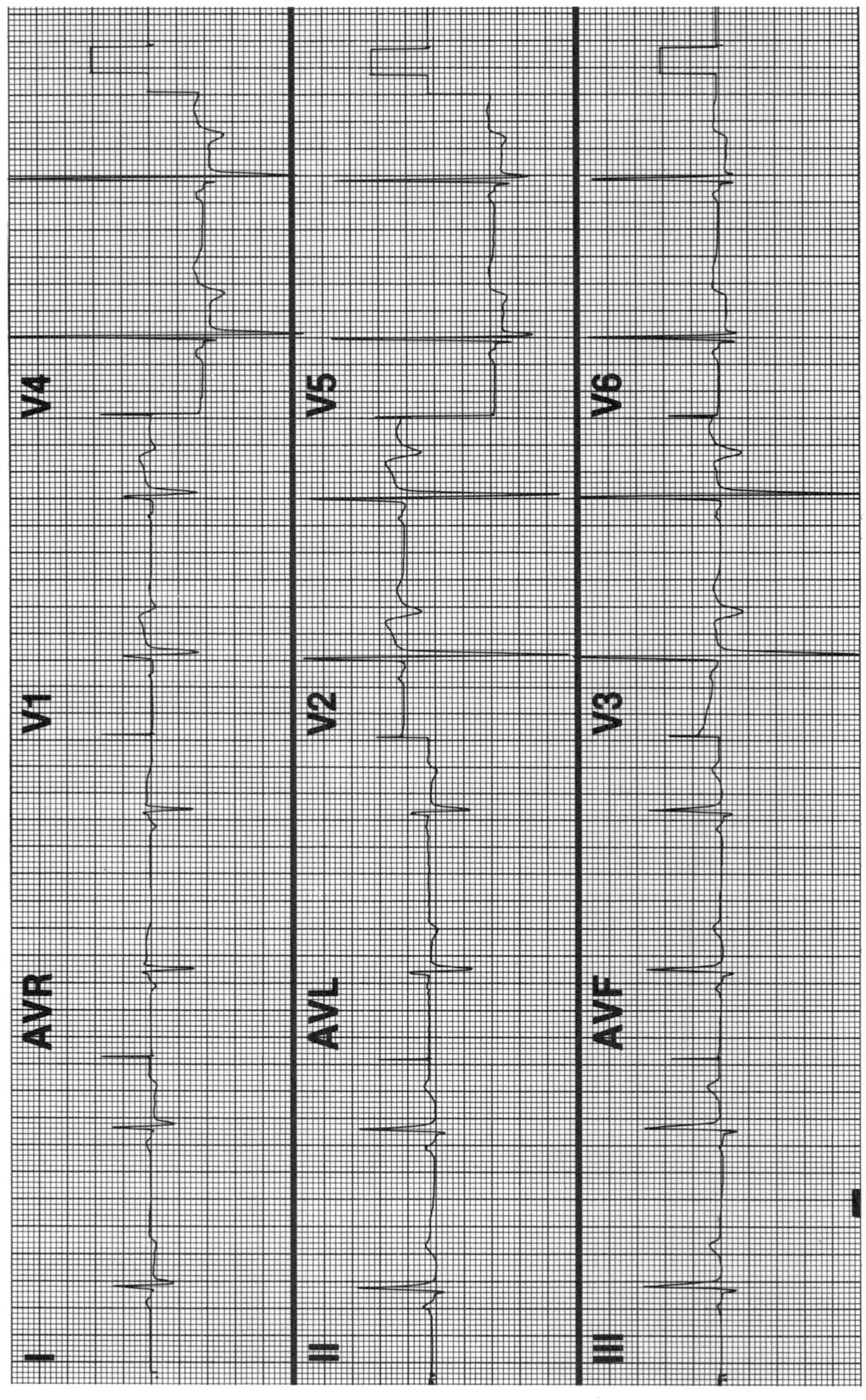
I
AVR
V1
V4
II
AVL
V2
V5
III
AVF
V3
V6

Electrocardiogram #94

Atrial Rate	52	**Beats/Minute**
Ventricular Rate	52	**Beats/Minute**
PR Interval	0.17	**Second**
QRS Duration	0.11	**Second**
QT-QTc	0.47–0.41	**Second**
QRS Complex Axis	80	**Degrees**

Rate: The atrial and ventricular rates are 52 beats per minute.

Rhythm: The PR interval is 0.17 second and constant. The rhythm is sinus bradycardia.

Conduction Abnormalities: The QRS is widened to 0.11 second. This is a nonspecific intraventricular conduction delay, as the specific QRS complex morphologies of right or left bundle branch block are not present.

QRS Complex Axis: The mean QRS complex axis is 80°.

Chamber Enlargement: The striking abnormalities in this electrocardiogram are the voltages of the QRS complexes. The S wave in lead V2 is 30 mm and the R wave in lead V6 is 23 mm, with their sum totaling 53 mm. Associated ST segment depression and T wave inversions are seen in the lateral leads. The diagnosis of left ventricular hypertrophy should be made.

Infarction: No criteria present in this electrocardiogram.

ST Segment and T Wave Abnormalities: The ST segment and T wave abnormalities are secondary repolarization abnormalities.

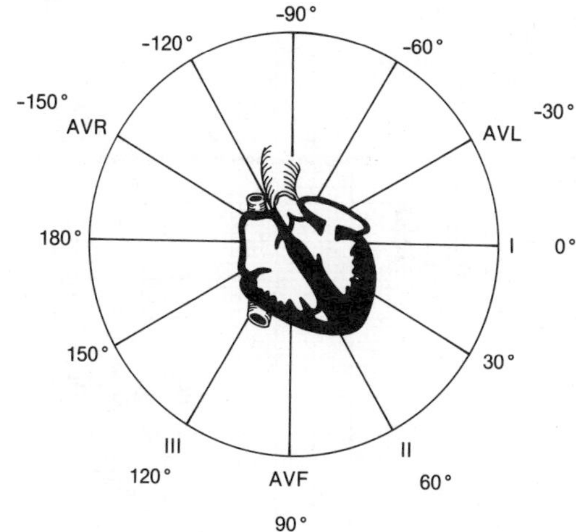

Summary

Marked sinus bradycardia

Left ventricular hypertrophy

Nonspecific intraventricular conduction delay

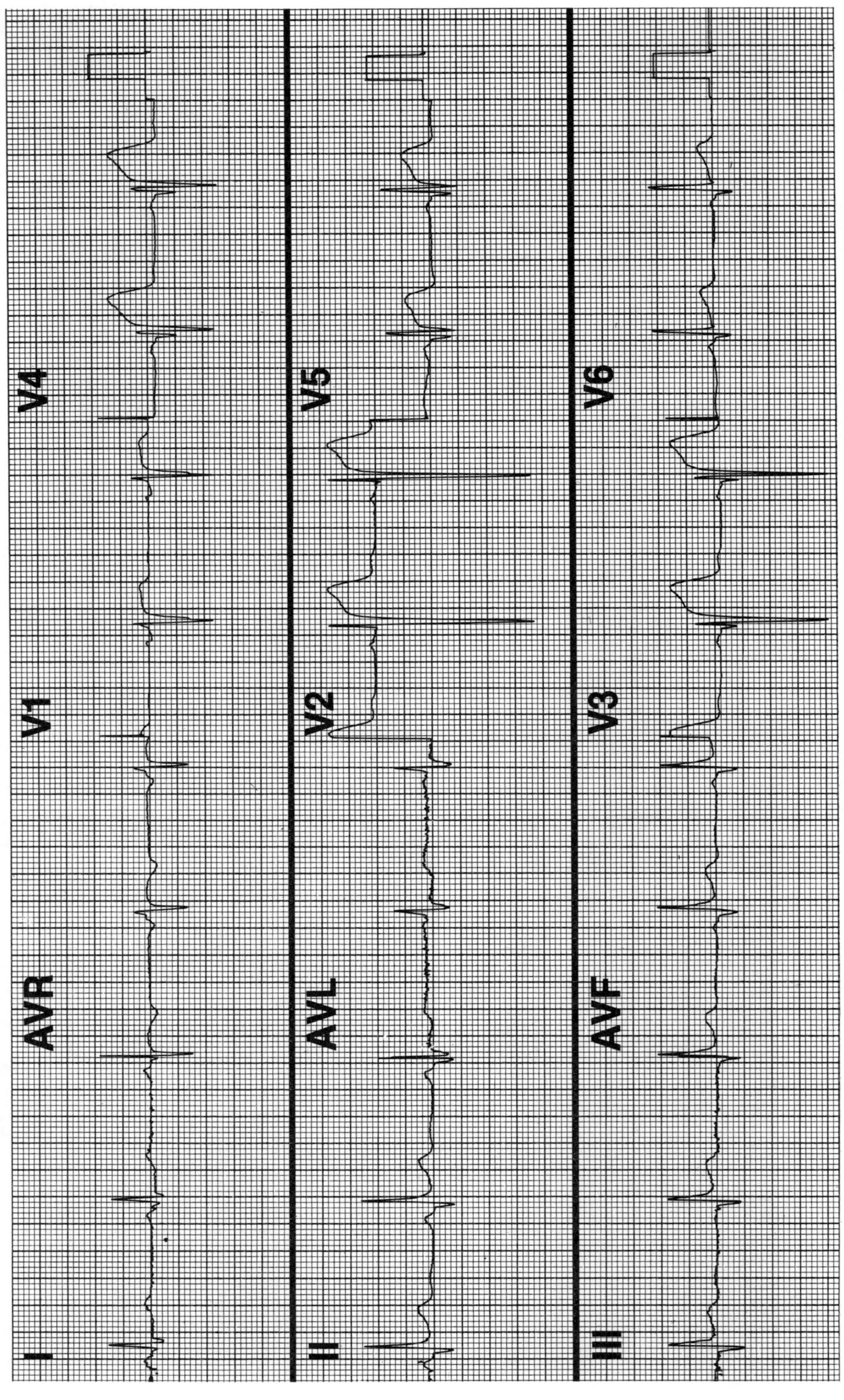
I
AVR
V1
V4
II
AVL
V2
V5
III
AVF
V3
V6

Electrocardiogram #95

Atrial Rate	56	Beats/Minute
Ventricular Rate	56	Beats/Minute
PR Interval	0.14	Second
QRS Duration	0.12	Second
QT-QTc	0.44–0.41	Second
QRS Complex Axis	60	Degrees

Rate: The atrial and ventricular rates are 56 beats per minute.

Rhythm: The PR interval is 0.14 second and constant. The rate is sinus bradycardia.

Conduction Abnormalities: No criteria present in this electrocardiogram.

QRS Complex Axis: The mean QRS complex axis is 60°, which is normal.

Chamber Enlargement: No criteria present in this electrocardiogram.

Infarction: The striking abnormality in this tracing is the ST segment elevation seen in leads V2 to V5. There is a 5 mm ST segment elevation in leads V2 to V4, and this is associated with a significant Q wave in leads V3 to V6. Therefore, the diagnosis of an anterolateral myocardial infarction should be made. In addition, there are significant Q waves in leads II, III and AVF, with a 1 mm ST segment elevation in these leads. This patient is a 64 year old who had a 1 day history of crushing chest pain. Compare this electrocardiogram with #94, which was taken 1 day prior. Notice the loss of R wave voltages in leads V3 to V6. The diagnosis of left ventricular hypertrophy can no longer be made, since the voltages have been reduced by the myocardial infarction.

ST Segment and T Wave Abnormalities: See the preceding discussion under infarction.

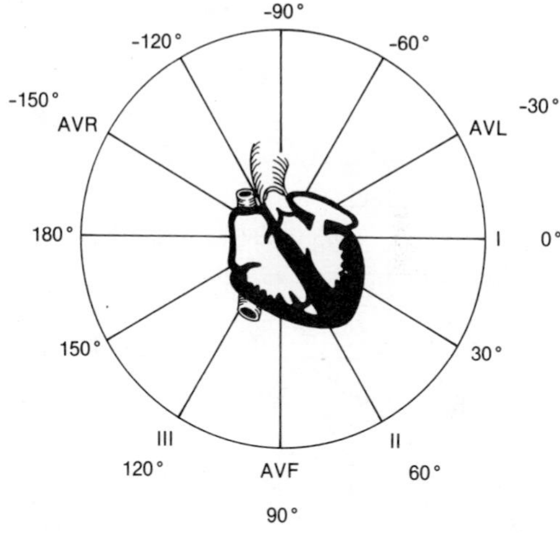

Summary

Sinus bradycardia

Inferior myocardial infarction, age undetermined

Anterolateral myocardial infarction, age undetermined

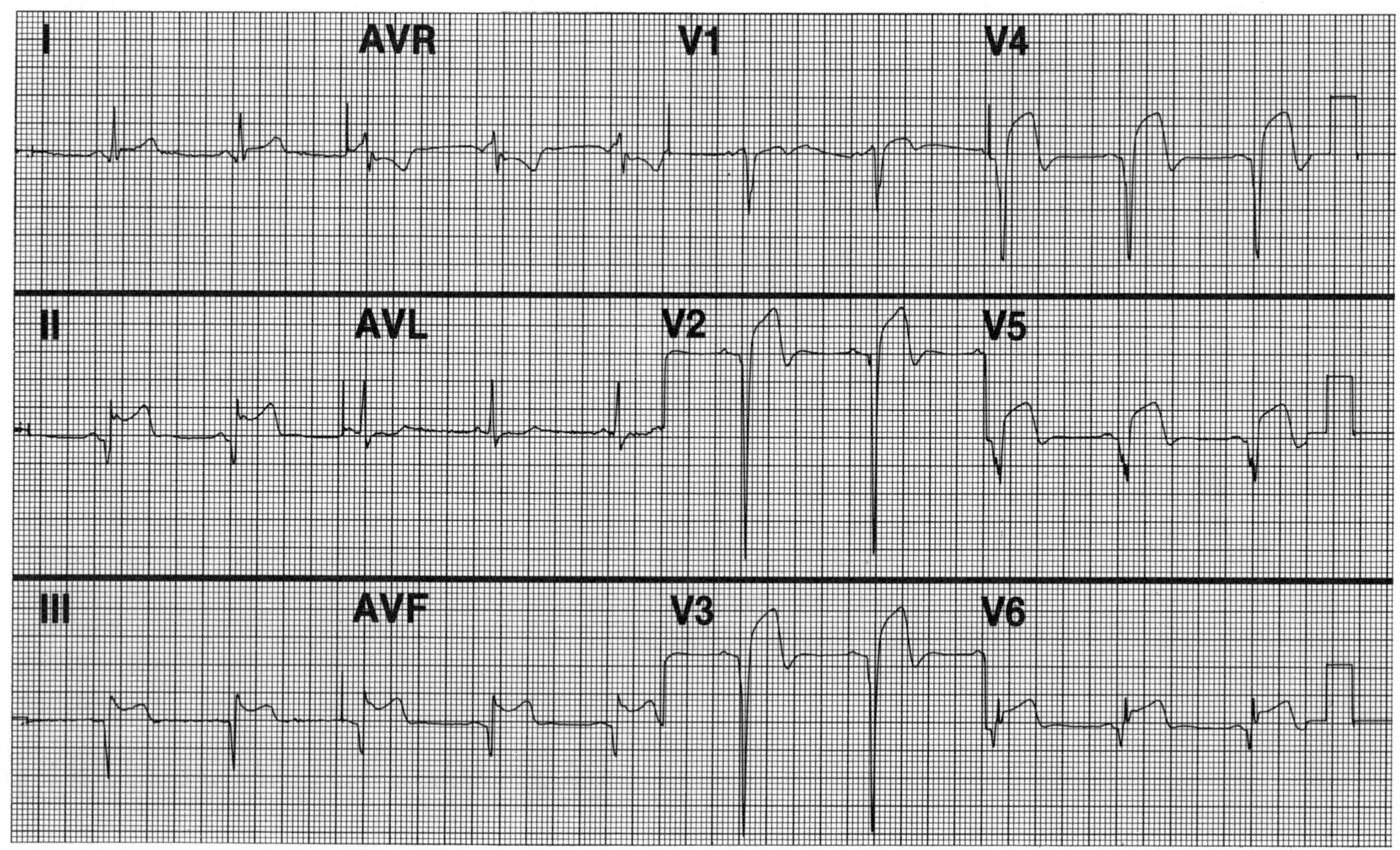
I
AVR
V1
V4
II
AVL
V2
V5
III
AVF
V3
V6

Electrocardiogram #96

Atrial Rate	63	Beats/Minute
Ventricular Rate	63	Beats/Minute
PR Interval	0.15	Second
QRS Duration	0.11	Second
QT-QTc	0.44–0.44	Second
QRS Complex Axis	−10	Degrees

Rate: The atrial and ventricular rates are 63 beats per minute.

Rhythm: The PR interval is 0.15 second and constant. The rhythm is normal sinus rhythm.

Conduction Abnormalities: No criteria present in this electrocardiogram.

QRS Complex Axis: The mean QRS complex axis is −10°.

Chamber Enlargement: No criteria present in this electrocardiogram.

Infarction: The striking abnormalities here are the QS complexes seen in leads V2 to V5 together with ST segment elevation and T wave inversions in the same leads. There are, in addition, significant Q waves in leads II, III and AVF together with a 3 mm ST segment elevation in these leads. This patient has suffered an anterolateral myocardial infarction with an inferior wall extension. Compare this electrocardiogram with #95, which was taken 6 hours earlier. This patient, who had suffered an anterolateral infarction, extended the infarction to involve the inferior wall. The occlusion of the right coronary artery or the left circumflex artery could have produced this extensive infarction. Notice the complete loss of R waves in leads V2 to V6 compared with the original electrocardiogram (#94).

ST Segment and T Wave Abnormalities: See the preceding discussion under Infarction.

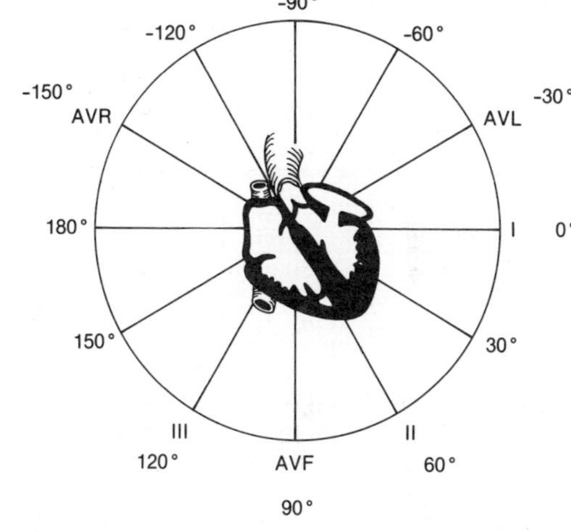

Summary

Normal sinus rhythm

Inferior myocardial infarction, possibly acute

Anterolateral myocardial infarction, possibly acute

I AVR V1 V4

II AVL V2 V5

III AVF V3 V6

Electrocardiogram #97

Atrial Rate	79	**Beats/Minute**
Ventricular Rate	79	**Beats/Minute**
PR Interval	0.08	**Second**
QRS Duration	0.11	**Second**
QT-QTc	0.38–0.42	**Second**
QRS Complex Axis	70	**Degrees**

Rate: The atrial and ventricular rates are 79 beats per minute.

Rhythm: The PR interval is 0.08 second and constant. The rhythm is normal sinus rhythm.

Conduction Abnormalities: The QRS interval is 0.11 second. The prolongation of the QRS complex is secondary to the initial widening of this complex by a delta wave, which is best seen in lead II. The short PR interval associated with the delta wave is diagnostic of ventricular pre-excitation—the Wolff-Parkinson-White syndrome.

QRS Complex Axis: The mean QRS complex axis is 70°.

Chamber Enlargement: No criteria present in this electrocardiogram.

Infarction: No criteria present in this electrocardiogram.

ST Segment and T Wave Abnormalities: No criteria present in this electrocardiogram.

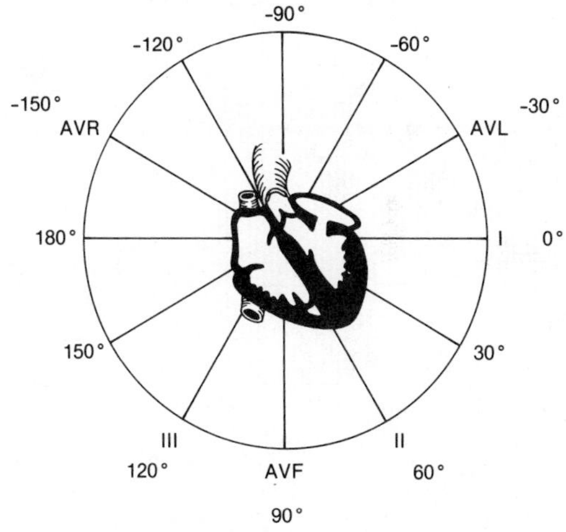

Summary

Normal sinus rhythm

Wolff-Parkinson-White syndrome, type B

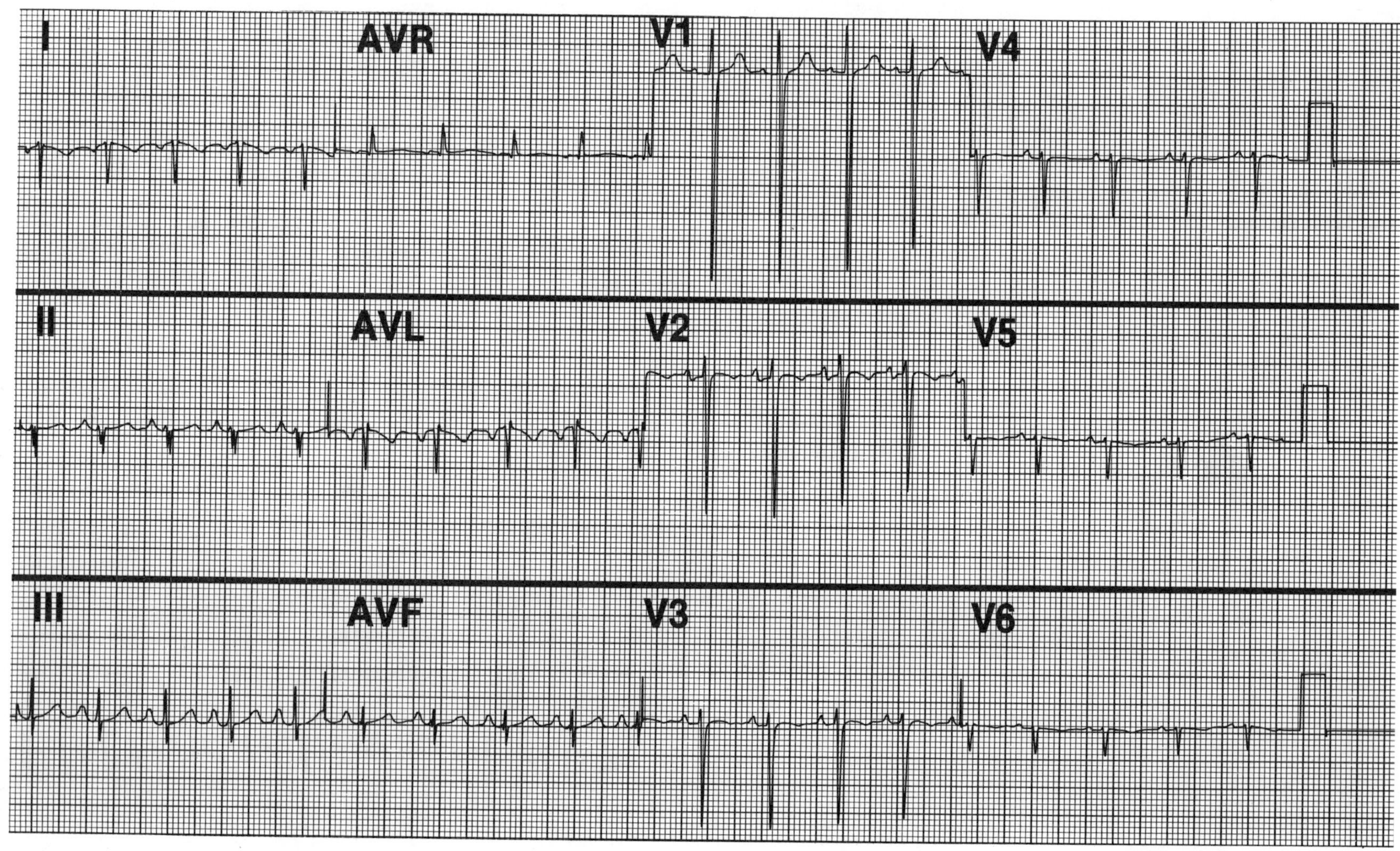

I
AVR
V1
V4
II
AVL
V2
V5
III
AVF
V3
V6

Electrocardiogram #98

Atrial Rate	**115**	**Beats/Minute**
Ventricular Rate	**115**	**Beats/Minute**
PR Interval	**0.14**	**Second**
QRS Duration	**0.08**	**Second**
QT-QTc	**0.29–0.40**	**Second**
QRS Complex Axis	**180**	**Degrees**

Rate: The atrial and ventricular rates are 115 beats per minute.

Rhythm: The PR interval is 0.14 second and constant. The rhythm is normal sinus rhythm.

Conduction Abnormalities: No criteria present in this electrocardiogram.

QRS Complex Axis: The QRS complex is negative in lead I and equiphasic in lead AVF. Therefore, the mean QRS complex axis is 180°, marked right axis deviation.

Chamber Enlargement: No criteria present in this electrocardiogram.

Infarction: No criteria present in this electrocardiogram.

ST Segment and T Wave Abnormalities: See Other Findings.

Other Findings: The striking abnormality in this tracing is the horizontal QRS axis to the *right*. The P waves are also inverted in leads I and AVL and are upright in lead AVR, making the P wave axis to the *right*. This indicates that either the arm leads are reversed or the heart is reversed in the patient's body—a condition called *dextrocardia*. When one evaluates the precordial leads, one notices that the R waves decrease as one goes from lead V1 to V6. Therefore, the diagnosis must be dextrocardia, since arm lead reversal would not change the precordial leads. In dextrocardia, lead V6 overlies the right ventricle. In order to better visualize the depolarization in dextrocardia, one can place additional electrodes on the right side of the chest, which are at mirror image positions to leads V5 and V6. These are called leads *V5R* and *V6R,* respectively, and are useful in diagnosing right ventricular hypertrophy or dextrocardia. In dextrocardia, leads V5R and V6R demonstrate a qR complex, which would represent an electrode overlying the left ventricular (leads V5 and V6 in a normal individual). Clinically, this patient had situs inversus, a condition in which all of his organs are reversed.

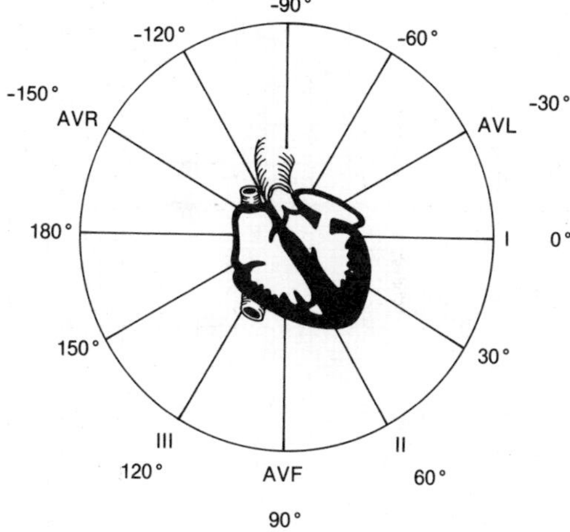

Summary

Normal sinus rhythm

Dextrocardia

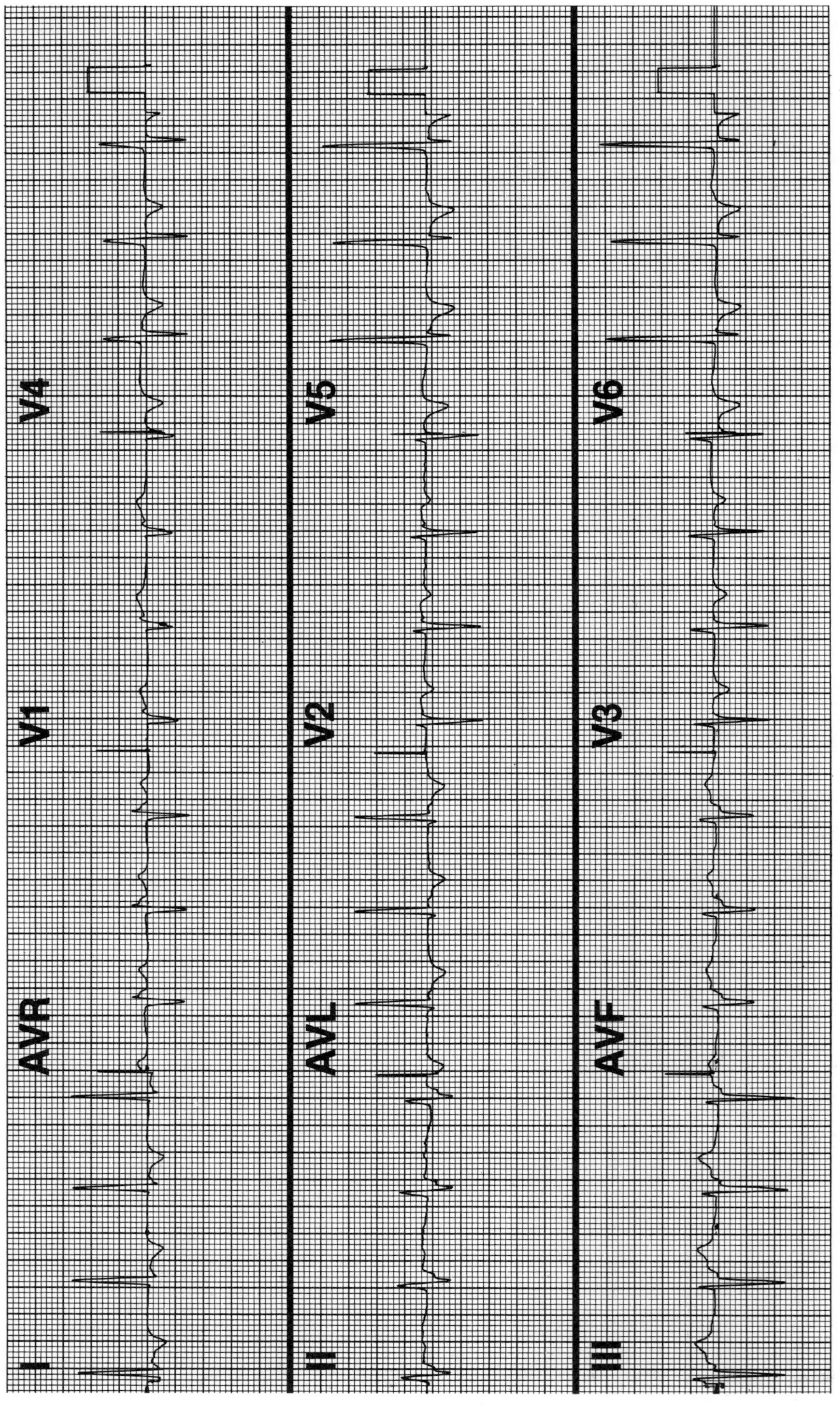
I
AVR
V1
V4
II
AVL
V2
V5
III
AVF
V3
V6

Electrocardiogram #99

Atrial Rate	**88**	**Beats/Minute**
Ventricular Rate	**88**	**Beats/Minute**
PR Interval	**0.11**	**Second**
QRS Duration	**0.09**	**Second**
QT-QTc	**0.37–0.42**	**Second**
QRS Complex Axis	**−30**	**Degrees**

Rate: The atrial and ventricular rates are 88 beats per minute.

Rhythm: The P waves are seen following the QRS complexes. The QRS complex is 0.09 second in duration. A slight deformation of the ST segment represents the retrograde P wave. These are best seen in leads AVL and V1 to V3. This rhythm is an accelerated junctional rhythm with retrograde activation of the atria and is frequently associated with digitalis toxicity.

Conduction Abnormalities: No criteria present in this electrocardiogram.

QRS Complex Axis: The mean QRS complex axis is −30°.

Chamber Enlargement: The R wave in lead AVL is 14 mm and is associated with ST segment depression in the same lead as well as in the anterolateral leads V4 to V6. The diagnosis of left ventricular hypertrophy should therefore be made.

Infarction: No criteria present in this electrocardiogram.

ST Segment and T Wave Abnormalities: The ST segment and T wave abnormalities seen in leads V4 to V6 are secondary repolarization changes.

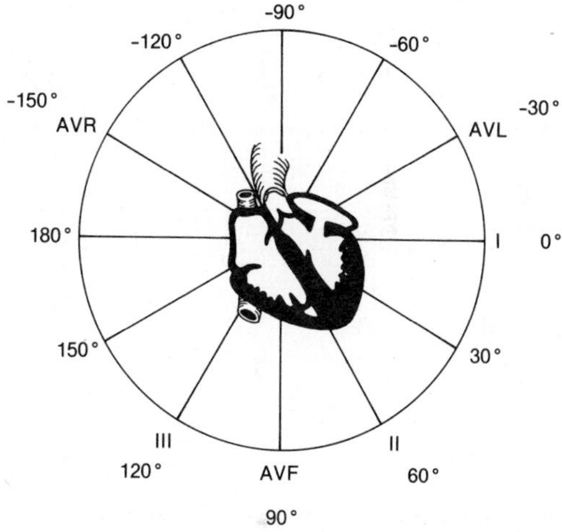

Summary

Accelerated junctional rhythm

Left ventricular hypertrophy

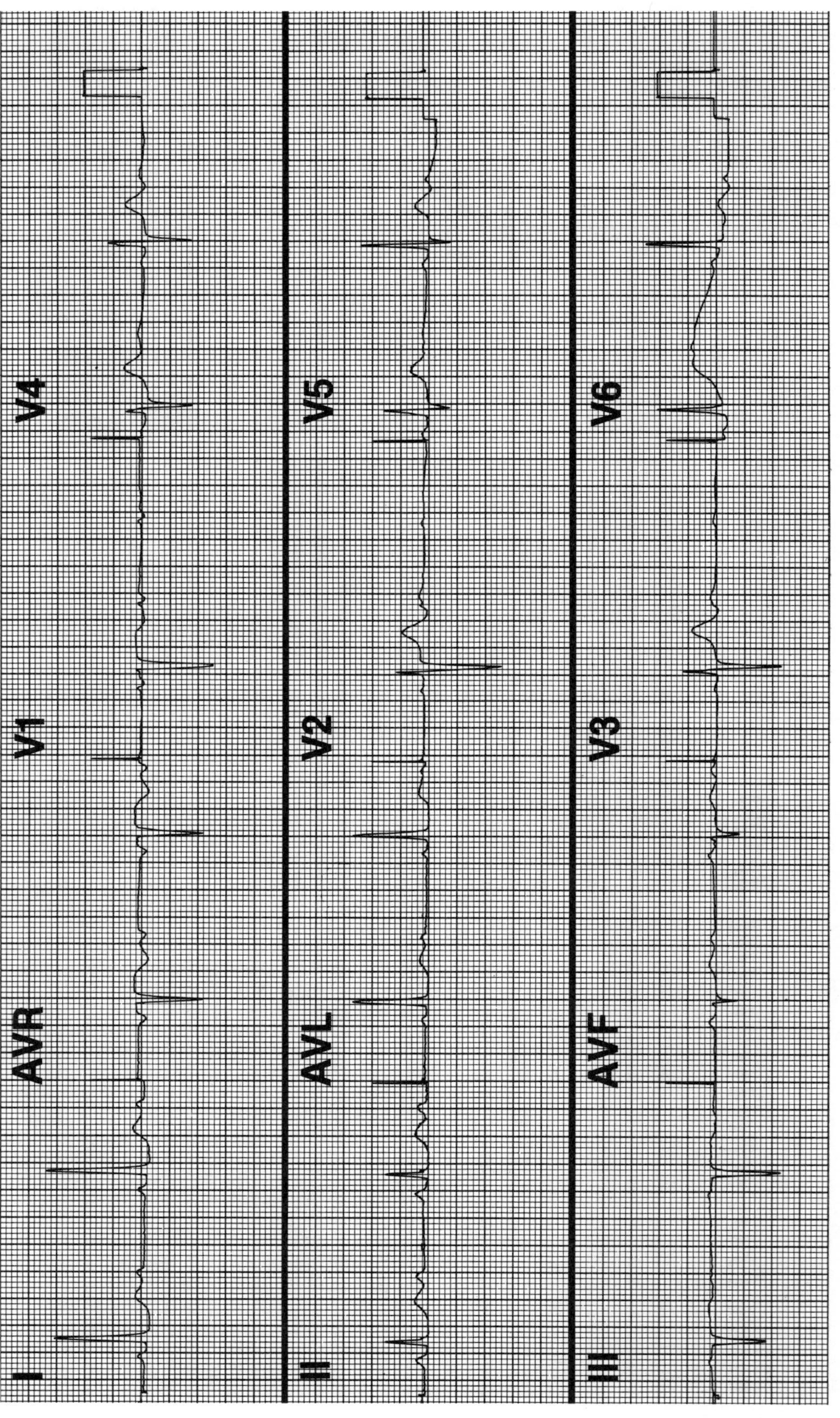
I
AVR
V1
V4
II
AVL
V2
V5
III
AVF
V3
V6

Electrocardiogram #100

Atrial Rate	**100**	**Beats/Minute**
Ventricular Rate	**49**	**Beats/Minute**
PR Interval	**0.17**	**Second**
QRS Duration	**0.10**	**Second**
QT-QTc	**0.50–0.42**	**Second**
QRS Complex Axis	**−5**	**Degrees**

Rate: The atrial rate is 100 beats per minute. The ventricular rate averages approximately 49 beats per minute.

Rhythm: If one measures the P-P intervals, they are regular; however, if one looks at leads I, II, III, AVR, AVL and AVF, one can clearly see that there are two P waves for every QRS complex. If one looks in leads V1, V2 and V3, there are three P waves for every QRS complex. Therefore, we are dealing with high-grade or advanced second degree atrioventricular block.

Conduction Abnormalities: No criteria present in this electrocardiogram.

QRS Complex Axis: The mean QRS complex axis is −5°.

Chamber Enlargement: The R wave in lead AVL is 13 mm, and the diagnosis of left ventricular hypertrophy should be made.

Infarction: No criteria present in this electrocardiogram.

ST Segment and T Wave Abnormalities: No criteria present in this electrocardiogram.

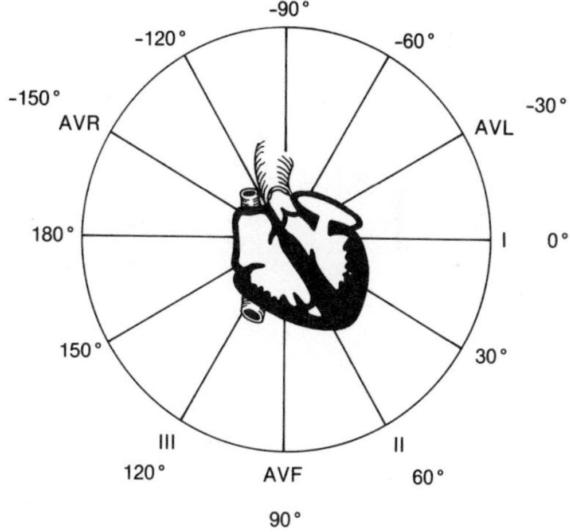

Summary

High grade second degree atrioventricular block

Left ventricular hypertrophy

Appendix A

Abbreviation	*Meaning*
A FIB	Atrial Fibrillation
AF	Atrial Fibrillation
AFL	Atrial Flutter
AIVR	Accelerated Idioventricular Rhythm
ALAD	Abnormal Left Axis Deviation
APB	Atrial Premature Beat
APC	Atrial Premature Contraction
ARAD	Abnormal Right Axis Deviation
AT	Atrial Tachycardia
AV	Atrioventricular
AVN	Atrioventricular Node
BBBB	Bilateral Bundle Branch Block
BOH	Bundle of His
CHB	Complete Heart Block
CI	Cardiac Index
CO	Cardiac Output
COPD	Chronic Obstructive Pulmonary Disease
IVCD	Intraventricular Conduction Delay
IVS	Interventricular Septum
JT	Junctional Tachycardia
LAD	Left Axis Deviation
LAE	Left Atrial Enlargement
LAHB	Left Anterior Hemiblock
LBB	Left Bundle Branch
LBBB	Left Bundle Branch Block
LGL	Lown-Ganong-Levine Syndrome
LPHB	Left Posterior Hemiblock
LVH	Left Ventricular Hypertrophy
MAT	Multifocal Atrial Tachycardia
MI	Myocardial Infarction
NSR	Normal Sinus Rhythm
NS-ST	Nonspecific ST Segment
NS-ST-T	Nonspecific ST Segment and T Wave
NS-T	Nonspecific T Wave
PAC	Premature Atrial Contraction
PAT	Paroxysmal Atrial Tachycardia
PE	Pulmonary Embolism
PH	Pulmonary Hypertension
PM	Pacemaker
PVC	Premature Ventricular Contraction
RAD	Right Axis Deviation
RAE	Right Atrial Enlargement
RBB	Right Bundle Branch
RBBB	Right Bundle Branch Block
RMP	Resting Membrane Potential
RVH	Right Ventricular Hypertrophy
SA	Sinoatrial
SAN	Sinoatrial Node
SB	Sinus Bradycardia
ST	Sinus Tachycardia
SVT	Supraventricular Tachycardia
TP	Threshold Potential
VF	Ventricular Fibrillation
V FIB	Ventricular Fibrillation
V TACH	Ventricular Tachycardia
VFL	Ventricular Flutter
VPB	Ventricular Premature Beat
VPC	Ventricular Premature Contraction
VT	Ventricular Tachycardia
WAP	Wandering Atrial Pacemaker
WPW	Wolff-Parkinson-White Syndrome

Appendix B

I. Review of rhythms
  A. Supraventricular rhythms
    1. Sinus
      a) Normal sinus rhythm: regular atrial and ventricular rates; all intervals normal and constant
      b) Sinus tachycardia: sinus rhythm with rate of greater than 100 beats per minute
      c) Sinus bradycardia: sinus rhythm with rate less than 60 beats per minute
    2. Atrial
      a) Atrial tachycardia: atrial pacemaker with regular atrial and ventricular rates between 200 ± 50 beats per minute; starts and stops abruptly
      b) Atrial flutter: regular atrial rate between 300 ± 50 beats per minute with "saw-toothed" baseline of "F" waves; usually 2:1, 3:1 or 4:1 atrioventricular block producing slower ventricular rates
      c) Atrial fibrillation: undulating baseline of "f" waves, irregular ventricular rate, absent P waves
      d) Wandering atrial pacemaker: different P wave configurations; PR and R-R intervals change as the site of impulse changes; multifocal atrial tachycardia occurs when at least three different P wave configurations are present
    3. Junctional rhythms: absent or retrograde (inverted) P waves that precede or follow the QRS complex; normal QRS configuration
      a) Junctional pacemaker: Junctional rhythm with regular ventricular rate of approximately 40 to 60 beats per minute
      b) Accelerated junctional pacemakers
        (1) Paroxysmal junctional tachycardia: regular rhythm with rate between 140 and 200 beats per minute; starts and stops abruptly
        (2) Nonparoxysmal junctional tachycardia: regular rhythm with rate between 70 and 130 beats per minute, often associated with digitalis toxicity
  B. Ventricular rhythms (caused by ectopic foci that produce bizarre, widened QRS complexes)
    1. Ventricular premature contraction
      a) Premature, bizarre, wide QRS complex usually greater than 3 small boxes
      b) ST segment and T waves directed opposite of the QRS complex
      c) Full compensatory pause
      d) Fusion beats
    2. Ventricular tachycardia
      a) Bizarre, widened QRS complexes greater than 3 small boxes
      b) Atrioventricular dissociation
      c) Regular ventricular rhythm
      d) RR′ complex in lead V1 and qR complex or QS complex in lead V6
      e) Fusion beats
      f) Capture beats
    3. Ventricular flutter
      a) A rapid ventricular tachycardia
      b) Widened QRS complex (greater than 3 small boxes)
      c) No obvious ST segment or T waves

4. Ventricular fibrillation
   a) Irregular, chaotic undulations of baseline
   b) No recognizable P waves, QRS complexes or T waves
5. Parasystole
   a) R-R intervals of the ectopic beats at multiples of the shortest inter-ectopic interval
   b) Variable coupling
   c) Fusion beats

C. Conduction Disturbances
1. Sinoatrial block
   a) Second degree sinoatrial block, type I (Wenckebach)
      (1) Decreasing P-P intervals followed by dropped P wave
   b) Second degree sinoatrial block, type II
      (1) Regular P-P interval with intermittently dropped P wave
2. Atrioventricular block
   a) First degree
      (1) Lengthening PR interval to greater than 0.20 second (5 small boxes)
   b) Second degree
      (1) Mobitz type I (Wenckebach)
         (a) Progressive lengthening of PR interval resulting in a dropped QRS complex
         (b) Shortening of the R-R interval
         (c) Regularly irregular rhythm
         (d) Normal configurations of P wave and QRS complex
      (2) Mobitz type II
         (a) Regular rhythm with rare period of irregularity due to dropped QRS complex
         (b) Constant PR interval
   c) Third degree (complete heart block)
      (1) Regular atrial rate
      (2) Atrioventricular dissociation
      (3) Regular ventricular rate, usually bradycardia
3. Ventricular block
   a) Right bundle branch block
      (1) Widened QRS complex (greater than 3 small boxes)
      (2) RSR′ or "M" patterns in lead V1
      (3) Deep slurred S wave in lead V6
      (4) Secondary T wave inversion in leads V1 to V3
   b) Left bundle branch block
      (1) Widened QRS (greater than 3 small boxes)
      (2) Absence of septal q wave
      (3) Broad monophasic QS wave in lead V1 and wide notched R wave in leads I and V6
      (4) Secondary T wave inversion in leads I and V6
   c) Intraventricular conduction delay
      (1) Widened QRS complex
      (2) No evidence of right or left bundle branch block
   d) Left anterior hemiblock
      (1) Left axis deviation
      (2) qR complex in lead I; rS complex in leads II, III, AVF
      (3) Normal QRS complex duration
      (4) No evidence of other conditions capable of producing the left axis deviation
   e) Left posterior hemiblock
      (1) Right axis deviation
      (2) rS complex in lead I; qR complex in leads II, III and AVF
      (3) Normal QRS complex duration
      (4) No evidence of right ventricular hypertrophy
   f) Wolff-Parkinson-White syndrome
      (1) Regular rhythm
      (2) Short PR interval
      (3) Delta wave
      (4) Widened QRS complex

II. Chamber enlargement

A. Left atrial enlargement
1. Wide, notched P wave in lead II
2. P wave duration in lead II greater than 3 small boxes
3. Biphasic P wave in lead V1 with a terminal component greater than 1 small box wide by 1 small box deep
4. Shift of P wave axis to the left

B. Right atrial enlargement
1. Tall, slender, peaked P waves in lead II
2. P wave height in lead II greater than 3 small boxes
3. Biphasic P wave in lead V1 with tall initial deflection equal to 2 small boxes high
4. Shift in P wave axis to the right

C. Biatrial enlargement
1. Terminal portion of P wave in V1 is greater than or equal to 1 small box wide
2. P wave in lead II is greater than or equal to 2.5 small boxes

D. Left ventricular enlargement
1. R wave in leads V5 or V6 plus S wave in lead V1 greater than 35 mm
2. R wave in lead I plus S wave in lead III greater than 25 mm
3. R wave in lead I greater than 15 mm
4. R wave in lead AVL greater than 11 mm

5. Intrinsicoid deflection in leads V3 to V6 greater than 0.05 second
6. Left axis deviation (occurs in only 50 per cent of cases)
7. Secondary ST segment and T wave changes

E. Right venticular enlargement
1. Right axis deviation greater than +110°
2. R/S ratio in V1 greater than 1
3. Deep S wave in leads V5 to V6, I and AVL
4. rSR′ complex in lead V1 with R′ greater than 10 mm
5. R wave in lead V1 plus S wave in lead V6 greater than 11 mm
6. Increased intrinsicoid deflection in lead V1 greater than or equal to 0.035 second
7. Secondary ST segment and T wave changes

III. Infarction (look for Q waves in the following areas)
A. Anteroseptal, leads V1 to V3
B. Anterolateral, leads V4 to V6
C. High lateral, leads I, AVL
D. Inferior (diaphragmatic), leads II, III, AVF
E. Posterior, tall R waves in leads V1 to V2
F. Subendocardial, ST segment and T wave changes only—no Q waves

IV. Pulmonary Pathology
A. Cor pulmonale
1. Tall peaked P waves
2. T wave inversions
3. ST segment changes
4. Right axis deviation
5. Right ventricular hypertrophy
6. Low voltages

B. Pulmonary embolus
1. Nonspecific
a) ST segment and T wave changes
b) Acute sinus tachycardia
2. Specific
a) Peaked P waves
b) Acute atrial fibrillation
c) S1-Q3-T3 pattern (deep S wave in lead I, deep Q wave in lead III and inverted T wave in lead III)
d) Acute right bundle branch block

V. Effects of drugs
A. Digitalis
1. Therapeutic dose
a) ST segment sagging
b) Prolonged PR interval
2. Toxic doses
a) Arrhythmias
(1) Premature ventricular contractions
(2) Ventricular tachycardia
(3) Paroxysmal atrial or nodal tachycardia with atrioventricular block
(4) Sinus bradycardia
b) Blocks
(1) Sinoatrial block
(2) Atrioventricular block

B. Quinidine
1. Therapeutic dose
a) Increased PR interval
b) Widened QRS complex
c) Prolonged QT interval
d) ST segment depression
2. Toxic dose
a) Sinoatrial block
b) Atrioventricular block
c) Intraventricular block
d) Ectopic beats
e) Ventricular tachycardia

VI. Electrolytes
A. Potassium
1. Hyperkalemia
a) Tall, peaked (tented) T waves
b) Intraventricular conduction delay
c) Decreased P wave amplitude
d) Absent P waves
e) Cardiac arrhythmias
f) Atrioventicular conduction delays
2. Hypokalemia
a) Prominent U waves
b) QRS complex prolongation
c) Decreased T wave amplitude
d) ST segment depression
e) Ventricular arrhythmias

B. Calcium
1. Hypercalcemia
a) Shortened QTc interval
b) Widened QRS complex
c) Conduction disturbances
d) Occasionally, premature ventricular contractions
2. Hypocalcemia
a) Prolonged QTc interval
b) Inverted T waves
c) Arrhythmias uncommon

Index

Note: Page numbers in *italics* refer to illustrations; page numbers followed by t refer to tables.